ADOLESCENT MEDICINE: STATE OF THE ART REVIEWS

Substance Use and Abuse Among Adolescents

GUEST EDITORS

Robert T. Brown, MD

Sheryl Ryan, MD

April 2014 • Volume 25 • Number 1

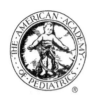

ADOLESCENT MEDICINE:
STATE OF THE ART REVIEWS
April 2014
Editor: Carrie Peters
Marketing Manager: Marirose Russo
Production Manager: Shannan Martin
eBook Developer: Houston Adams

Volume 25, Number 1
ISBN 978-1-58110-784-5
eISBN 978-1-58110-890-3
ISSN 1934-4287
MA0665
SUB1006

The recommendations in this publication do not indicate an exclusive course of treatment or serve as a standard of medical care. Variations, taking into account individual circumstances, may be appropriate.

Statements and opinions expressed are those of the author and not necessarily those of the American Academy of Pediatrics.

Products and Web sites are mentioned for informational purposes only. Inclusion in this publication does not imply endorsement by the American Academy of Pediatrics. The American Academy of Pediatrics is not responsible for the content of the resources mentioned in this publication. Web site addresses are as current as possible but may change at any time.

Every effort has been made to ensure that the drug selection and dosage set forth in this text are in accordance with the current recommendations and practice at the time of publication. It is the responsibility of the health care provider to check the package insert of each drug for any change in indications and dosage and for added warnings and precautions.

Adolescent Medicine: State of the Art Reviews is published three times per year by the American Academy of Pediatrics, 141 Northwest Point Blvd, Elk Grove Village, IL 60007-1019. Periodicals postage paid at Arlington Heights, IL.

POSTMASTER: Send address changes to American Academy of Pediatrics, Department of Marketing and Publications, Attn: AM:STARs, 141 Northwest Point Blvd, Elk Grove Village, IL 60007-1019.

Subscriptions: Subscriptions to Adolescent Medicine: State of the Art Reviews (AM:STARs) are provided to members of the American Academy of Pediatrics' Section on Adolescent Health as part of annual section membership dues. All others, please contact the AAP Customer Service Center at 866/843-2271 (7:00 am–5:30 pm Central Time, Monday–Friday) for pricing and information.

Adolescent Medicine: State of the Art Reviews

Official Journal of the American Academy of Pediatrics
Section on Adolescent Health

EDITORS-IN-CHIEF

VICTOR C. STRASBURGER, MD, Distinguished Professor of Pediatrics, Chief, Division of Adolescent Medicine, University of New Mexico, School of Medicine, Albuquerque, New Mexico

DONALD E. GREYDANUS, MD, Dr HC (ATHENS), Professor & Founding Chair, Department of Pediatric & Adolescent Medicine, Western Michigan University School of Medicine, Kalamazoo, Michigan

GUEST EDITORS

ROBERT T. BROWN, MD, Professor of Pediatrics, Adolescent Medicine, Cooper Medical School of Rowan University, Camden, New Jersey

SHERYL RYAN, MD, Associate Professor Pediatrics, Chief, Section of Adolescent Medicine, Yale University School of Medicine, New Haven, Connecticut

CONTRIBUTORS

SETH AMMERMAN, MD, Clinical Professor, Division of Adolescent Medicine, Department of Pediatrics, Stanford University, Lucile Packard Children's Hospital, Stanford, California

DAVID BENNETT, MBBS, Clinical Professor in Adolescent Medicine, University of Sydney; Senior Staff Specialist, Department of Adolescent Medicine, The Children's Hospital at Westmead; Senior Clinical Adviser, Youth Health and Wellbeing, NSW Kids and Families, Sydney, Australia

CORA COLLETTE BREUNER, MD, MPH, Professor Adolescent Medicine Section, Department of Pediatrics, Adjunct Professor Orthopedics and Sports Medicine, Seattle Childrens Hospital University of Washington, Seattle, Washington

JOANNA D. BROWN, MD, MPH, Assistant Professor (Clinical) of Family Medicine, Alpert Medical School of Brown University; Medical Director, Rhode Island Training School; Division of Adolescent Medicine, Hasbro Children's Hospital, Providence, Rhode Island

CONSUELO C. CAGANDE, MD, Associate Professor of Psychiatry, Department of Psychiatry, Cooper University Hospital and Cooper Medical School of Rowan University, Camden, New Jersey

DEEPA CAMENGA, MD, MHS, Yale School of Medicine, Department of Pediatrics, New Haven, Connecticut

RACHEL S-D FORTUNE, MD, Instructor, Adolescent Medicine, Yale University School of Medicine, Department of Pediatrics, New Haven, Connecticut

PAMELA K. GONZALEZ, MD, MS, Adjunct Assistant Professor, Department of Psychiatry, University of Minnesota, St. Paul, Minnesota

CHRISTOPHER J. HAMMOND, MD, Child Study Center, Yale University, School of Medicine; Department of Psychiatry, Yale University School of Medicine, Connecticut Mental Health Center, New Haven, Connecticut

SION KIM HARRIS, PhD, CPH, Center for Adolescent Substance Abuse Research, Boston Children's Hospital, Boston, Massachusetts

ELIZABETH JANOPAUL-NAYLOR, BS, Alpert Medical School of Brown University, Providence, Rhode Island

ALAIN JOFFE, MD, MPH, Director, Student Health and Wellness Center, Johns Hopkins University; Associate Professor of Pediatrics, Johns Hopkins University School of Medicine, Baltimore, Maryland

JOHN R. KNIGHT, MD, Center for Adolescent Substance Abuse Research, Boston Children's Hospital, Boston, Massachusetts

SHARON LEVY, MD, MPH, Director, Adolescent Substance Abuse Program, Children's Hospital Boston; Assistant Professor of Pediatrics, Harvard Medical School, Boston, Massachusetts

JENNIFER LOUIS-JACQUES, MD, MPH, Craig Dalsimer Division of Adolescent Medicine, The Children's Hospital of Philadelphia, Philadelphia, Pennsylvania

ELIZABETH A. LOWENHAUPT, MD, Assistant Professor (Clinical), Department of Psychiatry and Human Behavior, Alpert Medical School of Brown University; Associate Training Director, Child Psychiatry Fellowship & Triple Board Residency and Director, Medical Student Education in Child & Adolescent Psychiatry, Rhode Island Hospital/Alpert Medical School of Brown University; Director of Psychiatric Services, Rhode Island Training School, Providence, Rhode Island

LESLIE H. LUNDAHL, PhD, Assistant Professor, Department of Psychiatry and Behavioral Neurosciences, Wayne State University School of Medicine, Detroit, Michigan

LINDA C. MAYES, MD, Child Study Center, Yale University, School of Medicine, New Haven, Connecticut

MARC N. POTENZA, MD, PhD, Child Study Center, Yale University, School of Medicine; Department of Psychiatry, Yale University School of Medicine, Connecticut Mental Health Center; Department of Neurobiology, Yale University School of Medicine, New Haven, Connecticut

BASANT K. PRADHAN, MD, Assistant Professor of Psychiatry, Department of Psychiatry, Cooper University Hospital and Cooper Medical School of Rowan University, Camden, New Jersey

ANDRES J. PUMARIEGA, MD, Professor and Chair, Psychiatry, Department of Psychiatry, Cooper University Hospital and Cooper Medical School of Rowan University, Camden, New Jersey

STEWART STUBBS, BSS (PSYCH), MHS (CHILD & ADOLESCENT HEALTH), Parenting Research Project Coordinator, NSW Centre for the Advancement of Adolescent Health, The Children's Hospital at Westmead, Sydney, Australia

MARINA TOLOU-SHAMS, PhD, Assistant Professor (Research), Alpert Medical School of Brown University; Staff Psychologist, Rhode Island Hospital, Bradley Hasbro Children's Research Center; Director, Rhode Island Family Court, Mental Health Clinic and Director of Substance Abuse Treatment Services, Rhode Island Training School, Bradley Hasbro Children's Research Center, Providence, Rhode Island

JANET F. WILLIAMS, MD, Professor of Pediatrics, Distinguished Teaching Professor, Department of Pediatrics, Associate Dean for Faculty and Diversity, School of Medicine Office of the Dean, University of Texas Health Science Center, San Antonio, Texas

MARTHA J. WUNSCH, MD, Medical Director, Addiction Medicine, Kaiser Permanente–GSAA, Chemical Dependency Recovery Program, Union City, California

CONTENTS

Substance use is a major public health burden in the United States. Typically, onset occurs during childhood or adolescence. Pediatric and adolescent medicine physicians are uniquely positioned to address substance use in children across the pediatric age range and into young adulthood. Substance use can play a role in every aspect of health and health care, so physicians must be cognizant of the scope of its prevalence and effects when documenting the patient's social, personal, and family medical history; conducting the physical examination; discerning diagnoses; and providing patient and parent advice, anticipatory guidance, care management, referral, and continuity of services.

Psychoactive substance and nonsubstance/behavioral addictions are major public health concerns associated with significant societal cost. Adolescence is a period of dynamic biologic, psychological, and behavioral changes. Adolescence is also associated with an increased risk for substance use and addictive disorders. During adolescence, developmental changes in neural circuitry of reward processing, motivation, cognitive control, and stress may contribute to vulnerability for increased levels of engagement in substance use and nonsubstance addictive behaviors. Current biologic models of adolescent vulnerability for addictions incorporate existing data on allostatic changes in function and structure of the midbrain dopaminergic system, stress-associated neuroplasticity, and maturational imbalances between cognitive control and reward reactivity. When characterizing adolescent vulnerability, identifying subgroups of adolescents at high risk for addictive behaviors is a major goal of the addiction field. Genetics, epigenetics, and intermediate phenotypes/ endophenotypes may assist in characterizing children and adolescents at risk. Improved understanding of the neurobiology of adolescence and addiction vulnerability has the potential to refine screening, enhance prevention and intervention strategies, and inform public policy.

Although cigarette smoking is the predominant form of tobacco use in the United States, adolescents are increasingly using alternative tobacco products such as cigars, smokeless tobacco products (eg, chewing tobacco, snus, and dissolvables), hookah (ie, waterpipes), and electronic cigarettes. This article provides an update on cigarette smoking in adolescents and reviews the epidemiology of noncigarette tobacco use in youth, existing evidence on the health effects of noncigarette tobacco use, and clinical and policy implications.

In the western world, regular alcohol use in young people is trending down, risky binge drinking is trending up, and young women's drinking is matching that of young men. Young people's drinking, with all of its health and behavioral correlates, continues to challenge health professionals, health educators, and policymakers worldwide, not only because of the potential harm to the individual young person, both immediately and well into future life, but also because of the frustrating barriers to effective prevention and intervention often experienced. Fortunately, as we gain better insights into the contexts and cultural influences that predicate drinking trends in adolescents and young adults, our efforts to contain the damage through a range of contextual responses hold some promise. From both Australian and international perspectives, this review explores our contemporary understanding of what drinking means to young people, what shapes, sustains, and reinforces their drinking behavior, and current thinking about the breadth of responses and approaches available to address problematic drinking during adolescence and early adulthood.

Marijuana is one of the drugs most commonly used by adolescents. Medical marijuana is now legal in 20 states and the District of Columbia, and recreational use of marijuana by adults is now legal in Colorado and Washington State. Physicians are likely to be consulted by both adolescents and their parents regarding the possible benefits and risks of marijuana use. This article reviews definitions related to the marijuana plant and its components; epidemiology of current use patterns among adolescents; potential side effects; adolescent brain development and marijuana use; medical and recreational marijuana; marijuana delivery methods; medical marijuana and potential effects on adolescent use of recreational marijuana; comparisons between marijuana, alcohol, and tobacco; social justice issues; driving under the influence; adolescent use of medical marijuana; parental guidance; and counseling the adolescent patient.

A small but significant proportion of adolescents report the use of prescription stimulants without a physician's direction or the use of prescription stimulants in ways or dosages not intended by the prescribing physician. Compared to adolescents not reporting such use, those misusing prescription stimulants are more likely to display evidence of undiagnosed mood disorders or attention-deficit/hyperactivity disorder (ADHD) and have higher rates of other substance abuse. Physicians who prescribe ADHD medications should do so only after performing a comprehensive assessment, including screening for substance abuse and other comorbidities. Careful monitoring of refill requests may identify youth who are inadequately treated or diverting their medication. Misuse of these medications might be reduced by public health campaigns for adolescents and parents emphasizing that the use of prescription stimulants without a physician's direction can pose health risks.

Nonmedical use of prescription drugs remains a serious concern among adolescents. Prescription opioids are most frequently used, but stimulants and sedative-hypnotics also are involved. Medications often are received or stolen from family or peers, but many youth initiate nonmedical use from their own prescription leftovers. Nonmedical use contributes to drug poisonings and deaths. More commonly, nonmedical use is associated with alcohol and other drug use, and younger age at initiation of nonmedical use is linked with higher likelihood of developing substance use disorder. This article reviews the background and scope of the problem and offers the adolescent medicine physician some simple approaches to prevention and safer prescribing practices in this vulnerable group.

A performance-enhancing substance is any substance used by a person to perform better on the field, on the stage, or in the classroom. Use of performance-enhancing substances in children and adolescents is increasing, and this is a definite health concern. The increase is likely caused by a rise in popularity of team sports, easy availability of performance-enhancing substances via the Internet, focus on thinness or muscular bodies, parental and coach pressure, and a propensity for adolescents to engage in risk-taking behaviors. In this article, performance-enhancing substances available to adolescents are discussed, including steroids, steroid precursors, growth hormone, supplements, stimulants, and beta-blockers.

Adolescent screening and brief intervention (SBI) in general medical settings have the potential to greatly enhance our ability to prevent, identify, and treat substance abuse and its associated harms. Widespread implementation of SBI within such settings depends on the availability of practical and effective tools. This review describes recent developments in evidence-informed clinical practice guidelines that are designed to promote delivery of SBI through provision of structured algorithms and practical tools. An updated review of research on adolescent SBI shows increasing support for its feasibility and utility in general medical settings, particularly with the aid of computer technology.

Adolescents who use drugs before age 15 are at the greatest risk for developing long-lasting patterns of substance use. A comprehensive evaluation of biologic, psychological, and social factors should be considered when choosing an appropriate and effective treatment plan for adolescents. Different levels of care for treatment and prevention in this population are discussed in this article. Medications do not necessarily treat the substance use directly, but they can address underlying psychiatric disorders. An integrated collaborative plan of care involving primary care physicians, child and adolescent psychiatrists or addiction psychiatrists, and other addiction and mental health professionals is essential for treatment of this population.

Substance abuse and its consequent sequelae in youth is a complex and significant public health issue that has immediate and long-term consequences. Racial/ethnic diversity and the issues associated with substance abuse make the problem even more complex. Symptom expression, risk factors, stigma, and the process of evaluation and treatment become even more challenging with culturally diverse youth and hence require added expertise and unique approaches. This article presents an overview of adolescent substance abuse in diverse populations, including recent trends in epidemiology and risk factors in diverse youth. It presents various culturally informed treatment approaches.

There is an evolving and diverse array of substances that are popular among adolescents and young adults. These include substances in a number of classes: club drugs, dissociative anesthetics, hallucinogens, and inhalants. The substances within each of these classes differ in their pharmacology, effects, and routes of use, but they share the similarity for which their class is named. Given this variety of effect and pharmacology, the management of intoxication, overdose, and withdrawal is challenging and unique to each type of substance. This article reviews the epidemiology, detection, and acute and long-term management of club drugs and of additional classes of emerging substances. The specific substances to be discussed include flunitrazepam, gamma-hydroxybutyrate (GHB), phencyclidine, ketamine, lysergic acid diethylamide (LSD), inhalants, salvia, methylenedioxymethamphetamine (MDMA), methamphetamine, and the newer synthetic cathinones (bath salts) and synthetic cannabinoids.

Substance use is highly prevalent among juvenile offenders. This article reviews the current literature on screening methods and treatment modalities for youth involved in the juvenile justice system and discusses the role of drug courts and evidence-based community reentry programs. Although some interventions may improve outcomes among young offenders, their implementation has not occurred as widely as their effectiveness would warrant. Overall rates of recidivism and substance use in the juvenile justice population remain high. There is a continued need to better understand ways to prevent substance use relapse and associated reoffending in this population.

Adolesc Med 025 (2014) xv–xvi

Foreword

It seems that being an adolescent, which has always been challenging, is getting even tougher. Adolescents already are hardwired to seek novelty and take risks, but now they must navigate an environment crisscrossed with increasingly treacherous avenues for channeling those otherwise desirable traits. One of the most worrisome trends in this context is the growing variety and availability of legal and illegal psychoactive substances. These substances can compromise adolescents' physical, cognitive, and social health and push them onto a path to addiction.

Consequently, neuroscientists and addiction researchers, who have made adolescents the focus of their work, perform a doubly important function in the promotion of public health. Their combined contributions have transformed our understanding of the specific risks that affect this particularly vulnerable population, paving the way for more effective prevention and clinical interventions.

Consider, for example, the cross-sectional imaging study that uncovered the maturational imbalance between the prefrontocortical and limbic regions of the brain during an adolescent's development. That landmark observation helped explain much of a young person's penchant for engaging in risky behaviors, including substance use. This understanding added a critical new dimension to the epidemiologic evidence linking early initiation of substance use to a significantly higher incidence of substance use disorders later in life. Although we do not yet fully understand the roots of this connection, a large body of evidence suggests that the high malleability of neural circuits undergoing experience-dependent maturation at this stage plays a big role. A case in point is the recent study showing nicotine's time-restricted ability to epigenetically sensitize the adolescent rat brain to the behavioral effects of cocaine.

It is data such as these that have prompted the National Institute on Drug Abuse (NIDA) to recognize adolescence as a focal point in its overarching mission. Hence, NIDA has made a commitment to support a robust and multidisciplinary research portfolio geared toward understanding the unique constellation of interacting biologic and environmental factors that shape a young person's substance use trajectory.

The contributions that make up this special issue of *Adolescent Medicine: State of the Art Reviews (AM:STARs)* are particularly exciting because they convey a sense that actionable progress has been made in the field of adolescent substance abuse research in recent years. This issue is also very timely because the challenges facing young people today are more complex and dynamic than ever before. The effects of many such challenges, such as the potential effect of around-the-clock online activity, are largely unpredictable. Others, such as the proliferation of new designer drugs of abuse or the widespread confusion over nationwide efforts to legalize marijuana use, can be expected to have profoundly negative public health implications.

We hope the articles in this issue of *AM:STARs* will illuminate some of these important debates and spur additional transformative research on how best to protect our young people.

Nora D. Volkow, MD
NIDA Directior
National Institute on Drug Abuse

Ruben D. Baler, PhD
Health Scientist
National Institute on Drug Abuse

Preface

Substance Use and Abuse Among Adolescents

Substance abuse continues to be a significant health problem for adolescents and young adults in the United States and elsewhere. Up-to-date information on the many facets of this issue is essential for physicians who care for these young people. This issue of *Adolescent Medicine: State of the Art Reviews (AM:STARs)* provides reviews of and insights into the latest information on the various substances that adolescents use and how they use them. Articles ranging from overviews of current use data to facts about specific substances such as alcohol, marijuana, prescription stimulants, and opioids, use by different cultural groups, and various treatment options give an extensive and authoritative view of this significant adolescent health issue. We hope you find this issue of *AM:STARs* helpful in your care of adolescents and young adults.

Robert T. Brown, MD
Professor of Pediatrics, Adolescent Medicine
Cooper Medical School of Rowan University

Sheryl Ryan, MD
Associate Professor Pediatrics
Chief, Section of Adolescent Medicine
Yale University School of Medicine

Dedication

Dedicated to John R. Knight, MD and Peter D. Rogers, MD, who have inspired both of us to learn about, care for, and advocate for youth with substance abuse issues.

Adolesc Med 025 (2014) 1–14

Adolescent Substance Use: The Role of the Medical Home

Sharon Levy, MD, MPH[a]*; Janet F. Williams, MD[b]

[a]Director, Adolescent Substance Abuse Program, Children's Hospital Boston,
Assistant Professor of Pediatrics, Harvard Medical School, Boston, Massachusetts;
[b]Professor of Pediatrics, Distinguished Teaching Professor, Department of Pediatrics,
Associate Dean for Faculty and Diversity, School of Medicine Office of the Dean,
University of Texas Health Science Center, San Antonio, Texas

Providing excellent medical care to children includes obtaining a detailed family substance use history with every new patient and being prepared to counsel or refer parents whose substance use affects their children. Anticipatory guidance and age-appropriate substance use prevention counseling should be incorporated into routine medical home practices. Universal substance use screening should be part of the psychosocial history beginning in late childhood. Pediatricians should understand the neurodevelopmental effect of early initiation of alcohol, tobacco, or other drug use while the brain is still maturing. Physicians should be able to identify both specific toxicities and nonspecific symptoms that suggest a substance use disorder and should be prepared to assess and intervene accordingly. Abstinence from alcohol and other substance use should be the routine recommendation given to patients from childhood through adolescence. Physicians should be aware of local and national substance use epidemiology and develop a working relationship with area resources for information and referral. Through a range of services and materials, such as clinical practice guidelines, technical reports, policy statements, and educational tools about preventing, identifying, and managing substance use and substance use disorders, national institutes and professional societies serve as critical resources for health professionals and the public.

SCOPE OF THE PROBLEM

Childhood and adolescent substance use and substance use disorders (SUDs) have a substantial effect on American public health. In 2011, a nationally repre-

*Corresponding author:
Sharon.Levy@childrens.harvard.edu

sentative household survey found that adults rated drug abuse (tied with obesity) as their top health concern for youth from among a list of 23 health concerns.[1] These concerns were sufficiently significant to be included in the goals for *Healthy People 2020*, the current 10-year national objectives established by the US Department of Health and Human Services to improve the health of all Americans.[2]

The pattern of substance use among adolescents has changed significantly during the past 35 years. Before the late 1960s, adults were the predominant age group using alcohol and other psychoactive drugs, including tobacco (nicotine). Beginning in the late 1960s and early 1970s, substance use spread widely among adolescents and subsequently became popular among preadolescents. In 1981, about 66% of high school seniors reported having used an illegal drug at least once in their lives. By 2012, this percentage dropped substantially to 49%, likely representing the combined efforts of government, education, medical physicians, and community-based agencies.[3]

For any drug, the perceived risk, which varies over time, is inversely proportional to the rate of use. Other factors contributing to the changing patterns of substance use include availability of effective school-based prevention programs; media messages that glamorize alcohol, tobacco, and other substance use; patterns of parenting; and cultural messages that promote medication use.[4] For any new substance, perception of benefit always precedes perception of risk; thus, newly introduced drugs experience a relative "grace period of safety" before the risks become apparent, as has recently been seen with the introduction of "bath salts," synthetic cannabinoids, and the repackaging of the stimulant methylenedioxymethamphetamine (MDMA) as "Molly." A related phenomenon is the rediscovery of an older drug, such as lysergic acid diethylamide (LSD), by youths years after the original peak in popularity because the drug's negative effects are no longer remembered.[5,6] Popular sentiment that adolescent substance use is casual, experimental, recreational, or otherwise harmless, as frequently expressed in the current national conversation around marijuana policy, is also associated with increases in use rates among youths.[7]

EPIDEMIOLOGY

Three periodic surveys have long tracked national trends in alcohol, tobacco, and other drug use by adolescents: the annual Monitoring the Future (MTF) study of students in grades 8, 10, and 12[3]; the biannual Youth Risk Behavior Survey (YRBS) of students in grades 9 through 12[5]; and the annual National Survey on Drug Use and Health (NSDUH), a home-based computer-assisted interview of residents aged 12 years and older.[6] These surveys provide adolescent self-report of substance use within specific timeframes, quantified as daily, 2-week, 30-day, annual, and lifetime (ever) use.

Alcohol, tobacco, and marijuana remain the 3 substances most often used by children and adolescents in the United States. Thirty percent of students have tried alcohol by 8th grade, and 69% have done so by 12th grade. Thirteen percent of 8th-graders and more than half of 12th-graders have been drunk at least once in their life.[7] Alcohol is involved in more than one-third of deaths from unintentional injury, homicide, and suicide, which together account for three-fourths of mortality in the 15- to 19-year age group.[5] Heavy episodic or binge drinking is the most typical pattern of alcohol consumption among adolescents, comprising 90% of all alcohol consumed by this age group.[8] Binge drinking is typically defined as consuming 5 or more alcoholic drinks on one occasion, which is defined as a 2-hour period. By these criteria, 24% of adolescents binge drank in 2012. However, this definition is based on changes in blood alcohol level for the average adult male and may significantly underestimate the affect of alcohol on women and children. It has been proposed that binge drinking by children and adolescents is more accurately defined relative to average size and gender, that is, 3 or more alcoholic drinks for girls ages 9 to 17 and boys ages 9 to 13, 4 or more drinks for boys ages 14 to 15 years, and 5 or more drinks for boys older than 16 years.[9] Binge drinking with associated elevated blood alcohol concentration is particularly risky for adolescents who, compared to adults, are less likely to be sedated and are more likely to remain active despite impairment in coordination and judgment, thereby increasing their likelihood of engaging in activities such as driving.

Early initiation of tobacco use has a disproportionately large effect on health; it is predictive of other drug use, a greater variety of drug use, and poor health outcomes.[10] Teens who smoke cigarettes self-report poorer health during adolescence than their peers. Nicotine has high addiction liability; that is, a large proportion of individuals who initiate use will become addicted.[11,12] This process can progress rapidly during adolescence, which is a period of heightened vulnerability to the development of addictions. Some teens have reported becoming addicted after a single use of tobacco.[13] The average age for initiating tobacco use is 12 years and for becoming a regular smoker is 14 years. Most adults (80%) who smoke began doing so before age 18. Thus, pediatric care physicians are the front-line defense in the nation's smoking and other tobacco use prevention and cessation efforts.[10]

The rates of tobacco use by adolescents have fallen substantially in recent years. In 2012, daily cigarette smoking by 8th-graders fell to 1.9%, which is the lowest level since MTF began in 1975.[7] This improvement likely reflects effective public health efforts targeting tobacco prevention. However, there is more work to do because any tobacco use by children is unacceptable. Recently there has been an increase in use by adolescents of electronic (or E-) cigarettes, which are devices that deliver nicotine (without tobacco) via vapor. The product is available in flavors including cotton candy and bubble gum, which are attractive to children and teens. E-cigarettes are marketed as a safer alternative to smoking and a nicotine cessation device, but they may serve as the first exposure to nicotine for many teens. Given the health hazards, physicians should advise children and adolescents to avoid nicotine use in any form.

Although marijuana use rates have paralleled tobacco use during the past 4 decades, these rates have recently diverged, with marijuana use rising significantly. In 2011, marijuana use rates hit their highest level since 1981, peaking at 1.3%, 3.6%, and 6.6% of students in grades 8, 10, and 12, respectively.[14] A 2012 survey by the Partnership for a Drug-Free America found that 1 in 10 teens use marijuana nearly every day, an increase of 60% from rates of use in 2008.[15] The declining perceived risk of marijuana use, noted in *Monitoring the Future: National Results on Adolescent Drug Use: Overview of Key Findings, 2012*, correlates with the subsequent upswing in use.[3] A major influence likely has been the national conversations and state legislative actions regarding legalization, which often reinforce the portrayal of marijuana use as harmless. Although largely ignored, a growing body of literature has linked marijuana use in adolescence to a greater likelihood of addiction, to mood,[16,17] anxiety,[18] or thought disorders,[19,20] and to neurocognitive decline over time.[21] By paralleling the successful strategies used to address alcohol and tobacco use, physicians, particularly pediatric care physicians, can play an important role in educating the public about the known harms of marijuana even in states where use is now legal. The rising rates of adolescent marijuana use suggest that this important public health battle is far from being resolved, and much work remains to reverse these trends. Illicit drugs, prescription medications, over-the-counter (OTC) medications (eg, dextromethorphan), inhalants (or volatile substances ranging from solvents to whipped cream canister propellants), and herbal preparations (eg, *Salvia divinorum*) all are used as psychoactive substances by adolescents and by a growing number of preadolescents, with peak use rates in the late teens and early 20s.[14] New psychoactive substances and old ones in new forms (eg, alcohol/caffeine combination products) are constantly reaching the market. Substituted cathinones (stimulants with effects similar to methamphetamine) were purposely mislabeled as "bath salts" and sold legally through major commercial venues before their adverse effects were known.[22] Synthetic cannabinoids with marijuana-like effects and toxicity also were initially sold legally, making access to psychoactive substances more widespread.

The use of illicit substances other than alcohol, tobacco, and marijuana by adolescents and young adults remains less common, but an alarming new trend is misuse of prescription drugs, including stimulants and narcotic pain medications. Rates of amphetamine use in 12th-graders increased between 2008 and 2011 and started to plateau in 2012.[7] In 2012, past-year opioid use among 12th-graders was 7.9%, and lifetime use for the same age group was 12%.[7] In 2010, opioid pain medication misuse was responsible for 17.3% of all illicit drug use initiations, second only to marijuana.[6] Some adolescents who develop opioid dependence ultimately switch from pain medication to heroin to overcome tolerance because heroin is cheaper and more potent. The high rates of prescription medication diversion and misuse call for greater education of all physicians and other medical professionals on prescribing these medications and monitoring their use.

Research over the past decade has begun to elucidate the neurobiology of addiction as a chronic neurologic disease associated with changes in the brain's reward center.[23] Because of the significant brain development that occurs between the teen years and the mid-20s, adolescence is a developmentally vulnerable period for the onset of addiction.[24] Individuals who begin to use alcohol or marijuana in their teens are significantly more likely to develop an alcohol use disorder in their lifetime compared to those who delay initiation until early adulthood.[25,26]

THE ROLE OF PRIMARY CARE PHYSICIAN

Biopsychosocial History and Anticipatory Guidance

Anticipatory guidance regarding substance use should begin even before a child is born because prenatal exposure to alcohol, tobacco, and other drugs has profound acute and lifelong effects, such as fetal alcohol spectrum disorders (FASD), which is the main preventable cause of intellectual disability. A prenatal visit to the medical home where the child will receive primary care provides the opportunity to develop a rapport with the pregnant woman and other family members and to promote abstinence from alcohol, tobacco, and other drugs during pregnancy and breastfeeding.

An especially important factor in providing primary care for children and adolescents is identifying environmental substance use exposure and SUDs in family members. These are associated with a greater propensity for children to have behavioral problems, difficulties in school, or multiple somatic complaints and to use substances themselves. It is estimated that 1 in 5 children grows up in a home with someone who has an alcohol use disorder or uses illicit drugs, which places these children at risk environmentally and potentially indicates a genetic risk.[27] Inquiry regarding the use of tobacco, alcohol, or other drugs by family members should be a part of the routine history for every new patient. If this discussion reveals a family or home environment history of active substance use or possible dependence, the role of the physician includes recommending a substance use evaluation and management plan, including tobacco cessation, and facilitating patient and family member access to programs and coping mechanisms, such as Alanon.[28]

Anticipatory guidance regarding management of prescription and over-the-counter (OTC) medications is an important part of every well-child visit and should be included during acute care whenever possible. Patients and families need clear guidance about the appropriate use, storage, and disposal of both prescription and OTC medications. Physicians should be familiar with safe practice guidelines for prescribing medications having abuse potential and for educating others about safe medication use, storage, and disposal (eg, see http://www.fda.gov/Drugs/ResourcesForYou/Consumers/BuyingUsingMedicineSafely/EnsuringSafeUseofMedicine/SafeDisposalofMedicines/ucm186187.htm#MEDICINES for a list of medicines that can be disposed of by flushing).

Guidance to parents of young children can include education and encouragement to discuss and model healthful, substance-free means to express or resolve the normal range of emotions, feelings, and stress in order to counter unhealthy socio-cultural messages that encourage substance use, including binge drinking and intoxication. Parents and respected adults can influence children and teens posi-tively when they set high, yet attainable, expectations and model healthy choices regarding psychoactive substances. Using an open, supportive, and developmen-tally appropriate approach, parents should regularly discuss with their children of all ages the risks of substance use as well as healthy ways to avoid this and other risk activities. Teachable moments can help broach the topic in a guiding yet non-confrontational manner. For example, young children can be made aware of someone smoking nearby in a way that discourages future tobacco use. Parents should use all available sources, including print, Web, and entertainment media; advertisements; news; songs; and stories, to start a discussion. Conversations of this sort should encourage children to join the discussion, ask questions, and think critically about healthy life choices so that they become a matter of lifestyle. When healthy lifestyle role models in making choices, critical thinking, and problem-solving are a consistent part of family discussions, expectations, and boundary-setting, they become normal personal standards. Armed with knowledge, attitudes, and skills in understanding and avoiding risk, teenagers may be more likely to view risk situations as solvable, less enticing, and less threatening (see Table 1).

Beginning in late childhood, well-child care should include a psychosocial his-tory (comprising questions about family and peer relationships, academic prog-ress, extracurricular activities, self-esteem, mood, interests, and perceived degree of intra- and extrafamilial conflict or connectedness) obtained directly from the patient. Common acronyms that help physicians delve into the gamut of key psychosocial areas in the patient's life include HEADSS[29] and SSHADESS.[30] Adolescents usually provide honest health histories, even regarding personal matters, although, like patients of any age, their reported substance use may be minimized or occasionally exaggerated. The pediatrician should stay tuned to parental concerns, medical complaints, and contextual clues, such as mood, appearance, behavior, and other psychosocial issues, in order to fully assess usage patterns and health risks.

Part of the challenge in providing holistic health care to adolescents is educating patients and their parents about how assurance of confidentiality must be bal-anced with addressing health and safety needs. Minor consent laws vary by state and generally set a minimum age at which minors may be treated confidentially,

Table 1
Risk and protective factors associated with adolescent use of tobacco, alcohol, and other drugs[20-23]

	Risk factors	Protective factors
Individual	Attitude favorable to substance use	Perceived risk of substance use
	Low self-esteem or poor coping skills	Positive sense of self, assertiveness, social competence; good problem-solving skills
	Mental health disorders including depression and anxiety	Appropriate diagnosis and treatment of mental health disorders
	Attention-deficit/hyperactivity disorder	Pharmacotherapy for attention-deficit/hyperactivity disorder
	Sensation-seeking, impulsivity, distractibility	Resilient temperament; appropriate emotional regulation
Family	Permissive or authoritarian parenting	Authoritative parenting, parental monitoring of activities and supervision
	Parental and older sibling use of alcohol, tobacco, or other drugs	Clearly communicated parental expectation of nonuse and clear rules of conduct consistently enforced
	Family history of alcoholism	Parent in recovery
	High levels of family conflict	Positive, supportive relationships with family
	Child abuse and neglect or sexual abuse	Supportive relationships with adults; close connectedness
Peers	Friends who drink, smoke, or use other drugs	Friends who do not use substances
	Perceived peer drug use	Peer disapproval of substance use; peer resistance skills
School	Poor academic achievement and school failure	Good academic achievement and school success
	Limited interest in school and hobbies	High academic aspirations and involvement in prosocial activities
Community	Marketing of tobacco and alcohol	Media literacy
	Availability of licit and illicit drugs	Strict law enforcement
	Advertisement of licit substances	Comprehensive, theory-based antidrug education programs
	Availability of tobacco and alcohol	High taxes/cost of alcohol and tobacco

although these generally provide little guidance on when physicians should disclose a report of substance use received from minor patients. Ultimately physicians must rely on clinical judgment to manage the delicate balance between protecting a therapeutic relationship and ensuring safety. Practical guidance on discussing and managing confidentiality can be found in the *Alcohol Screening and Brief Intervention for Youth: A Practitioner's Guide* by the National Institute on Alcohol Abuse and Alcoholism (NIAAA).[31]

Screening and Brief Interventions

Given their often longstanding relationships with patients and their families, pediatricians may be the first or only health care professionals in a position to recognize problems with substance use and intervene as they develop. The American Academy of Pediatrics (AAP) and the NIAAA, among others, have recommended universal screening, brief intervention, and referral to treatment (SBIRT) as part of routine health care for all adolescents and have provided policy guidance to support physicians.[31,32,33]

A teen's experience with substances can be viewed as occurring on a spectrum, ranging from abstinence to severe SUD, which includes loss of control and compulsive use.[33] The goal of screening is to discriminate between different levels of substance use in order to provide advice or appropriate intervention. Of note, most substance-related morbidity and mortality occur in patients who do not meet the diagnostic criteria for addiction and often occur in those who do not have an SUD. Routine health advice for teens should include a clear recommendation to abstain from alcohol, tobacco, and other substance use because of their associated acute risk, their ability to impair decision-making regarding other high-risk behaviors, and their negative long-term effects on health and functioning.

The publication of DSM-5[34] changed the terminology used to describe substance use disorders (SUD) from the previous, "substance abuse" and "substance dependence" in DSM-IV to mild, moderate, or severe substance use disorder. This renaming reduces the threshold for diagnosing an SUD and eliminates "diagnostic orphans" or individuals who met 1 or 2 criteria for a diagnosis of substance dependence but none for substance abuse and thus could not be diagnosed with a substance use disorder despite in some cases striking symptoms. Using DSM-5 (Table 2), mild SUD is diagnosed when 2 to 3 criteria are met and suggests that

Table 2
DSM-5 Substance Use Disorders Features

- Persistent desire or unsuccessful efforts to cut down or control use of the substance
- Continued use of the substance despite knowledge of having a persistent or recurrent physical or psychological problem that is likely to have been caused or exacerbated by the substance
- Substance often taken in larger amounts or over longer periods than was intended
- Withdrawal experienced
- Great deal of time spent in activities necessary to obtain the substance, use the substance, or recover from its effects
- Recurrent use of the substance in situations where it is physically hazardous
- Important social, occupational, or recreational activities given up or reduced because of use of the substance
- Tolerance to increasing amounts of the substance experienced
- Craving or a strong desire or urge to use the substance experienced
- Recurrent use of the substance resulting in a failure to fulfill major role obligations at work, school, or home
- Continued use of the substance despite having persistent or recurrent social or interpersonal problems caused or exacerbated by the effects of its use

American Psychiatric Association. *Diagnostic and Statistical Manual for Mental Disorders.* 5th ed. Arlington, VA: American Psychiatric Association; 2013. Reprinted with permission.

an individual has begun to have problems associated with use. Moderate SUD is diagnosed when 4 to 5 criteria are met and indicates more significant problems, but without loss of control and compulsive use associated with severe SUD, which is diagnosed when 6 or more criteria are met. Unlike *DSM-IV*, in *DSM-5* the same modifiers (mild, moderate, severe) are used for tobacco use disorders as other substances. *DSM-5* does not include caffeine use disorders but poses study questions to better define this entity in future versions.

Beyond Screening

Adolescent SUDs are among the most commonly missed diagnoses in pediatric and adolescent medicine. Increased rates of routine screening can help to address this problem, although all primary care physicians as well as medical and surgical subspecialists must maintain awareness of the gamut of medical and behavioral presentations that may indicate substance use even when use is denied. An SUD should be considered in the differential diagnosis whenever an adolescent presents with academic problems, legal problems, sudden changes in behavior or peer group, or abrupt onset of mental health symptoms, such as anxiety or attention problems, mood swings, or disordered thoughts. An SUD should be suspected when any of these nonspecific symptoms occurs coincident with possession of alcohol, drugs, or drug paraphernalia or with second-hand report of substance use. When an SUD is part of a differential diagnosis, the adolescent should be referred for evaluation by a mental health or addiction specialist who is experienced in working with adolescents. All adolescents who are referred for treatment should undergo follow-up in their medical home in order to monitor and guide treatment as necessary.

Although substance use commonly has characteristic behavioral manifestations, pediatricians should be equally familiar with recognizing medical manifestations. Trauma, chronic cough or congestion, chest pain, poorly controlled asthma, abdominal complaints, chronic pain, or recurrent flu-like symptoms all may be signs of substance use or substance withdrawal. When asked about substance use, patients respond best to open-ended questions and an empathic, nonjudgmental style of interviewing, which help build an honest and open physician-patient rapport and relationship. Whenever an adolescent reports substance use, the adolescent SBIRT guidelines[32] can help determine the degree of associated risk and the appropriate level of intervention.[35] Even experienced physicians tend to underestimate the degree of associated problems when relying on clinical impressions alone.[35]

Continually updated Web sites (Table 3) can be useful sources for obtaining general substance use information; following local, national, and global trends; and identifying drugs by their "street names," which often vary by geographic region. Engaging in community- or school-based projects is another means for physicians to stay abreast of local trends from the police and other professionals who work with children, such as school counselors.

Table 3
Internet resources

American Academy of Pediatrics:
  Committee on Substance Abuse: www.aap.org/en-us/about-the-aap/Committees-Councils-
  Sections/Pages/Committee-on-Substance-Abuse.aspx
Government agencies:
  National Institute on Drug Abuse: www.drugabuse.gov
  National Institute on Alcohol Abuse and Alcoholism: www.niaaa.nih.gov
  Substance Abuse and Mental Health Services Administration: www.samhsa.gov
National surveys:
  Monitoring the Future: www.monitoringthefuture.org
  Youth Risk Behavior Surveillance System: www.cdc.gov/nccdphp/dash/yrbs
  National Survey on Drug Use and Health: http://oas.samhsa.gov/nhsda.htm
Street drug names:
  Office of National Drug Control Policy: www.streetlightpublications.net/misc/ondcp.htm
Drug trends and updates:
  National Institute on Drug Abuse: www.nida.nih.gov/infofacts/hsyouthtrends.html
  The Partnership for a Drug-Free America Join Together: www.drugfree.org/join-together
  MedlinePlus: www.nlm.nih.gov/medlineplus/drugabuse.html
Support:
  Above the Influence: www.abovetheinfluence.com/

Drug Testing

Laboratory testing for substances of abuse should be considered part of emergency or acute care when an adolescent presents with altered mental status or symptoms of a toxidrome, suggesting recent use of a particular substance. As with any other laboratory test results, drug test results should be interpreted within the context of the history and physical examination. Permission, confidentiality, and chain of evidence each must be considered when testing for drugs of abuse. Patients should never be tested for drugs without their explicit knowledge and consent, unless they are in an emergency circumstance. If an adolescent refuses to be tested, the physician should explore the reasons for refusal. Guidelines from the AAP,[36] in conjunction with issues of consent and confidentiality,[37] should be considered when deciding whether to use drug testing in a nonemergency diagnosis and or in the management of substance use.

Drug testing may be useful as part of an assessment of nonspecific signs and symptoms that possibly could be ascribed to drug use even when the history is negative, but its role is limited because of several significant limitations inherent to each of the different types of drug testing procedures. For most drug use, a single drug test is likely to be negative even in the context of ongoing sporadic drug use because timing is crucial and most substances cannot be detected 48 to 72 hours after the last use (see Table 4). Multipanel tests detect only a select sample of substances, and some substances are not easily detected or cannot be detected at all in biologic matrices. Being knowledgeable about the test panel

Table 4
Approximate duration of detectability and common cutoffs for selected drugs

Drug	Metabolite	Window of detection	Comments
Alcohol	Alcohol	7-12 hr	Ethylsuccinate and ethyl glucuronide can persist in the urine up to 5 d after heavy alcohol use; however, use of hand sanitizer, mouthwash, cough syrup, etc, can result in low levels without "alcohol use"
	Ethylsuccinate	Up to 5 d	
	Ethyl glucuronide		
Amphetamines			
Amphetamine (AMP)	MAMP	1-3 d	Note that methylphenidate is not detected on a routine amphetamine panel; therefore, a positive amphetamine test cannot be explained by use of a methylphenidate preparation
Methamphetamine (MAMP)	>100 ng/mL of AMP + MAMP	1-2 d	
3,4-MethylenediozyAMP	MDA	1-2 d	
3,4-MethylenediozyMAMP	MDMA	1-2 d	
Barbiturates			
Pento/Secobarbital	Secobarbital	Short-acting, 4-6 d	
Butalbital	Secobarbital	Intermediate, 3-8 d	
Phenobarbital	Secobarbital	Long-acting, 10-30 d	

Table 4
Approximate duration of detectability and common cutoffs for selected drugs (continued)

Drug	Metabolite	Window of detection	Comments
Benzodiazepines			
Triazolam	Hydroxyethyl-flurazepam	Short-acting, 1 d	Most benzodiazepines screens identify oxazepam and so will not pick up *all* benzodiazepines; if evaluating a patient for benzodiazepine use it is important to find the specific medication on the test panel or speak with laboratory personnel
Clonazepam	7-Amino clonazepam	Intermediate, 1-12.5 d	
Diazepam	Oxazepam	Long-acting, 5-8 d	
Chronic use		Can last 30 d after last use	
Cocaine	Benzoylecgonine	1-3 d	
Cannabinoids	Carboxy-THC	Single use, 1-3 d; Moderate use, 4 d; heavy use, 10 d; Chronic, 3-5 wk after last use	Note that synthetic cannabinoids will not be picked up on a cannabinoid screen; if use of synthetic cannabinoids is suspected, speak to laboratory personnel regarding availability of tests for these substances
Lysergic acid Diethylamide (LSD)	Nor-LSD	4 hr	
Methadone	Methadone & metabolite EDDP	1 d-1 wk	
Opiates			
Morphine (M)	Morphine	1-2 d	
Codeine (C)	Morphine & codeine	1-2 d	
Semisynthetic opiates	Hydrocodone	1-2 d	
	Hydromorphone	1-2 d	
	Oxycodone	1-3 d	
	Oxymorphone	1.5-2.5 d	
Heroin	6-Acetylmorphine + M	<24 hr; 1-2 d for morphine	6-Acetylmorphine is pathognomonic for heroin use but has a very narrow time window and most often is *not* detected on a drug test; a test that is positive for morphine outside of the use of prescribed morphine is suggestive of heroin use
Phencyclidine (PCP)	Phencyclidine	Casual use, 2-10 d; Chronic use, several wk	

used, detection windows, and common sources of false-positive and false-negative results is necessary to prevent errors in interpreting test results.[38]

SUMMARY

Given the continued high rates of substance use by adolescents and young adults, it should be among the topics addressed at every health care visit in the medical home. Primary care physicians should counsel and refer parents for substance use assessment, counseling, and cessation management when pediatric or adolescent patients are environmentally exposed to substances and substance use. The role of the medical home includes providing parents, children, and adolescents with anticipatory guidance, drug use screening, health advice, brief intervention, and referral for further assessment and treatment when an SUD is suspected. Clinical and technical reports, policy statements, and educational materials provided by national institutes and health professional societies assist those caring for children and adolescents by assuring best practices in detailed guidance and developmentally appropriate strategies related to alcohol, tobacco, and other substance use across the pediatric age range.

References

1. University of Michigan. *Drug Abuse Now Equals Childhood Obesity as Top Health Concern for Kids.* Ann Arbor: University of Michigan, CS Mott Children's Hospital; 2011
2. US Department of Health and Human Services. *Healthy People 2020: Substance Abuse Objectives.* Washington, DC: US Government Printing Office; 2011
3. Johnston LD, O'Malley PM, Bachman JG, Schulenberg JE. *Monitoring the Future: National Results on Adolescent Drug Use: Overview of Key Findings, 2012.* Ann Arbor, MI: Institute for Social Research, The University of Michigan; 2013
4. Strasburger VC. Alcohol advertising and adolescents. *Pediatr Clin North Am.* 2002;49(2):353–376, vii
5. Eaton DK, Kann L, Kinchen S, et al. Youth risk behavior surveillance—United States, 2009. *MMWR Surveill Summ.* 2010;59(5):1–142
6. Substance Abuse and Mental Health Services Administration. *Results from the 2010 National Household Survey on Drug Abuse: Summary of National Findings.* Rockville, MD: Substance Abuse and Mental Health Services Administration; 2011
7. Johnston LD, O'Malley PM, Bachman JG, Schulenberg JE. *Monitoring the Future: National Survey Results on Drug Use, 1975-2012. Volume I: Secondary School Students.* Ann Arbor, MI: Institute for Social Research, The University of Michigan; 2013
8. Office of Juvenile Justice and Delinquency Prevention. *Drinking in America: Myths, Realities, and Prevention Policy.* Washington, DC: US Department of Justice; 2005
9. Donovan JE. Estimated blood alcohol concentrations for child and adolescent drinking and their implications for screening instruments. *Pediatrics.* 2009;123(6):e975–e981
10. Sims TH; Committee on Substance Abuse. From the American Academy of Pediatrics: Technical report—Tobacco as a substance of abuse. *Pediatrics.* 2009;124(5):e1045–e1053
11. Johnson PB, Richter, L. The relationship between smoking, drinking, and adolescents' self-perceived health and frequency of hospitalization: analyses from the 1997 National Household Survey on Drug Abuse. *J Adolesc Health.* 2002;30(3):175–183
12. Vingilis ER, Wade TJ, Seeley JS. Predictors of adolescent self-rated health. Analysis of the National Population Health Survey. *Can J Public Health.* 2002;93(3):193–197

13. DiFranza JR, Richmond JB. Let the children be heard: lessons from studies of the early onset of tobacco addiction. *Pediatrics.* 2008;121(3):623–624

14. Johnston LD, O'Malley PM, Bachman JG, JE S. *Monitoring the Future: National Results on Adolescent Drug Use: Overview of Key Findings, 2011.* Ann Arbor: Institute for Social Research, The University of Michigan; 2012

15. *2012 Partnership Attitude Tracking Study: Teens and Parents.* Available at: www.drugfree.org/wp-content/uploads/2013/04/PATS-2012-FULL-REPORT2.pdf. Accessed February 28, 2014

16. Degenhardt L, Hall W, Lynskey MT. Exploring the association between cannabis use and depression. *Addiction.* 2003;98:1493–1504

17. de Graaf R, Radovanovic M, van Laar M, et al. Early cannabis use and estimated risk of later onset of depression spells: epidemiologic evidence from the population-based World Health Organization World Mental Health Survey Initiative. *Am J Epidemiol.* 2010;172(2):149–159

18. Patton GC, Coffey C, Carlin JB, et al. Cannabis use and mental health in young people: cohort study. *BMJ.* 2002;325(7374):1195–1198

19. Bossong MG, Niesink RJM. Adolescent brain maturation, the endogenous cannabinoid system and the neurobiology of cannabis-induced schizophrenia. *Prog Neurobiol.* 2010;92(3):370–385

20. Sugranyes G, Flamarique I, Parellada E, et al. Cannabis use and age of diagnosis of schizophrenia. *Eur J Psychiatry.* 2009;24:282–286

21. Meier MH, Caspi A, Ambler A, et al. Persistent cannabis users show neuropsychological decline from childhood to midlife. *Proc Natl Acad Sci U S A.* 2012;109(40):E2657–E2664

22. Ross EA, Watson M, Goldberger B. "Bath salts" intoxication. *N Engl J Med.* 2011;365(10):967–968

23. Lee AM, Messing RO. Protein kinases and addiction. *Ann N Y Acad Sci.* 2008;1141:22–57

24. Lubman DI, Yucel M, Hall WD. Substance use and the adolescent brain: a toxic combination? *J Psychopharmacol.* 2007;21(8):792–794

25. Hingson RW, Zha W. Age of drinking onset, alcohol use disorders, frequent heavy drinking, and unintentionally injuring oneself and others after drinking. *Pediatrics.* 2009;123(6):1477–1484

26. Chen CY, O'Brien MS, Anthony JC. Who becomes cannabis dependent soon after onset of use? Epidemiological evidence from the United States: 2000-2001. *Drug Alcohol Depend.* 2005;79(1):11–22

27. Eigen LD, Rowden DW. A methodology and current estimate of the number of children of alcoholics. In: Adger H Jr, Black C, Brown S, et al, eds. *Children of Alcoholics: Selected Readings.* Rockville, MD: National Association for Children of Alcoholics; 1995:77–97

28. Wilson CR, Harris SK, Sherritt L, et al. Parental alcohol screening in pediatric practices. *Pediatrics.* 2008;122(5):e1022–e1029

29. Goldenring J, Cohen G. Getting into adolescent heads. *Contemp Pediatr.* 1988;5(7):75–90

30. Ginsburg K. Viewing our adolescent patients through a positive lens. *Contemp Pediatr.* 2007;24:65–76

31. National Institute on Alcohol Abuse and Alcoholism. *Alcohol Screening and Brief Intervention for Youth: A Practitioner's Guide.* Bethesda, MD: National Institute on Alcohol Abuse and Alcoholism, National Institutes of Health; 2011. NIH publication 11-7805

32. American Academy of Pediatrics Committee on Substance Abuse. Substance use screening, brief intervention, and referral to treatment for pediatricians. *Pediatrics.* 2011;128(5):e1330–e1340

33. Wilson CR, Sherritt L, Gates E, Knight JR. Are clinical impressions of adolescent substance use accurate? *Pediatrics.* 2004;114(5):e536–e540

34. American Psychiatric Association. *Diagnostic and Statistical Manual of Mental Disorders.* 5th ed. Arlington, VA: American Psychiatric Association; 2013

35. Levy SJ, Kokotailo PK. Substance use screening, brief intervention, and referral to treatment for pediatricians. *Pediatrics.* 2011;128(5):e1330–e1340

36. American Academy of Pediatrics Committee on Substance Abuse. Testing for drugs of abuse in children and adolescents. *Pediatrics.* 1996;98(2 Pt 1):305–307

37. Clark DB, Gordon AJ, Ettaro LR, Owens JM, Moss HB. Screening and brief intervention for underage drinkers. *Mayo Clin Proc.* 2010;85(4):380–391

38. Casavant MJ. Urine drug screening in adolescents. *Pediatr Clin North Am.* 2002;49(2):317–327

Adolesc Med 025 (2014) 15–32

Neurobiology of Adolescent Substance Use and Addictive Behaviors: Treatment Implications

Christopher J. Hammond, MD[a,b*];
Linda C. Mayes, MD[a]; Marc N. Potenza, MD, PhD[a,b,c]

[a]Child Study Center, Yale University, School of Medicine, New Haven, Connecticut;
[b]Department of Psychiatry, Yale University School of Medicine, Connecticut Mental Health Center,
New Haven, Connecticut; [c]Department of Neurobiology, Yale University School of Medicine,
New Haven, Connecticut

*Corresponding author:
christopher.hammond@yale.edu

Funding Source: This research was supported in part by grants RL1 AA017539, R01 DA018647, and P20DA027844 from the National Institutes of Health, Bethesda, MD; the Connecticut State Department of Mental Health and Addiction Services, Hartford, CT; the Yale Center for Clinical Investigation, New Haven, CT; and a Center of Excellence in Gambling Research Award from the National Center for Responsible Gaming and its Institute for Research on Gambling Disorders. The funding agencies did not provide input or comment on the content of the manuscript, and the content of the manuscript reflects the contributions and thoughts of the authors and do not necessarily reflect the views of the funding agencies. Conflict of Interest and Financial Disclosures: The authors report no conflicts of interest with respect to the content of this article. Dr. Hammond has received support from the American Psychiatric Association Child & Adolescent Fellowship; an unrestricted education grant supported by Shire Pharmaceuticals; and the American Academy of Child & Adolescent Psychiatry Pilot Research Award for Junior Investigators supported by Lilly USA, LLC. Dr. Potenza has consulted for and advised Boehringer Ingelheim, Ironwood, and Lundbeck; has consulted for and had financial interests in Somaxon; has received research support from the National Institutes of Health, Veteran's Administration, Mohegan Sun Casino, National Center for Responsible Gaming and its affiliated Institute for Research on Gambling Disorders, Forest Laboratories, Ortho-McNeil, Oy-Control/Biotie, Glaxo-SmithKline, and Psyadon Pharmaceuticals; has participated in surveys, mailings, and telephone consultations related to drug addiction, impulse control disorders, and other health topics; has consulted for law offices and the federal public defender's office on issues related to impulse control disorders; provides clinical care in the Connecticut Department of Mental Health and Addiction Services Problem Gambling Services Program; has performed grant reviews for the National Institutes of Health and other agencies; has guest-edited journal sections; has given academic lectures in grand rounds, CME events, and other clinical or scientific venues; and has generated books or book chapters for publishers of mental health texts. Dr. Mayes reports no disclosures. The authors alone are responsible for the content and writing of this manuscript.
Contributor's Statements: All authors have participated in the concept and design, analysis and interpretation of data, and drafting or revising of this article. Dr. Hammond conceptualized and designed the article, drafted the initial article, and approved the final article as submitted. Dr. Mayes conceptualized and designed the article, critically reviewed, edited, and revised drafts of this article, and approved the final article as submitted. Dr. Potenza conceptualized and designed the article, critically reviewed, edited, and revised drafts of this article, and approved the final article as submitted.

INTRODUCTION

Adolescence is marked by dramatic biologic, psychological, and behavioral changes, including physical maturation and puberty, identity formation and individuation, increased independence and responsibility, increased salience of social and peer interactions including romantic interests, and increased exploratory behavior.[1] Although adolescence is one of the healthiest periods with regard to acute and chronic diseases, it is also associated with a 2- to 3-fold increase in morbidity and mortality compared to childhood and adulthood.[2] The primary causes of death during adolescence include motor vehicle crashes, suicides, and homicides. All are related to cognitive control and impulsive/risky behaviors that may be exacerbated by substance use.

Recent studies suggest that more than 80% of adolescents experiment with drugs or alcohol before adulthood.[3] Psychoactive drug initiation, progression into more severe use patterns, and dependency rates peak during adolescence and young adulthood, and adolescents have higher rates of substance use and addictive disorders compared to children and older adults.[4] Early use of psychoactive drugs robustly predicts later drug addiction, psychopathology, and deficits in social and occupational functioning.[5,6] Similar to substance use, other appetitive behaviors are also elevated during adolescence and, in some individuals, may represent nonsubstance/behavioral addictions.[7] Understanding the neurobiologic basis of addiction may facilitate identification of teenagers who are at risk for addiction and its associated health consequences and promote development of effective treatment and prevention strategies. Additionally, understanding the neurobiologic basis of addiction in adolescence may inform policy and public health initiatives relevant to this developmental period.

In this article, we examine the neurobiologic correlates of substance use and addictive behaviors during adolescence and different biologic models of addiction. We discuss biologic risk factors for drug initiation and progression to addiction in adolescence and the neurotoxic effects of specific drugs. Finally, we review implications for treatment, prevention, and policy.

ADDICTIONS: SUBSTANCE AND NONSUBSTANCE/BEHAVIORAL

Addiction comes from the Latin *addicere* meaning "enslaved by" or "bound."[8] Central features of addiction include compulsive engagement in a behavior (eg, drug use), a craving or appetitive urge state immediately preceding engagement in the behavior, diminished control over the behavior, and continued engagement in the behavior despite adverse consequences.[9] Significant debate continues over whether the term *addiction* should be expanded to include nonsubstance appetitive behaviors that are compulsive or excessive in nature. Nonsubstance appetitive behaviors (eg, gambling, eating, sex, shopping, Internet usage, and video gaming) share commonalities in their rewarding properties and propensity for habit formation similar to those of psychoactive substances.[7] Although most people gamble, use the Internet, play video games, and shop adaptively, in a subgroup of people, particularly those with poor impulse control, these activities may constitute behavioral/nonsubstance addictions with associated adverse consequences.[7]

These appetitive behaviors in adolescence may follow parallel developmental trajectories to psychoactive substance use behaviors, with elevated rates of engagement and addiction in adolescence compared to adulthood. Rates of problem and pathologic gambling are 2- to 4-fold higher in adolescents compared to adults, and problematic video gaming, Internet usage, and shopping all have been found to occur in adolescents and are associated with adverse measures of health and functioning.[10-13] Obesity rates among children and adolescents also have risen dramatically over the past several decades, driven in part by overconsumption of palatable foods.[14] Furthermore, the levels of engagement in appetitive behaviors and substance use may be important, especially in adolescence, when subsyndromal levels of engagement that do not meet full threshold for an addiction are still associated with impairments in health and functioning.[15]

BIOLOGIC MODELS OF ADDICTION

Multiple biologic models may explain substance use and addictive disorders and vulnerability to addictions.[9] Most models are not mutually exclusive but rather are complementary; they examine different facets of addictive behaviors, especially as they relate to dopaminergic circuits. The mesolimbic dopaminergic system is a neural circuit involving the nucleus accumbens (located in the ventral striatum), which receives dopaminergic inputs from the ventral tegmental area.[16] This neural circuit is a common neural pathway of reward. Activity with dopamine release in the nucleus accumbens is associated with reward responsiveness to both substance-related rewards (eg, cocaine) and "natural" rewards (eg, sex, video gaming).[17] Reward-centric models of addiction have focused on reward processing and the reinforcing aspect of drug using. One model posits that repeated exposures to a drug or appetitive behavior in susceptible individuals may prime these neurocircuits and shift the hedonic set-point (allostatic loading).[18] Thus, over time addictive behaviors may hijack the brain's natural reward system, in effect making it more responsive to the primary drug of abuse and less responsive to other natural reinforcers/rewards.

Dopamine is not the only neurotransmitter of importance, nor is the midbrain dopaminergic system the only brain region of importance to addiction models. Addictive disorders are associated with dysfunction in the expression and function of a broad range of neurotransmitters and neuropeptides, including glutamate, gamma-aminobutyric acid (GABA), serotonin, norepinephrine, and acetylcholine, as well as corticotrophin-releasing factor, opioids, cannabinoids, oxytocin, vasopressin, and neuropeptide Y.[19] Different brain regions also have been linked to different stages of the addiction cycle (see Figure 1).[9] Whereas the midbrain dopaminergic system and associated dorsal striatum seem to be relevant to binging and intoxication, stress-related neurocircuitry encompassing the extended amygdala (bed nucleus of the stria terminalis, central nucleus of the amygdala) and the central and peripheral noradrenergic systems seem to be relevant to negative affect and withdrawal states. Prefrontal cortex (PFC) (orbitofrontal, medial prefrontal, anterior cingulate), basolateral amygdalar, insular, and hippocampal contributions are linked to craving states.

Recent studies have sorted psychological components of reward processing into domains of reward anticipation and valuation, reinforcement learning, salience attribution (ie, assigning degree of relevance to stimuli), and loss/punishment processing.[20-22] Berridge and Robinson[20] proposed an incentive salience model of addiction, which suggests that "liking" (the affective response of experiencing pleasure) and "wanting" (stimulus-driven incentive motivation) can be dissociated anatomically and chemically. The "reward deficiency syndrome" is another reward-centric model of addiction vulnerability positing that hyporesponsiveness of the midbrain dopaminergic system may lead individuals at risk for substance dependence and addictive disorders to seek out and engage in addictive behaviors in order to compensate for underarousal.[23] The reward deficiency model is consistent with self-medication theories of addiction.[24] Different biologic models may explain temporally dissociated components of the addiction cycle. For example, preadolescent hypoactive dopamine signaling (reward deficiency) may lead to earlier onset of drug use, and repeated drug exposures during adolescence may lead to drug-induced priming of reward circuitry and

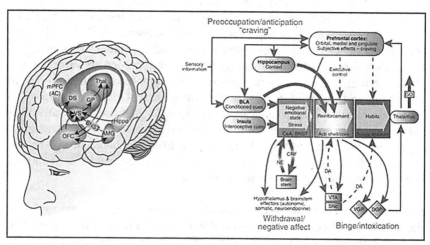

Fig 1. Neurocircuitry schematic illustrating the combination of neuroadaptations in the brain circuitry for the 3 stages of the addiction cycle: 1) binge/intoxication; 2) withdrawal/negative affect; 3) reoccupation/anticipation 'craving'. (From Koob GF, Volkow ND. Neurocircuitry of addiction. *Neuropsychopharmacology.* 2010;35(1):217-238. Reprinted with permission from Macmillan Publishers Ltd.)

progression to dependence. These biologic components contribute to vulnerability at different developmental stages.

Motivation is a process that initiates, guides, and maintains goal-oriented behaviors.[25] Motivation-based models of addiction incorporate elements of motivation, cognitive control, and decision-making. They posit that addictive disorders may represent misdirected motivation in which relatively greater priority is given to appetitive behaviors, such as drug use, and less is given to other behaviors such as work, school, and family care.[26-28] Thus, the motivation to engage in appetitive behaviors overpowers other motivational goals. These models incorporate the neuroeconomic concept of temporal discounting: the selecting of smaller immediate rewards over larger delayed rewards. These decisional pathways are associated with discrete brain regions and circuits.[29] Biologically, the choice of smaller immediate rewards seems to be associated with activity in the ventral striatum and ventromedial PFC. In contrast, the choice of larger delayed rewards seems to be associated with dorsal prefrontal regions, although the subjective value of the immediate or delayed reward may influence neural response.[29,30] Differences in temporal discounting can be found across and within developmental stages, according to severity of addiction. Adolescents are more likely than adults to choose smaller immediate rewards over larger delayed rewards (ie, discount rewards more rapidly).[31] Adults and adolescents with addictive disorders discount rewards more rapidly than do age-matched controls.[29,32,33]

These findings highlight the importance of cognitive control and executive functioning in risk/reward decision-making. Developmentally, the PFCs (the brain regions particularly relevant to exerting "top-down" cognitive control) are among the last brain regions to reach maturation (often not occurring until young adulthood), and this may contribute in part to the specific vulnerability of adolescents to addictions, risk behaviors, and other forms of psychopathology.[1]

ADOLESCENT BRAIN DEVELOPMENT AND ADDICTION VULNERABILITY

Dynamic shifts in brain morphology, fiber architecture, and biochemistry occur during adolescence. Neurodevelopmental morphology studies indicate that gray matter volume and cortical thickness follow an inverted parabolic curve across the lifespan, with a peak occurring in early adolescence (ages 12-14 years) followed by a decline.[34-36] Regional brain morphology shows temporal variance. It follows a caudal-to-rostral pattern, with maturation occurring in the occipital and sensorimotor cortices and striatum at an earlier stage of development than the PFC and association cortices, which are among the last to reach adult levels (see Figure 2).[35,37,38] In contrast to gray matter volumes, white matter pathways show more linear growth and fiber tract enhancement across adolescence, and they reach a plateau in adulthood.[39-41] More recently, diffusion tensor imaging (DTI) has permitted in vivo assessments of white matter architecture by relying on diffusion of water molecules through fiber tracts.[42] Fractional anisotropy (FA), a DTI variable that describes the directional variance of motion, provides an index for fiber tract organization and integrity. FA increases during adolescence and young adulthood, with the most robust changes occurring in the tracts of the superior longitudinal fasciculus, superior corona radiate, thalamic radiations, and posterior limb of the internal capsule.[40,41,43] Parallel to the temporal lag of gray matter decline, fronto-temporal white matter tracts seem to mature at a later stage in development.[44,45] Multiple biochemical changes that also occur during adolescence include altera-tions in dopaminergic and GABAergic neurotransmitter systems and pubertal maturation with its associated neuroendocrine changes.[46-49]

Different neurodevelopmental models postulate why adolescents are prone to experimenting with drugs and alcohol and engaging in other risky behaviors. A developmental imbalance between "top-down" cognitive control systems and "bottom-up" incentive-reward systems has been proposed.[26,50,51] The ability to resist temptation in favor of long-term goal-oriented behavior is one form of cognitive control.[52] Cognitive control improves in a relatively linear fashion from childhood through adulthood and is associated with maturation of the dorsolateral PFC and anterior cingulate, which are components of a top-down executive system.[34] A bottom-up subcortical system, including the striatum and midbrain dopaminergic system, is important in reinforcement learning and

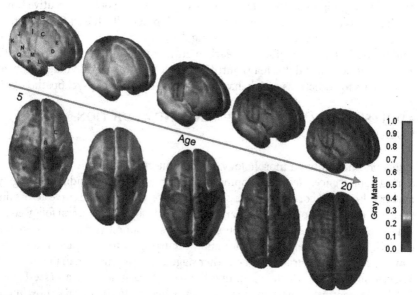

Fig 2. Dynamic sequence of Cortical Gray Matter Maturation from childhood through early adulthood from right lateral and top views. (From Gogtay N, Giedd JN, Lusk L, et al. Dynamic mapping of human cortical development during childhood through early adulthood. *Proc Natl Acad Sci U S A.* 2004;101(21):8174–8179. Copyright 2004 National Academy of Sciences USA.)

matures at an earlier stage of development than a top-down system.[34,35,50] Taken together as a circuit, the imbalance between immature top-down cognitive control processes and mature (and possibly hyperactive) bottom-up incentive-reward processes during adolescence may allow incentive modulation to supersede cognitive control, leading to increased susceptibility to the motivational properties of psychoactive substances and appetitive behaviors.[50]

A triadic model explains adolescent addiction and risky behavior involving the interface of 3 neurobiologic systems: a control/regulatory system involving the medial and ventral PFCs; a reward (approach) system involving the ventral striatum and midbrain dopaminergic system; and a threat (harm-avoidance) system involving the amygdala.[51] In this model, an inefficient regulatory system, a strong reward system, and a weak harm-avoidance system contribute to increased engagement in substance use and other risky behaviors.[51] Another developmental model of motivation neurocircuitry separates the brain into primary and secondary motivational neurocircuits.[26] The primary neurocircuit involves the PFC, striatum, and thalamus (including cortico-striatal-thalamic-cortical loops) and subserves neural processes of decision-making and the selection of discrete goal-oriented behaviors, including those seen in addictions.[26] This model of appetitive and motivated behavior is applicable to both substance and nonsubstance addictions.[26,53] The primary motivational system influencing motivated decision-making is supported by a secondary motivational neurocircuitry that provides multimodal inputs from other brain circuits (sensory, affective, memory, hormonal/homeostatic).[26] Multiple factors likely influence vulnerability to drug use and addictive behavior; they include internal states (eg, emotional distress) and external influences (eg, peer influence, access, media, parental monitoring).[54] Consistent with this model, the interaction of brain regions that modulate the relationship between the primary reward neurocircuitry and different cognitive processes may be dysfunctional in individuals with addictive disorders and in vulnerable at-risk adolescents. These regions include the amygdala in affective states,[55,56] hippocampus and temporal cortices in memory,[56] hypothalamus and septum in homeostatic processes (hunger, thirst),[57] and the insula and parietal cortex in sensing physical and somatic states and attention.[58] Because these bottom-up secondary motivational systems mature at different temporal rates, their relative influence on the primary motivational systems changes across the lifespan. Thus, during adolescence, when these maturational imbalances are the greatest, adolescents may not be able to regulate motivational or emotional states in the same way as adults, which may explain the onset and elevated rates of both addictive and affective disorders during this developmental period.[26,50,51,59]

Controversy remains as to how reward processing and midbrain dopaminergic functioning contribute to addiction vulnerability and addictive disorders in adolescence and whether hyper- or hypo-activation of dopamine functioning conveys risk.[20,60-62] Some studies of typically developing adolescents have demonstrated increased reward responses in the striatum,[63,64] whereas others have shown diminished activation.[65,66] Similar to adults with addictive disorders, adolescents who meet criteria for substance use and addictive disorders show diminished ventral striatal activation during reward anticipation compared to matched controls.[67-69] Similar patterns of ventral striatal hypo-activation apply to impulsivity and risk-taking in adults and adolescents with addictive disorders.[70] These conflicting results underscore the importance of examining individual differences within adolescents. Whereas adolescents in general may express hyperactivation of ventral striatal circuitry during reward processing, those who demonstrate blunted striatal responses may be more vulnerable with respect to development of addictive disorders.[70]

When considering adolescent vulnerability to addictive disorders, the extent to which findings suggest normal development versus aberrant development or pathology currently is unknown. However, behaviors considered developmentally appropriate or normative during adolescence (eg, drug experimentation and risk-taking behaviors) are associated with negative outcomes and real-life measures of adverse functioning.[71,72] Thus, although considered normative, these behaviors are not without individual, familial, and societal cost. Future research should aim to characterize neural substrates that individually predict why some teens but not others are vulnerable to developing substance use and addictive disorders in order to develop targeted interventions and preventions for specific at-risk subgroups.

AFFECT OF DRUG EXPOSURE OR ADDICTIVE PROCESSES ON BRAIN STRUCTURE AND FUNCTION

Characterizing differences in brain structure and function among adolescents is complicated, especially among those who are using alcohol and other drugs. Biologic changes may represent part of normal development,[34,73] relate to addictive processes,[26,74] or reflect neuroadaptation or neurotoxicity related to recent or long-term drug or alcohol exposure that may or may not be central to addictive processes.[75] Further complicating these findings are differences in samples and study design and other confounding variables, such as comorbid psychiatric disorders and polysubstance use, both of which are the norm rather than the exception in adolescents with addictive disorders.[76]

Animal models suggest that the brain is more vulnerable to the effects of psychoactive substances during adolescence.[77] Adolescent alcohol and cannabis use may differentially affect the developing brain, with substance-related differences found in brain morphology, white matter integrity, and activation during cognitive tasks.[78] Among adolescents, differing levels of engagement ranging from alcohol use disorders (AUDs) to binge-pattern drinking for as few as 1 to 2 years have been associated with structural and functional deficits. Alterations have been found in white matter and in regional brain morphology in the hippocampus, PFC, corpus callosum, and cerebellum of adolescents who use alcohol and cannabis compared to those who do not.[79,80] Hippocampal volumes are smaller among adolescents with heavy alcohol use patterns compared to adolescents with co-occurring alcohol and cannabis use and to nonsubstance-using adolescents.[79,81-83] Smaller hippocampal volume also has been associated with age at alcohol onset and duration of dependence.[79] PFC volume seems to be smaller among adolescents with AUD compared to nondrinking controls, and the findings vary by gender. Female adolescents with AUDs had significantly smaller PFC volumes compared to female nondrinkers, whereas male adolescents with AUDs had significantly larger PFC volumes compared to male nondrinkers.[80] No differences in PFC volume were observed between adolescent cannabis users and nonusers.[84] Among adolescent cannabis users, the cerebellar vermis was significantly larger than that in matched control subjects.[84] Using DTI techniques, binge-drinking and alcohol-using adolescents demonstrated lower FA than control subjects across multiple white matter pathways, including the corpus callosum, superior longitudinal fasciculus, corona radiata, internal and external capsules, and commissural, limbic, brainstem, and cortical projection fibers.[85-87] Cannabis use among adolescents was associated with lower FA in the superior longitudinal fasciculus, postcentral gyrus, and inferior longitudinal fasciculus compared to control subjects[86,88] but was associated with increased FA compared to binge-drinking adolescents.[86] Neurocognitive deficits can be found in alcohol- and cannabis-using adolescents across the domains of attentional, visuospatial, and speeded information processing, memory, and executive functioning.[84,89-91] Using functional magnetic resonance imaging techniques, activation patterns during go/no-go, spatial working memory, and word-pair learning tasks differentiated adolescents who use cannabis and alcohol from those who do not.[92-94] These structural and functional abnormalities seem to occur across brain regions that subserve neuropsychological capacities (ie, hippocampus: memory; PFC: executive functions, planning).

Many of these studies are cross-sectional and preclude the ability to draw causality. Longitudinal studies in adolescents with carefully assessed measures of substance use that control for comorbid psychiatric disorders and co-occurring substance use will help to further clarify the extent to which group differences may reflect preexisting characteristics of at-risk youth compared to the sequelae of exposure to specific substances. Recent longitudinal studies suggest that differences in PFC morphology and hypo-activation of PFC during response inhibition in adolescents is associated prospectively with progression to heavier alcohol and drug use.[95-98]

Additionally, possible interactions between developmental stage and drug exposure should be considered. During adolescence, vulnerability windows may exist during which exposure to psychoactive drugs is more likely to affect long-term functioning.[99] Earlier age at onset of alcohol, cannabis, and other drug use has been associated with increased addiction severity and poorer outcomes. Animal models suggest that exposure to psychoactive substances during adolescence increases the risk for addictive behaviors by priming the reward system and making it more responsive.[100] Exposure to psychoactive substances during adolescence also seems to affect pursuit of natural rewards and may provide a link between substance and nonsubstance/behavioral addictions.[101]

GENETICS, EPIGENETICS, AND ENVIRONMENTAL CONTRIBUTIONS

The complex interface of genetic predisposition and early environmental exposures that predate the onset of drug use and addictive behaviors may generate brain-behavior relationships in adolescence that can promote subsequent vulnerability or protection.[102-104] Also, gene and environmental influences seem to vary across developmental epochs and stages of addiction.[105,106] Recent studies suggest that initiation and early patterns of drug use are strongly influenced by family and social factors, whereas progression to heavy and compulsive use is strongly influenced by genetics.[105,106]

Indeed, genetic contributions to addictive disorders are significant, although few studies in adolescents are available. Twin studies suggest that genetic factors account for 30% to 70% of the variance in substance addictions.[107] Emerging evidence also suggests a role for genetic factors in behavioral addictions, including gambling and Internet use disorders, as well as in childhood- and adolescent-onset obesity.[108-111] Genome-wide association studies have implicated several regions and genes in addictive disorders, but studies in adolescents are lacking.[112] Addictive disorders in adults are associated with genes and genetic loci involving a diverse array of neurobiologic processes, including neurotransmitter/neuropeptide transport and function (serotonin, dopamine, and norepinephrine transporters, dopamine receptor 2, μ-opioid receptor), drug metabolism (cytochrome P450 2A6, dopamine β-hydroxylase), growth factors (brain-derived neurotropic factor), and secondary messenger signaling.[103,112] A recent study found evidence that a polymorphism of the μ-opioid receptor encoding gene is associated with adolescent alcohol misuse.[113] Genetic susceptibility to addictions may be classified according to shared/common versus drug-specific genetic vulnerabilities.[107]

In the past decade, epigenetics and gene-by-environment (GXE) interaction studies have examined how the expression of common gene variants and early childhood environmental conditions may affect development of disease.[114] Understanding GXE interactions and how "nature" and "nurture" interact may have relevance for addictions and other psychiatric disorders. For example, a recent GXE study found an interaction between a variant in the gene coding for the corticotropin-releasing hormone receptor 1 (a receptor that contributes to the biologic response to stress) and stressful life events that influence drinking initiation and progression to heavy alcohol use among adolescents.[115] GXE studies also have been used to characterize the effect of adolescent drug exposure on adult functioning and psychopathology. A functional polymorphism of the gene coding for catechol-O-methyltransferase seems to influence the association between adolescent cannabis exposure and development of psychosis in adulthood, with the valine coding allele conveying increased risk.[116] Studies should clearly define the timing of exposure to environmental factors (eg, childhood trauma) in order to better characterize "vulnerability windows," especially in the context of dynamic brain changes that occur across childhood and adolescent development.[114]

PREVENTION, TREATMENT, AND POLICY IMPLICATIONS

Understanding the neurobiology of addiction vulnerability and addictive disorders in adolescents holds significant promise for improved prevention and treatments and for alterations in public policy. For example, such information could aid in the development of novel pharmacotherapies using intelligent drug designs that target specific neurotransmitter systems, neural regions and circuitry, receptor sites, and secondary messenger systems; additional avenues may involve gene therapies and drug vaccines.[117] Dopamine-blocking agents have shown limited efficacy and may exacerbate some nonsubstance addictive behaviors.[117,118] Instead, agents that modulate dopamine signaling within the reward pathways by way of glutamatergic (N-acetylcysteine, acamprosate) and opioid (naltrexone, buprenorphine) receptor systems have shown promise.[117,119-122] Few of these agents have been examined in adolescents, so studies are needed to clarify the safety and efficacy in adolescent samples.[119-122] Equally important is the common neurobiology of comorbid psychiatric and addictive disorders and the potential effect of concurrent treatment of co-occurring psychiatric disorders and addictive disorders on addiction severity and psychiatric symptomatology. Preliminary evidence from comorbid substance use disorders (SUDs) and major depressive disorder or attention-deficit/hyperactivity disorder suggests that remission of mood and attentional symptoms is associated with reductions in drug use.[123,124] Finding common neurobiologic targets for drug development may represent another pathway to new psychopharmacologic treatments.

A major challenge for the field of addiction moving forward is developing biobehavioral markers for early identification of vulnerability to substance use and addictive behaviors. Characterizing the biologic factors related to addiction vulnerability compared to the neurotoxic/neuroadaptive effects of drug exposure is key to developing targeted prevention programs for at-risk youth. Intermediate phenotypes, including delay discounting,[29] impulsivity,[125] and stress-reactivity/responsiveness,[126,127] warrant consideration as markers for risk. In vivo neuroimaging "challenge" studies involving behavioral challenges that require cognitive control in the presence of appetitive cues or affective stimuli may be useful assays for determining those adolescents who have elevated cognitive control to reward activity imbalance or elevated affective reactivity that potentially conveys enhanced risk for addictive behaviors.[64,128,129]

Prevention and interventional strategies should take into account the specific biologic vulnerabilities and strengths of adolescents. Because adolescents are biologically more responsive to rewards and are less responsive to aversive stimuli/losses compared to adults, programs that utilize positive reinforcement rather than punishment or negative reinforcement may be more effective. Rather than trying to eliminate "stimulating" risky behaviors, providing access to exciting activities under controlled settings may help replace or limit harmful risk-taking opportunities.[50] Incorporating contingency management with positive reinforcers (ie, rewards) for prosocial behavior, engagement, and reduction in drug use (ie, negative urine drug tests) has been successfully utilized in treatment of adolescents with SUDs.[130] Alternatively, attempting to enhance cognitive control by cognitive training or cognitive behavioral therapy has been effective for addictive disorders in adolescents.[131-134] Preliminary evidence suggests that the effect of cognitive therapies is related to changes in function/activity in neural circuitry of motivation and cognitive control.[133-134] Recent epidemiologic and phenomenologic data also suggest that adolescent females have different protective factors and risk profiles and may be more likely to abuse illicit substances compared with adolescent males.[135,136] Thus, clarifying the role of gender in treatment response and development of gender-informed interventions may improve outcomes in adolescents.

Public policy and legislation also should be neurodevelopmentally informed. Tax strategies targeting tobacco products have been an effective deterrent to both adult and adolescent smoking behaviors, and taxation of hyperpalatable calorie-dense foods such as sugared sodas warrants exploration.[137,138] Additionally, limiting sugared sodas and unhealthy food choices in school cafeterias and vending machines may influence obesity rates. Adolescents are arguably "hyperconsumers" of media, and a better understanding of the influence of advertising/marketing of appetitive/hedonic products (eg, alcohol, tobacco, palatable foods) on adolescent addictions is warranted, especially in the realm of nonsubstance appetitive behaviors.[139-141]

CONCLUSION

Addictive disorders, including both substance and behavioral addictions, remain among the most costly diseases in society, and adolescence is a critical developmental period for protecting the next generation and curbing future social costs. Emerging evidence on the neurobiology of addictive disorders and addiction vulnerability has the potential to advance the field by enhancing prevention and treatment and influencing public policy.

References

1. Casey BJ, Getz S, Galvan A. The adolescent brain. *Dev Rev.* 2008;28(1):62–77
2. Eaton LK, Kann I, Kinchen S, et al. Youth risk behavior surveillance-United States, 2007, surveillance summaries. *MMWR Morb Mortal Wkly Rep.* 2008;57(SS04):1–131
3. Johnston LD, O'Malley PM, Bachman JG, Schulenberg JE. *Monitoring the Future: National Survey Results on Drug Use, 1975-2012. Volume II: College Students and Adults Ages 19-50.* Ann Arbor, MI: Institute for Social Research, The University of Michigan; 2013

4. Wagner FA, Anthony JC. From first drug use to drug dependence—developmental periods of risk for dependence upon marijuana, cocaine, and alcohol. *Neuropsychopharmacology.* 2002;26(4): 479–488

5. McGue M, Lacono WG. The association of early adolescent problem behavior with adult psychopathology. *Am J Psychiatry.* 2005;162(6):1118–1124

6. Grant BF, Dawson DA. Age of onset of drug use and its association with DSM-IV drug abuse and dependence: results from the national longitudinal alcohol epidemiologic survey. *J Subst Abuse.* 1998;10(2):163–173

7. Grant JE, Potenza MN, Weinstein A, Gorelick DA. Introduction to behavioral addictions. *Am J Drug Alcohol Abuse.* 2010;36:233–241

8. Maddux JF, Desmond DP. Addiction or dependence? *Addiction.* 2000;95:661–665

9. Koob GF, Volkow ND. Neurocircuitry of addiction. *Neuropsychopharmacology.* 2010;35:217–238

10. Shaffer HJ, Hall MN, Vander Bilt J. Estimating the prevalence of disordered gambling behavior in the United States and Canada: a research synthesis. *Am J Public Health.* 1999;89(9):1369–1376

11. Desai RA, Krishnan-Sarin S, Cavallo D, Potenza MN. Video-gaming among high school students: health correlates, gender differences and problematic gaming. *Pediatrics.* 2010;126:e1414–e1424

12. Liu TC, Desai RA, Krishnan-Sarin S, et al. Problematic internet use and health in adolescents: data from a high school survey in Connecticut. *J Clin Psychiatry.* 2011;72:836–845

13. Grant JE, Potenza MN, Krishnan-Sarin S, et al. Shopping problems among high school students. *Comp Psychiatry.* 2011;52:247–252

14. Volkow ND, Wang GJ, Baler RD. Reward, dopamine, and the control of food intake: implications for obesity. *Trends Cogn Sci.* 2011;15(1):37–46

15. Yip SW, Desai RA, Steinberg MA, et al. Health/functioning characteristics, gambling behaviors and gambling related motivations in adolescents stratified by gambling severity: findings from a high school risk survey. *Am J Addict.* 2011;20:495–508

16. Sulzer D. How addictive drugs disrupt presynaptic dopamine neurotransmission. *Neuron.* 2011;69:628–649

17. Kenny PJ. Reward mechanisms in obesity: new insights and future directions. *Neuron.* 2011;69:664–679

18. George O, Le Moal M, Koob GF. Allostasis and addiction: role of the dopamine and corticotropin-releasing factor systems. *Physiol Behav.* 2012;106:58–64

19. Robbins TW, Everitt BJ, Nutt DJ. *The Neurobiology of Addictions: New Vistas.* New York: Cambridge University Press; 2010

20. Berridge KC, Robinson TE. Parsing reward. *Trends Neurosci.* 2003;26(9):507–513

21. Berridge KC. The debate over dopamine's role in reward: the case for incentive salience. *Psychopharmacology (Berl).* 2007;191:391–431

22. Schultz W. Potential vulnerabilities of neuronal reward, risk and decision mechanisms to addictive drugs. *Neuron.* 2011;69:603–617

23. Blum K, Cull JG, Braverman ER, et al. Reward deficiency syndrome. *Am Sci.* 1996;84:132–145

24. Khantzian EJ. The self-medication hypothesis of addictive disorders: focus on heroin and cocaine dependence. *Am J Psychiatry.* 1985;142:1259–1264

25. Dalley JW, Everitt BJ, Robbins TW. Impulsivity, compulsivity, and top-down cognitive control. *Neuron.* 2011;69:680–694

26. Chambers RA, Taylor JR, Potenza MN. Developmental neurocircuitry of motivation in adolescence: a critical period of addiction vulnerability. *Am J Psychiatry.* 2003;160:1041–1052

27. Chambers RA, Bickel WK, Potenza MN. A scale-free systems theory of motivation and addiction. *Neurosci Biobehav Rev.* 2007;31:1017–1045

28. Kalivas PW, Volkow ND. The neural basis of addiction: a pathology of motivation and choice. *Am J Psychiatry.* 2005;162:1403–1413

29. Stanger C, Elton A, Ryan SR, et al. Neuroeconomics and adolescent substance abuse: individual differences in neural networks and delay discounting. *J Am Acad Child Adolesc Psychiatry.* 2013; 52(7):747–755

30. Kable JW, Glimcher PW. The neural correlates of subjective value during intertemporal choice. *Nat Neurosci.* 2007;10(12):1625–1633

31. Steinberg L, Graham S, O'Brien L, et al. Age differences in future orientation and delay discounting. *Child Dev.* 2009;80(1):28–44

32. Petry NM. Substance abuse, pathological gambling, and impulsiveness. *Drug Alcohol Depend.* 2001;63(1):29–38

33. Field M, Christiansen P, Cole J, et al. Delay discounting and the alcohol Stroop in heavy drinking adolescents. *Addiction.* 2007;102(4):579–586

34. Giedd JN, Blumenthal J, Jeffries NO, et al. Brain development during childhood and adolescence: a longitudinal MRI study. *Nat Neurosci.* 1999;2:861–863

35. Gogtay N, Giedd JN, Lusk L, et al. Dynamic mapping of human cortical development during childhood through early adulthood. *Proc Natl Acad Sci U S A.* 2004;101(21):8174–8179

36. Sowell ER, Peterson BS, Thompson PM, et al. Mapping cortical change across the human life span. *Nat Neurosci.* 2003;6(3):309–315

37. Sowell ER, Thompson PM, Mattson SN, et al. Regional brain shape abnormalities persist into adolescence after heavy prenatal alcohol exposure. *Cereb Cortex.* 2002;12(8):856–865

38. Sowell ER, Trauner DA, Gamst A, Jernigan TL. Development of cortical and subcortical brain structures in childhood and adolescence: a structural MRI study. *Dev Med Child Neurol.* 2002;44(1):4–16

39. Giedd JN. The teen brain: insights from neuroimaging. *J Adolesc Health.* 2008;42(4):335–343

40. Lebel C, Walker L, Leemans A, Phillips L, Beaulieu C. Microstructural maturation of the human brain from childhood to adulthood. *Neuroimage.* 2008;40(3):1044–1055

41. Barnea-Gorlay N, Menon V, Eckert M, et al. White matter development during child and adolescence: a cross sectional diffusion tensor imaging study. *Cereb Cortex.* 2005;15(12):1848–1854

42. Roberts TP, Schwartz ES. Principles and implementation of diffusion-weighted and diffusion tensor imaging. *Pediatr Radiol.* 2007;37(8):739–748

43. Bava S, Jacobus J, Mahmood O, Yang TT, Tapert SF. Neurocognitive correlates of white matter quality in adolescent substance users. *Brain Cogn.* 2010;72(3):347–354

44. Tamnes CK, Ostby Y, Fjell AM, et al. Brain maturation in adolescence and young adulthood: regional age-related changes in cortical thickness and white matter volume and microstructure. *Cereb Cortex.* 2009;20(3):534–548

45. Schneiderman JS, Buchsbaum MS, Haznedar MM, et al. Diffusion tensor anisotropy in adolescents and adults. *Neuropsychobiology.* 2007;55(2):96–111

46. Spear LP. Heightened stress responsivity and emotional reactivity during pubertal maturation: implications for psychopathology. *Dev Psychopathol.* 2009;21(1):87–97

47. Jucaite A, Forssberg H, Karlsson P, Halldin C, Farde L. Age-related reduction in dopamine D1 receptors in the human brain from late childhood to adulthood, a positron emission tomography study. *Neuroscience.* 2010;167(1):104–110

48. Cunningham MG, Bhattacharyya S, Benes FM. Increasing interaction of amygdalar afferents with GABAergic interneurons between birth and adulthood. *Cereb Cortex.* 2008;18(7):1529–1535

49. Spear LP. The adolescent brain and age-related behavioral manifestations. *Neurosci Biobehav Rev.* 2000;24(4):417–463

50. Casey BJ, Jones RM. Neurobiology of the adolescent brain and behavior: implications for substance use disorders. *J Am Acad Child Adolesc Psychiatry.* 2010;49(12):1189–1201

51. Ernst M, Pine DS, Hardin M. Triadic model of the neurobiology of motivated behavior in adolescence. *Psychol Med.* 2006;36:299–312

52. Somerville LH, Casey B. Developmental neurobiology of cognitive control and motivational systems. *Curr Opin Neurobiol.* 2010;20(2):236–241

53. Brewer JA, Potenza MN. The neurobiology and genetics of impulse control disorders: relationships to drug addictions. *Biochem Pharmacol.* 2008;75:63–75

54. Sinha R. Chronic stress, drug use, and vulnerability to addiction. *Ann N Y Acad Sci.* 2008;1141:105–130

55. Metcalfe J, Mischel W. A hot/cool-system analysis of delay of gratification: dynamics of willpower. *Psychol Rev.* 1999;106:3–19

56. Belujon P, Grace AA. Hippocampus, amygdala, and stress: interacting systems that affect susceptibility to addiction. *Ann N Y Acad Sci.* 2011;1216:114–121

57. Davidson S, Lear M, Shanley L, et al. Differential activity by polymorphic variants of a remote enhancer that supports galanin expression in the hypothalamus and amygdala: implications for obesity, depression and alcoholism. *Neuropsychopharmacology.* 2011;36:2211–2221

58. Naqvi NH, Bechara A. The hidden island of addiction: the insula. *Trends Neurosci.* 2009;32:56–67

59. Casey BJ, Jones RM, Levita L, et al. The storm and stress of adolescence: insights from human imaging and genetics. *Dev Psychobiol.* 2010;52(3):225–235

60. Gardner EL. The neurobiology and genetics of addiction: implications of the "reward deficiency syndrome" for therapeutic strategies in chemical dependency. In: Elster J, ed. *Addiction: Entries and Exits.* New York: Russell Sage; 1999:57–119

61. Volkow ND, Swanson JM. Variables that affect the clinical use and abuse of methylphenidate in the treatment of ADHD. *Am J Psychiatry.* 2003;160(11):1909–1918

62. Robinson TE, Berridge KC. Addiction. *Annu Rev Psychol.* 2003;54:25–53

63. Galvan A, Hare TA, Parra CE, et al. Earlier development of the accumbens relative to orbitofrontal cortex might underlie risk-taking behavior in adolescents. *J Neurosci.* 2006;26:6885–6892

64. Somerville LH, Hare TA, Casey BJ. Frontostriatal maturation predicts behavioral regulation failures to appetitive cues in adolescence. *J Cogn Neurosci.* 2011;23(9):2123–2134

65. Bjork JM, Smith AR, Chen G, Hommer DW. Adolescents, adults and rewards: comparing motivational neurocircuitry recruitment using fMRI. *PLoS ONE.* 2010;5:e11440

66. Bjork JM, Knutson B, Fong GW, et al. Incentive-elicited brain activation in adolescents: similarities and differences from young adults. *J Neurosci.* 2004;24:1793–1802

67. Wrase J, Schlagenhauf F, Kienast T, et al. Dysfunction of reward processing correlates with alcohol craving in detoxified alcoholics. *Neuroimage.* 2007;35:787–794

68. Balodis IM, Kober H, Worhunsky PD, et al. Diminished frontostriatal activity during processing of monetary rewards and losses in pathological gambling. *Biol Psychiatry.* 2012;71:749–757

69. Beck A, Schlagenhauf F, Wüstenberg T, et al. Ventral striatal activation during reward anticipation correlates with impulsivity in alcoholics. *Biol Psychiatry.* 2009;66:734–742

70. Schneider S, Peters J, Bromberg U, et al. Risk taking and the adolescent reward system: a potential common link to substance abuse. *Am J Psychiatry.* 2012;169:39–46

71. Lejuez CW, Aklin WM, Jones HA, et al. The balloon analogue risk taking task (BART) differentiates smokers and nonsmokers. *Exp Clin Psychopharmacol.* 2003;11:26–33

72. Lejuez CW, Aklin WM, Zvolensky MJ, Pedulla CM. Evaluation of the balloon analogue risk task (BART) as a predictor of adolescent real-world risk taking behaviours. *J Adolesc.* 2003;26:475–479

73. Giedd JN. Structural magnetic resonance imaging of the adolescent brain. *Ann N Y Acad Sci.* 2004;1021:77–85

74. Koob GF, Le Moal M. Drug addiction, dysregulation of reward, and allostasis. *Neuropsychopharmacology.* 2001;24:97–129

75. Beveridge TJ, Gill KE, Hanlon CA, et al. Parallel studies of cocaine related neural and cognitive impairment in humans and monkeys. *Philos Trans R Soc Lond B Biol Sci.* 2008;363:3257–3266

76. Tims FM, Dennis ML, Hamilton N, et al. Characteristics and problems of 600 adolescent cannabis abusers in outpatient treatment. *Addiction.* 2002;97(Suppl 1):46–51

77. Monti PM, Miranda R Jr, Nixon K, et al. Adolescence: booze, brains, and behavior. *Alcohol Clin Exp Res.* 2005;29(2):207–220

78. Squeglia LM, Jacobus J, Tapert SF. The influence of substance use on adolescent brain development. *Clin EEG Neurosci.* 2009;40:31–38

79. De Bellis MD, Clark DB, Beers SR, et al. Hippocampal volume in adolescent onset alcohol use disorders. *Am J Psychiatry.* 2000;157(5):737–744

80. Medina KL, McQueeny T, Nagel BJ, et al. Prefrontal cortex volumes in adolescents with alcohol use disorders: unique gender effects. *Alcohol Clin Exp Res.* 2008;32(3):386–394

81. Nagel BJ, Schweinsburg AD, Phan V, et al. Reduced hippocampal volume among adolescents with alcohol use disorders without psychiatric comorbidity. *Psychiatry Res.* 2005;139(3):181–190

82. Medina KL, Schweinsburg AD, Cohen-Zion M, et al. Effects of alcohol and combined marijuana and alcohol use during adolescence on hippocampal volume and asymmetry. *Neurotoxicol Teratol.* 2007;29(1):141–152

83. Medina KL, Hanson K, Schweinsburg AD, et al. Neuropsychological functioning in adolescent marijuana users: subtle deficits detectable after 30 days of abstinence. *J Int Neuropsychol Soc.* 2007;13(5):207–220

84. Medina KL, Nagel BJ, Tapert SF. Abnormal cerebellar morphometry in abstinent adolescent marijuana users. *Psychiatry Res.* 2010;182(2):152–159

85. McQueeny T, Schweinsburg BC, Schweinsburg AD, et al. Altered white matter integrity in adolescent binge drinkers. *Alcohol Clin Exp Res.* 2009;33(7):1278–1285

86. Jacobus J, McQueeny T, Bava S, et al. White matter integrity in adolescents with histories of marijuana use and binge drinking. *Neurotoxicol Teratol.* 2009;31(6):349–355

87. Tapert SF, Theilmann RJ, Schweinsburg AD. Reduced fractional anisotropy in the splenium of adolescents with alcohol use disorder. *Proc Intl Soc Magn Reson Med.* 2003;11(8217):2241

88. Bava S, Frank LR, McQueeny T, et al. Altered white matter microstructure in adolescent substance users. *Psychiatry Res.* 2009;173(3):228–237

89. Brown SA, Tapert SF, Granholm E, Delis DC. Neurocognitive functioning of adolescents: effects of protracted alcohol use. *Alcohol Clin Exp Res.* 2000;24(2):164–171

90. Tapert SF, Brown SA. Substance dependence, family history of alcohol dependence and neuropsychological functioning in adolescence. *Addiction.* 2000;95(7):1043–1053

91. Tapert SF, Granholm E, Leedy NG, Brown SA. Substance use and withdrawal: neuropsychological functioning over 8 years in youth. *J Int Neuropsychol Soc.* 2002;8(7):873–883

92. Tapert SF, Schweinsburg AD, Drummond SP, et al. Functional MRI of inhibitory processing in abstinent adolescent marijuana users. *Psychopharmacology (Berl).* 2007;194(2):173–183

93. Tapert SF, Schweinsburg AD, Barlett VC, et al. Blood oxygen level dependent response and spatial working memory in adolescents with alcohol use disorders. *Alcohol Clin Exp Res.* 2004;28(10):1577–1586

94. Schweinsburg AD, McQueeny T, Nagel BJ, Eyler LT, Tapert SF. A preliminary study of functional magnetic resonance imaging response during verbal encoding among adolescent binge drinkers. *Alcohol.* 2010;44(1):111–117

95. Norman AL, Pulido C, Squeglia LM, et al. Neural activation during inhibition predicts initiation of substance use in adolescence. *Drug Alcohol Depend.* 2011;119:216–223

96. Mahmood OM, Goldenberg D, Thayer R, et al. Adolescents' fMRI activation to a response inhibition task predicts future substance use. *Addict Behav.* 2013;38:1435–1441

97. Rando K, Chaplin TM, Potenza MN, Mayes L, Sinha R. Prenatal cocaine exposure and gray matter volume in adolescent boys and girls: relationship to substance use initiation. *Biol Psychiatry.* 2013;74:482–289

98. Cheetham A, Allen NB, Whittle S, et al. Orbitofrontal volumes in early adolescence predict initiation of cannabis use: a 4-year longitudinal and prospective study. *Biol Psychiatry.* 2012;71(8):684–692

99. Lisdahl KM, Gibart ER, Wright NE, Shollenberger S. Dare to delay? The impact of adolescent alcohol and marijuana use onset on cognition, brain structure, and function. *Front Psychiatry.* 2013;4:1–16

100. Pisitis M, Perra S, Pillolla G, et al. Adolescent exposure to cannabinoids induces long-lasting changes in the response to drugs of abuse of rat midbrain dopamine neurons. *Biol Psychiatry.* 2004;56:86–94

101. Fattore L, Melis M, Fadda P, Pistis M, Fratta W. The endocannabinoid system and nondrug rewarding behaviors. *Exp Neurol.* 2010;224:23–36

102. Rutter R, Moffitt TE, Caspi A. Gene-environment interplay and psychopathology: multiple varieties but real effects. *J Child Psychol Psychiatry.* 2006;47:226–261

103. Kreek MJ, Nielsen DA, Butelman ER, LaForge KS. Genetic influences on impulsivity, risk taking, stress responsivity and vulnerability to drug abuse and addiction. *Nat Neurosci.* 2005;8:1450–1457

104. Swendsen J, Le Moal M. Individual vulnerability to addiction. *Ann N Y Acad Sci.* 2011;1216:73–85

105. Kendler KS, Schmitt E, Aggen SH, Prescott CA. Genetic and environmental influences on alcohol, caffeine, cannabis, and nicotine use from early adolescence to middle adulthood. *Arch Gen Psychiatry.* 2008;65(6):674–682

106. Pagan JL, Rose RJ, Viken RJ, et al. Genetic and environmental influences on stages of alcohol use across adolescence and into young adulthood. *Behav Genet.* 2006;36(4):483–497

107. Tsuang MT, Lyons MJ, Meyer JM, et al. Co-occurrence of abuse of different drugs in men: the role of drug-specific and shared vulnerabilities. *Arch Gen Psychiatry.* 1998;55:967–972

108. Lobo DS, Kennedy JL. The genetics of gambling and behavioral addictions. *CNS Spectr.* 2006;11(12):931–939

109. Lobo DS, Vallada HP, Knight J, et al. Dopamine genes and pathological gambling in discordant sib-pairs. *J Gambl Stud.* 2007;23:421–433

110. Montag C, Kirsch P, Sauer C, Markett S, Reuter M. The role of CHRNA4 gene in internet addiction: a case-control study. *J Addict Med.* 2012;6(3):191–195

111. Zametkin AJ, Zoon CK, Klein HW, Munson S. Psychiatric aspects of child and adolescent obesity: a review of the past 10 years. *J Am Acad Child Adolesc Psychiatry.* 2004;43(2):134–150

112. Li MD, Burmeister M. New insights into the genetics of addiction. *Nat Rev Genet.* 2009;10;225–231

113. Miranda R, Ray L, Justus A, et al. Initial evidence of an association between OPRM1 and adolescent alcohol misuse. *Alcohol Clin Exp Res.* 2010;34(1):112–122

114. Caspi A, Sugden K, Moffitt TE, et al. Influence of life stress on depression: moderation by a polymorphism in the 5-HTT gene. *Science.* 2003;301:386–389

115. Schmid B, Blomeyer D, Treutlein J, et al. Interacting effects of CRHR1 gene and stressful life events on drinking initiation and progression among 19-year olds. *Int J Neuropsychopharmacol.* 2010;13:703–714

116. Caspi A, Moffitt TE, Cannon M, et al. Moderation of the effect of adolescent-onset cannabis use on adult psychosis by a functional polymorphism in the catechol-o-methyltransferase gene: longitudinal evidence of a gene x environment interaction. *Biol Psychiatry.* 2005;57:1117–1127

117. Potenza MN, Sofuoglu M, Carroll KM, Rounsaville BJ. Neuroscience of behavioral and pharmacological treatments for addictions. *Neuron.* 2011;69:695–712

118. Zack M, Poulos CX. A D2 antagonist enhances the rewarding and priming effects of a gambling episode in pathological gamblers. *Neuropsychopharmacology.* 2007;32:1678–1686

119. Grant JE, Kim SW, Odlaug BL. N-acetyl cysteine, a glutamate-modulating agent, in the treatment of pathological gambling: a pilot study. *Biol Psychiatry.* 2007;62:652–657

120. Deas D, May K, Randall C, Johnson N, Anton R. Naltrexone treatment of adolescent alcoholics: an open-label pilot study. *J Child Adolesc Psychopharmacol.* 2005;15(5):723–728

121. Woody GE, Poole SA, Subramaniam G, et al. Extended vs short-term buprenorphine-naloxone for treatment of opioid-addicted youth. *JAMA.* 2008;300(17):2003–2011

122. Gray KM, Carpenter MJ, Baker NL, et al. A double-blind randomized controlled trial of N-acetyl-cysteine in cannabis-dependent adolescents. *Am J Psychiatry.* 2012;169(8):805–812

123. Riggs PD, Mikulich-Gilbertson SK, Davies RD, et al. A randomized controlled trial of fluoxetine and cognitive behavioral therapy in adolescents with major depression, behavior problems, and substance use disorders. *Arch Pediatr Adolesc Med.* 2007;161:1026–1034

124. Riggs PD, Winhusen T, Davies RD, et al. Randomized controlled trial of osmotic-release methylphenidate with CBT in adolescents with ADHD and substance use disorders. *J Am Acad Child Adolesc Psychiatry.* 2011;50(9):1–19

125. Verdejo-Garcia A, Lawrence AJ, Clark L. Impulsivity as a vulnerability marker for substance-use disorders: review of findings from high-risk research, problem gamblers, and genetic association studies. *Neurosci Biobehav Rev.* 2008;32:777–810

126. De Wit H, Vicini L, Childs E, Sayla MA, Terner J. Does stress reactivity or response to amphetamine predict smoking progression in young adults? A preliminary study. *Pharmacol Biochem Behav.* 2007;86:312–319

127. Van Leeuwen AP, Creemers HE, Greaves-Lord K, et al. Hypothalamic-pituitary-adrenal axis reactivity to social stress and adolescent cannabis use: the TRAILS study. *Addiction.* 2011;106:1484–1492

128. Van Leijenhorst L, Moor BG, Op de Macks ZA, et al. Adolescent risky decision making: neurocognitive development of reward and control regions. *Neuroimage.* 2010;51:345–355

129. Figner B, Mackinlay RJ, Wilkening F, Weber EU. Affective and deliberative processes in risky choice: age differences in risk taking in the Columbia Card Task. *J Exp Psychol Learn Mem Cogn.* 2009;35(3):709–730

130. Stanger C, Budney AJ, Kamon JL, Thostensen J. A randomized trial of contingency management for adolescent marijuana abuse and dependence. *Drug Alcohol Depend.* 2009;105:240–247

131. Dennis M, Godley SH, Diamond G, et al. The cannabis youth treatment (CYT) study: main findings from two randomized trials. *J Subst Abuse Treat.* 2004;27:197–213

132. Bickel WK, Yi R, Landes RD, et al. Remembering the future: working memory training decreases delay discounting among stimulant addicts. *Biol Psychiatry.* 2011;69:260–265

133. Devito EE, Worhunsky PD, Carroll KM, et al. A preliminary study of the neural effects of behavioral therapy for substance use disorders. *Drugs Alcohol Depend.* 2012;22:228–235

134. Riggs PD, Thompson LL, Tapert SF, et al. Advances in neurobiological research related to interventions in adolescents with substance use disorders: research to practice. *Drug Alcohol Depend.* 2007;91:306–311

135. Nolen-Hoeksema S. Gender differences in risk factors consequences for alcohol use and problems. *Clin Psychol Rev.* 2004;24(8):981–1010

136. Lynch WJ, Potenza MN, Cosgrove KP, et al. Sex differences in vulnerability to stimulant abuse: a translational perspective. In: Brady KT, Back S, Greenfield SF, eds. *Women and Addiction.* New York: Guilford Press; 2009:407–418

137. Bader P, Boisclair D, Ferrence R. Effects of tobacco taxation and pricing on smoking behavior in high risk populations: a knowledge synthesis. *Int J Environ Res Public Health.* 2011;8:4118–4139

138. Brownell KD, Farley T, Willett WC, et al. The public health and economic benefits of taxing sugar-sweetened beverages. *N Engl J Med.* 2009;361:1599–1605

139. Brown JA, Witherspoon EM. The mass media and American adolescent's health. *J Adolesc Health.* 2002;31:153–170

140. Dalton MA, Sargent JD, Beach ML, et al. Effect of viewing smoking in movies on adolescent smoking initiation: a cohort study. *Lancet.* 2003;362:281–285

141. Primack BA, Kraemer KL, Fine MJ, Dalton MA. Association between media exposure and marijuana and alcohol use in adolescents. *Subst Use Misuse.* 2009;44(5):722–739

Adolesc Med 025 (2014) 33–49

"The New Cigs on the Block": An Update on Conventional and Novel Tobacco Products

Deepa Camenga, MD, MHS*

Yale School of Medicine, Department of Pediatrics, New Haven, Connecticut

OVERVIEW

Tobacco use is a pervasive public health problem and is the leading cause of preventable morbidity and mortality in the United States. The well-known deleterious effects of tobacco use lead to 1 in 5 deaths in the United States and result in more than $193 billion in annual health care costs and lost productivity.[1] Tobacco use has its roots in adolescence, and 90% of adult smokers began using tobacco before age 18.[2] Overall, with the implementation of tobacco policies such as youth access laws, cigarette taxation, and regulation of advertising, tobacco use among youths has declined over the past decade.[3] However, despite great advances in tobacco control, 6.7% of middle school students and 23.3% of high school students report current tobacco use.[4] Although cigarette smoking is the predominant form of tobacco use in the United States, rates of use of other tobacco products, such as cigars, smokeless tobacco products (eg, chewing tobacco, snus, and dissolvables), and hookah (ie, waterpipes), by adolescents is remaining steady or increasing.[4] This article provides a brief update on cigarette smoking in adolescents and reviews the epidemiology of noncigarette tobacco use in youths, existing evidence on the health effects of noncigarette tobacco use, and clinical and policy implications.

CIGARETTES

Prevalence of Use in Youths

Adolescent cigarette smoking continues to be a substantial public health priority. Although rates of cigarettes use have declined in the past decade, in 2011 14.0% of high school students and 3.5% of middle school students reported cur-

---

*Corresponding author:
deepa.camenga@yale.edu

rent cigarette use (Figure 1). Overall, rates of adolescent cigarette smoking have decreased since 1991 but have plateaued in recent years.[5] Every day, approximately 3200 youths younger than 18 years of age initiate cigarette smoking, and 700 youths begin daily smoking.[6] Most youths (65.7%) perceive great risk from smoking a pack or more of cigarettes per day.[6]

Health Effects: Causal Associations

The 2012 Surgeon General report *Preventing Tobacco Use Among Youth and Young Adults* provided an update on the evidence supporting the causal relationship between adolescent tobacco use and adverse health outcomes.[2] It specifically reported strong causal associations between active cigarette smoking in young people and addiction to nicotine, reduced lung function and lung growth, asthma, and early abdominal aortic atherosclerosis.[2]

Clinical Implications: Guidelines for Treatment of Tobacco Use in Adolescents

Many professional organizations endorse the importance of cigarette smoking prevention and cessation counseling in primary care. Both the 2008 US Department of Health and Human Services clinical practice guideline on treating tobacco use and dependence and the 2009 American Academy of Pediatrics (AAP) policy statement on tobacco recommend that all physicians ask pediatric and adolescent patients about tobacco use and provide a strong message regarding the importance of total abstinence from tobacco use.[7] These guidelines are

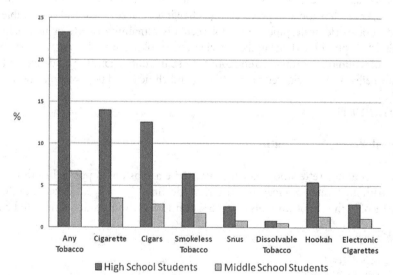

Fig 1. Prevalence of current tobacco use in high school and middle school students, 2012. (From 2012 National Youth Tobacco Survey. Tobacco product use among middle and high school students—United States, 2011 and 2012. *MMWR Morb Mortal Wkly Report.* 2013;62(45):893-897.)

supported by a large body of evidence as outlined by the 2010 Surgeon General Report *How Tobacco Smoke Causes Disease: The Biology and Behavioral Basis for Smoking-Attributable Disease,* which demonstrates that there is no risk-free level of exposure to tobacco smoke.[1]

In 2013 the US Preventive Services Task Force reviewed the literature pertaining to the efficacy of primary care–relevant interventions aimed at reducing tobacco use among children and adolescents.[8] The task force identified 10 good/fair-quality studies that evaluated the effectiveness of smoking prevention interventions.[9-19] Six of the studies were home based,[9,13-16,19] 2 were primary care based,[10,20] and the remaining 2 were dental clinic based.[11,17] Nine studies were included in the pooled meta-analysis examining smoking initiation in baseline nonsmokers. The meta-analysis, which included 26,624 children and adolescents, found a statistically significant reduction in smoking initiation in youths who received the intervention at a 6- to 36-month follow-up compared with the control group (risk ratio, 0.81 [95% confidence interval (CI), 0.70-0.93]). This resulted in a 2% absolute risk reduction of smoking initiation.[18]

The task force also examined 7 studies evaluating the efficacy of interventions to promote smoking cessation.[9-12,20-22] The resulting meta-analysis, which included 2328 children and adolescents, found a small but statistically insignificant effect at a 6- to 12-month follow-up (risk ratio, 0.96 [95 CI%, 0.90-1.02]).[18] Additionally, the task force identified 2 other studies evaluating bupropion for adolescent smoking cessation and did not find a statistically significant benefit of this pharmacotherapy.[23,24] Interestingly, they could not identify any controlled trials conducted in health care settings that evaluated nicotine replacement therapy or varenicline. Therefore, although the task force found insufficient evidence to determine whether behavioral-based interventions or pharmacotherapy for cessation is effective, they did recommend that primary care physicians provide interventions to prevent initiation of tobacco use in school-aged children and adolescents.

Regulating Cigarettes: The Family Smoking Prevention and Tobacco Control Act

In 2009 the United States passed the Family Smoking Prevention and Tobacco Control Act (FSPTCA), which gives the US Food and Drug Administration (FDA) authority to regulate the manufacturing, distribution, and marketing of tobacco products to protect the public's health.[25,26] Before the enactment of this legislation, tobacco products were largely exempted from other public health regulatory requirements, except for product labeling and marketing restrictions. The FSPTCA gives the FDA the authority to regulate all products made or derived from tobacco products and intended for human consumption; this includes cigarettes, smokeless tobacco products, and roll-your-own tobacco.[27] The first tobacco product standard issued was a ban on flavoring in cigarettes (other than menthol), which is intended to reduce the appeal of tobacco products in youth.[28] The FDA authority over tobacco products has several limitations. For example, the FDA cannot require the elimination of nicotine from tobacco products, it cannot ban tobacco sales in particular sales outlets, and it cannot regulate tobacco farming.[25] Although the FSPTCA regulates cigarettes, cigars are notably excluded from the regulations.

CIGARS, LITTLE CIGARS, AND CIGARILLOS

Cigars are the second most common tobacco product used by youths ages 12 to 17 years.[4] The US Department of the Treasury defines cigars as "any roll of tobacco wrapped in leaf tobacco or in any substance containing tobacco."[29] In contrast to cigarettes, which contain tobacco that is air-cured and is wrapped in paper or a substance that does not contain tobacco, cigars are made with tobacco that is both air-cured and fermented, which leads to their strong aroma and flavor. The US Department of Agriculture recognizes 3 types of cigars: (1) little cigars (weighing less than 3 lb per thousand); (2) cigarillos (weighing 3-10 lb per thousand); and (3) large cigars (weighing more than 10 lb per thousand) (Figure 2). Little cigars are comparable to cigarettes with regard to shape and size, and they often have a filter.[30] The tobacco industry has promoted little cigars as a lower-cost alternative to cigarettes.[31] Cigarillos are larger than cigarettes and little cigars, and they are longer slimmer versions of the large cigar.[30] From 1993 to 2006, unit sales of both little cigars and cigarillos increased, whereas sales of large cigars dropped[32]; however, sales of large cigars have recently increased.[33]

Prevalence of Use in Youths

Currently there are no national prevalence data for little cigar or cigarillo products because most national surveys do not distinguish between these products

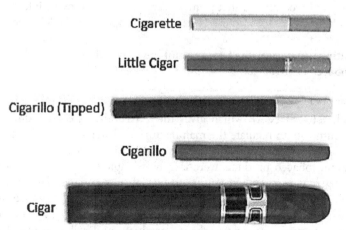

Fig 2. Cigars, little cigars, and cigarillos. (From The Legacy Foundation. Understanding the similarities and differences between little cigars and cigarillos. Available at: www.legacyforhealth.org/newsletters/2010/Jan/1102972476712.html. Reprinted with permission.)

and large cigars. According to the 2012 National Youth Tobacco Survey, 12.6% of high school students and 3.5% of middle school students reported current (past month) cigar use.[4] The prevalence of current cigar use among high school males (16.7%) was approximately double that of high school females (8.4%), and approximated current cigarette use in high school males (16.3%).[4] Cigarette use is a strong predictor of cigar use. A study of adolescent smokers found that cigar, little cigar, and cigarillo use was highly prevalent: 76.7% reported ever trying any type of cigar and 40.7% reported past month use.[33] Furthermore, the Centers for Disease Control and Prevention recently reported that between 2011 to 2012, cigar use increased, particularly among non-Hispanic black high school students, from 11.7% to 16.7%, which indicates the increasing popularity of cigar use in this population.[4]

Health Effects

Similar to cigarette smoking, cigar smoking is associated with increased risk of lung, oral, laryngeal, and esophageal cancers, and chronic obstructive pulmonary disease.[34] Large cigars, in particular, have more tobacco per unit and therefore generate more smoke than cigarettes.[35] Furthermore, secondhand cigar smoke has higher levels of carbon monoxide and polycyclic aromatic hydrocarbons than cigarettes.[36]

Clinical and Policy Implications

There are several opportunities to promote decreased cigar use in youths. Although the deleterious health effects of cigarettes are widely disseminated to the public, youths in particular seem less educated about the effects of cigars. Cigar use increases the risk of cancer and cardiovascular disease; however, youths may view cigars as less harmful than traditional cigarettes. Physicians, health educators, and public health officials all can play an important role in educating youths about the health consequences of cigar smoking and secondhand cigar smoke. Because most states do not tax large cigars at the same rates as cigarettes, cigars are cheaper than cigarettes.[29,37] Given that little cigars and cigarillos are generally less expensive than cigarettes and manufacturers can still sell individually wrapped cigars, a practice that appeals to price-sensitive populations such as youths and young adults, another opportunity to prevent cigar use may be to increase taxation or regulate packaging. Regulating the flavoring in cigars may reduce their appeal among youths. Flavors can mask the natural harshness and taste of tobacco,[38] thus increasing the appeal of cigars and their ease of use among youth.[39,40] An analysis of the 2011 National Youth Tobacco Survey demonstrated that 35.9% of high school current cigar smokers reported using flavored cigars.[41] Although flavored cigarettes are prohibited from sale through the 2009 FSPTCA,[42] mentholated cigarettes and other flavored products, such as flavored cigars, cigarillos, and little cigars, still can be manufactured, distributed, and legally sold.

SMOKELESS TOBACCO PRODUCTS

Despite recent declines in cigarette use among youths, declines in smokeless tobacco use have stalled in recent years.[2] In the United States, smokeless tobacco usually is consumed as either chewing tobacco or moist snuff (Figure 3). Chewing tobacco is composed of long strands of tobacco. Snuff tobacco is a fine-grain product that comes in a moist blend that usually is used orally.[2]

Within the last 10 years, novel smokeless tobacco products such as snus and dissolvables have become available. Snus are made of nonfermented, heat-cured, finely grained tobacco with additives such as water, sodium carbonate, sodium chloride, moisturizers, and, in some commercial types, flavors.[43] Snus are spit-free and consumed via pouches, which are placed between the cheek and gum. Snus have been used in Sweden since the early 19th century. They were introduced to the US market in 2006 when major US cigarette manufacturers acquired smokeless tobacco companies and started marketing snus with cigarette brand names (eg, Marlboro Snus, Camel Snus).[44] Dissolvables are another novel smokeless tobacco product that comes in pellets, strips, or sticks. They are designed to be held and dissolved in the mouth for between 3 (strips) and 30 (sticks) minutes.[45] Similar to snus, dissolvables were recently introduced in US markets and bear cigarette brand names (eg, Camel Orbs, Camel Strips).[46]

Prevalence of Use

In 2011, 6.4% of high school students and 1.7% of middle school students reported current smokeless tobacco use,[4] and most used chew/dip.[47] White males have the highest prevalence of smokeless tobacco use as measured by mul-

Product		Description	Common Brands	Use
Loose leaf chewing tobacco		Air cured tobacco usually treated with sugar and licorice.	Red Man, Levi Garrett	Requires spitting.
Moist snuff		Ground tobacco with a high moisture and salt content. Some moist snuff is sold in porous pouches (e.g., Skoal Bandits).	Copenhagen, Skoal, Grizzly	Requires spitting.
Snus		Finely ground oral tobacco packaged in small porous pouches; placed between gum and lip. "Snus" name refers to a traditional Swedish product, which is produced with a different manufacturing process (including pasteurization and storage in refrigeration) that reduces tobacco-specific nitrosamines linked to oral cancer.	Camel Marlboro	Tobacco-laden saliva is swallowed.
Dissolvable tobacco		Dissolvable pellets, strips, or sticks either made fully from tobacco or consisting of wooden dowels coated with tobacco. Designed to be held and dissolved in the mouth for between 3 (strips) and 30 (sticks) minutes.	Camel	Tobacco-laden saliva is swallowed.
Electronic cigarettes		A device comprising a battery, a heater, and a cartridge filled with a solution of nicotine, propylene glycol, and other chemicals. This solution is vaporized by the heater and inhaled.	blu, V2, Smokestik	Vapor is inhaled.

Fig 3. Smokeless tobacco products and electronic cigarettes. (From Popova L, Ling PM. Alternative tobacco product use and smoking cessation: a national study. *Am J Public Health.* 2013;103(5): 923-930. Reprinted with permission.)

tiple national surveys, including the National Survey on Drug Use and Health,[48] Monitoring the Future, and the National Youth Tobacco Survey.[4] Overall, more than 20% of white males report ever using smokeless tobacco.[2] Predictors of smokeless tobacco use include increasing age, male gender, cigarette smoking, and perceived friend approval.[49] In general, adolescents perceive that conventional smokeless tobacco product use is less risky than cigarette use.[50]

The prevalence of both snus and dissolvable use currently is quite low. In 2012, 2.5% of high schools students and 0.8% of middle school students reported current snus use. During the same year, only 0.8% of high school students and 0.5% of middle school students reported current dissolvable use.[4]

Health Effects

Conventional smokeless tobacco use has been associated with increased risk for oral and oropharyngeal cancer.[51] More than 30 carcinogens exist in smokeless tobacco, including volatile and tobacco-specific nitrosamines (TSNAs), nitrosamine acids, and polycyclic aromatic hydrocarbons.[51,52] Smokeless tobacco is one of the highest known nonoccupational sources of carcinogenic nitrosamines.[51] Both snus[53] and dissolvables have lower levels of TSNAs and do not require users to spit out their contents. Given these lower levels of nitrosamines, some argue that these novel tobacco products provide some harm reduction compared to traditional tobacco products. However, this holds true only if individuals exclusively use novel smokeless tobacco without conventional smokeless tobacco or traditional cigarettes. Unfortunately, almost 80% of snus/dissolvables users in the United States also smoke combustible tobacco products such as cigarettes,[47] suggesting that the harm-reducing properties of these products are limited.

Clinical Implications

Many professional organizations endorse the importance of smokeless tobacco prevention cessation counseling in primary care. Both the 2008 US Department of Health and Human Services clinical practice guideline on treating tobacco use and dependence and the 2009 American Academy of Pediatrics (AAP) policy statement on tobacco recommend that all physicians ask pediatric and adolescent patients about tobacco use and provide a strong message regarding the importance of total abstinence from tobacco use.[7] Therefore, it is important to screen for all forms of tobacco use (including smokeless tobacco), educate patients about the health consequences of use, and be familiar with the physical signs of smokeless tobacco use.

HOOKAH

Hookah, also known as narghile, hubble-bubble, shisha, and waterpipe, is a form of tobacco that commonly is flavored and delivered through a waterpipe

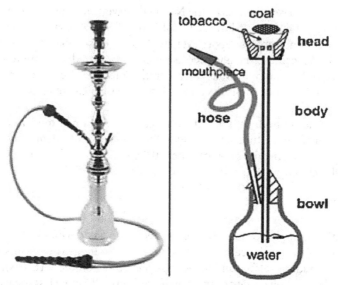

Fig 4. Hookah. (From Maziak W. The waterpipe: an emerging global risk for cancer. *Cancer epidemiology.* 2013;37(1):1-4. Reprinted with permission.)

(Figure 4). During the smoking process, the flavored tobacco (or shisha) is wrapped in aluminum foil and heated with charcoal. Inhaling through the waterpipe pulls smoke through the waterpipe's water reservoir and then through a tube to which the mouthpiece is attached.[54]

Prevalence of Use in Youths

In 2012, 5.4% of high school students and 1.3% of middle school students reported current hookah use,[4] with rates increasing between 2011 and 2012. Hookah use increases with age and has increased in popularity among young adults. A 2008 to 2009 survey of 82,155 college students attending 148 colleges found that 22% of college students ever used hookah, and 9.6% of college students reported hookah use within the past month.[55]

A systematic review of 56 studies evaluating risk factors for hookah found that socializing, relaxation, pleasure, and entertainment motivated both adults and adolescents to use hookah.[56] Predictors of hookah smoking in college and high school students include peer pressure/social acceptability,[57,58] the perception that hookah is not harmful or addictive,[58,59] the presence of a family member who uses hookah,[60] and curiosity.[57] A study of female college freshman initiating hookah use additionally found that concurrent alcohol and marijuana use predicted initiation and frequency of hookah use.[61]

Health Effects

A few well-designed epidemiologic studies have evaluated the health risks of hookah smoking. A recent systematic review of 24 studies evaluating health outcomes found that hookah smoking increased the odds of several deleterious health consequences, including lung cancer, respiratory illness, low birth weight, periodontal disease, and heart disease; however, the quality of the evidence was rated as low.[62] In addition, the act of smoking through a shared mouthpiece of the waterpipe may increase the risk of acquiring infectious diseases, such as tuberculosis and herpes[63]; however studies have not evaluated this association thoroughly. The smoke from one hookah session contains up to 40 times the tar,[64] 30 to 50 times the carcinogenic polycyclic aromatic hydrocarbons,[65] 2 times the nicotine,[64] and 10 times the carbon monoxide[64] of the smoke from a single cigarette. Hookah smokers have higher levels of carbon monoxide exposure than traditional cigarette smokers, presumably because of charcoal burning.[66] At least one case of carbon monoxide poisoning secondary to hookah use has been reported.[54] Hookah produces a tremendous amount of smoke, and a hookah smoking session produces 40 times the smoke of a cigarette smoking session of the same length.[67] A study of patrons of hookah bars who did not smoke hookah found that secondhand hookah smoke exposure resulted in elevated carbon monoxide levels in these people.[68] Additionally, a study examining the air quality of 10 hookah lounges in Oregon found that the particulate matter from hookah smoke resulted in air quality rated as "unhealthy" or "hazardous" by the Environmental Protection Agency.[69]

Clinical and Policy Implications

Given the growing body of evidence demonstrating the health risks of hookah use, physicians should consider advising their patients that because waterpipe tobacco smoking exposes them to some of the same toxicants as cigarette smoking, the 2 tobacco-smoking methods likely share some of the same health risks.[66] Given the relatively lax tobacco control environment surrounding hookah use, some argue that tobacco control policies that have been shown to effectively curb cigarette smoking among youths also should be implemented for hookah use prevention.[70] For example, youths are highly sensitive to price, and increasing the taxation of shisha (the tobacco smoked in hookah) may deter its use. Shisha is considered a type of pipe tobacco for which the current federal tax is $2.83 per pound, which is nearly $22 per pound less than the tax on roll-your-own (loose) cigarette tobacco.[29] The 2009 FSPTCA banned flavored cigarettes with the exception of menthol; however, this regulation does not extend to pipe tobacco (and therefore shisha). Given the appeal of flavors in youths, a ban on flavored shisha may deter hookah smoking initiation in youth. Another potential opportunity for tobacco control of hookah is extending smoke-free laws to hookah smoking lounges.[70] Primack et al[71] reviewed municipal, county, and state legal texts applicable to the 100 largest US cities and found that although 75% of the 100 cities prohibited cigarette smoking in bars, 90% of cities allowed indoor hookah tobacco smoking via legal exemptions. The presence of hookah lounges in a community is associated with increased youth usage rates. In 2010 the Oregon Tobacco Prevention and Education Program conducted a study of hookah lounges in that state. The program found that from 2008 to 2009 the prevalence of hookah use increased significantly from 2.7% to 5.1% among 8th-grade students in counties with hookah lounges compared to a smaller increase from 1.6% to 1.9% in counties without hookah lounges.

ELECTRONIC CIGARETTES

Electronic cigarettes (E-cigarettes) are battery-operated devices that deliver nicotinized or denicotinized vapor through inhalation. Most E-cigarettes are manufactured to resemble cigarettes, cigars, or pipes; however, some resemble everyday items such as pens. E-cigarettes contain cartridges filled with liquid containing propylene glycol, glycerin, and nicotine. Puffing the E-cigarettes activates a heating element in the atomizer, and the liquid in the cartridge is vaporized into a mist that is inhaled.[72] The act of inhaling is sometimes called "vaping," and E-cigarettes do not combust tobacco and therefore do not produce smoke. Not all E-cigarettes contain nicotine, and cartridges with nicotine typically contain 6 to 24 mg of nicotine per milliliter of solution.[73,74] Therefore, a 5-mL vial of a 20 mg/mL solution contains 100 mg of nicotine, which, if inappropriately ingested, would result in a lethal dose of nicotine.[74] However, the act of inhaling the vaporized cartridge solution results in blood and saliva cotinine levels similar to, or lower than, those achieved by smoking a cigarette.[75-79] About 200 different brands of E-cigarettes are available for purchase, and sales total $1.7 billion per year in the United States (compared to >$90 billion in cigarettes sales).[80] Currently, convenience stores are an important distribution point for E-cigarettes, although Internet marketing is growing and potentially increasing exposure of the product to adolescents.[81]

Prevalence of Use

In 2012, 2.8% of high school students and 1.1% of middle school students reported current E-cigarette use. However, from 2011 to 2012 the prevalence of ever E-cigarette use doubled among both middle school and high school students, indicating increased experimentation.[4,63] During 2011 and 2012, among all students in grades 6 to 12, ever use of E-cigarettes increased from 3.3% to 6.8%.[63] Emerging evidence indicates that E-cigarettes especially appeal to cigarette smokers. Although many adolescents are aware of E-cigarettes, adolescent smokers are more willing to try E-cigarettes than nonsmokers[82] and have increased odds of current use.[83] The increasing prevalence of E-cigarette use may be attributed to heavy marketing and advertising in youth-dominated media outlets such as social networking and Internet sites,[84] their low price, and perceptions that E-cigarettes are a safer alternative to traditional cigarettes.

Health Effects

The absolute safety of E-cigarettes is unknown; however, some researchers argue that, when used as directed in adults, E-cigarettes are less harmful than cigarettes.[85,86] A 2011 review of 15 studies that analyzed the liquid used in E-cigarettes concluded that E-cigarettes contain only 0.07% to 0.2% of the TSNAs present in cigarettes. This amount is similar to the concentration of TSNAs found in nicotine replacement products, such as the nicotine replacement patch.[85] Experimental studies evaluating comparing the cytotoxic potential of 21 E-cigarette vapors compared to conventional cigarette smoke found that E-cigarette vapor was significantly less cytotoxic than cigarette smoke when applied to murine fibroblasts[87] and cultured myocardial cells.[88] Another study supported these results by demonstrating that E-cigarette vapor contains much lower levels of the toxins (eg, nitrosamine) present in cigarette smoke.[89] Although E-cigarette cartridges typically contain nicotine (varying from 6-24 mg/mL solution), few data on the amount of nicotine actually delivered from the cartridges are available because of the relative novelty of the product. Experimental studies have shown that active[75] and passive[76] E-cigarette smoking results in blood and saliva cotinine levels similar to those obtained through traditional cigarette smoking. On the other hand, 3 small published studies of human subjects who used 1 of the products showed little delivery of nicotine to the bloodstream,[77-79] even when products that contained high nicotine levels were used. Overall, given the current state of the evidence, it is not possible to firmly conclude whether E-cigarettes are less harmful than cigarettes, although existing evidence does suggest E-cigarettes have lower levels of tobacco-containing toxicants.

Role of E-cigarettes in Smoking Cessation

Proponents of E-cigarettes argue that they help promote smoking cessation by allowing users to mimic smoking behaviors (ie, hand-to-mouth movement) without delivering high levels of toxins. E-cigarettes also may provide a coping mechanism for some of the rituals associated with smoking and for conditioned smoking cues (eg, smoking when eating).[90] Studies have shown that smoking denicotinized cigarettes reduces craving symptoms; this suggests that the reinforcing behaviors associated with smoking can suppress smoking urges independent of nicotine delivery.[91] To date, few studies have analyzed the effectiveness of E-cigarettes for smoking cessation in adults. Bullen et al[92] randomized 689 adult cigarette smokers who smoked more than 10 cigarettes per day to nicotine-containing (10-16 mg/mL) E-cigarettes, placebo (non-nicotine containing) E-cigarettes, or nicotine patch (21 mg in 24 hours). At 6 months, the biochemically verified continuous abstinence rate was 7.3% in the E-cigarette group, 5.8% in the patch group, and 4.1% in the placebo E-cigarette group. However, the study was not statistically powered to detect a difference in abstinence rates among the groups. An observational study of 2758 adults who called state quit-lines found that 30% had used E-cigarettes and that both ever and current

E-cigarette users were less likely than non–E-cigarette users to be abstinent at 7 months (30-day point prevalence quit rates: 21.7% and 16.6% vs 31.3%, $P <.001$).[93] The most frequently reported reasons for use were to help quit use of other tobacco products (51.3%) or to replace other tobacco products (15.2%). Similar to the data regarding the safety of E-cigarettes, it currently is not possible to determine whether E-cigarettes promote cessation from tobacco products.

Concerns with E-cigarettes and Policy Implications

Several concerns regarding the spread of E-cigarette use have emerged. Experts argue that E-cigarettes may serve as a gateway to use of other tobacco products, promote and sustain nicotine addiction, prevent adolescent smokers from quitting cigarettes, or promote nicotine exposure among youths who otherwise would have been nonsmokers.[63] There is additional concern that tobacco companies, which are increasingly entering the E-cigarette market, will target young consumers in an effort to counteract lower cigarette use with a new pool of nicotine users.[94] Although currently there is a lack of data supporting these concerns, most experts agree that it is critical to develop strategies to prevent marketing, sales, and use of E-cigarettes among youths.[63]

The 2009 FSPTCA[42] gives the FDA authority to regulate the manufacturing, distribution, and marketing of tobacco products to protect the public's health.[26] Therefore, the FDA may choose to issue standards that reduce the appeal of tobacco products to youths as well as reduce the amounts of potentially harmful constituents and thus the addictive potential of the products.[26] As of this time, the FDA Center for Tobacco Products (CTP) has reported its intention to regulate E-cigarettes, but it has not yet exerted its authority on this issue.[95]

CONCLUSION

Despite great advances in tobacco control that have resulted in recent declines in cigarette use among youths, adolescent rates of use of tobacco products such as cigars, hookah, smokeless tobacco, and E-cigarettes are remaining steady or are rising. Cigars and conventional smokeless tobacco products have well-documented deleterious health effects that often are underestimated by adolescents. Evidence continues to emerge about the safety of hookah and newer tobacco products such as snus, dissolvables, and E-cigarettes. Regardless, practice guidelines recommend that all physicians ask pediatric and adolescent patients about *all forms* of tobacco use and provide a strong message on the importance of total abstinence.

References

1. US Department of Health and Human Services. *How Tobacco Smoke Causes Disease: The Biology and Behavioral Basis for Smoking-Attributable Disease: A Report of the Surgeon General.* Atlanta, GA: Department of Health and Human Services, Centers for Disease Control and Prevention,

National Center for Chronic Disease Prevention and Health Promotion, Office on Smoking and Health; 2010

2. US Department of Health and Human Services, Centers for Disease Control and Prevention and National Center for Chronic Disease Prevention. *Preventing Tobacco Use Among Youth and Young Adults: A Report of the Surgeon General.* Atlanta, GA: Department of Health and Human Services, Centers for Disease Control and Prevention and National Center for Chronic Disease Prevention; 2012

3. Current tobacco use among middle and high school students—United States, 2011. *MMWR Morb Mortal Wkly Rep.* 2012;61(31):581–585

4. Tobacco product use among middle and high school students—United States, 2011 and 2012. *MMWR Morb Mortal Wkly Rep.* 2013;62(45):893–897

5. Centers for Disease Control and Prevention. Trends in the prevalence of selected risk behaviors and obesity for all students. National YRBS: 1991-2011. Available at: www.cdc.gov/healthyyouth/yrbs/pdf/us_summary_all_trend_yrbs.pdf. Published 1997. Accessed December 12, 2013

6. Substance Abuse and Mental Health Services Administration. *Results from the 2012 National Survey on Drug Use and Health: Summary of National Findings.* Rockville, MD: Substance Abuse and Mental Health Services Administration; 2013

7. American Academy of Pediatrics. Policy statement—tobacco use: a pediatric disease. *Pediatrics.* 2009;124(5):1474–1487

8. Moyer VA. Primary care interventions to prevent tobacco use in children and adolescents: U.S. preventive services task force recommendation statement. *Pediatrics.* 2013;132(3):560–565

9. Bauman KE, Ennett ST, Foshee VA, et al. Influence of a family program on adolescent smoking and drinking prevalence. *Prevent Sci.* 2002;3(1):35–42

10. Hollis JF, Polen MR, Whitlock EP, et al. Teen reach: outcomes from a randomized, controlled trial of a tobacco reduction program for teens seen in primary medical care. *Pediatrics.* 2005;115(4):981–989

11. Lando HA, Hennrikus D, Boyle R, et al. Promoting tobacco abstinence among older adolescents in dental clinics. *J Smok Cessat.* 2007;2:23–30

12. Pbert L, Flint AJ, Fletcher KE, et al. Effect of a pediatric practice-based smoking prevention and cessation intervention for adolescents: a randomized, controlled trial. *Pediatrics.* 2008;121(4):e738–e747

13. Ausems M, Mesters I, Van Breukelen G, De Vries H. Short-term effects of a randomized computer-based out-of-school smoking prevention trial aimed at elementary schoolchildren. *Prevent Med.* 2002;34(6):581–589

14. Curry SJ, Hollis J, Bush T, et al. A randomized trial of a family-based smoking prevention intervention in managed care. *Prevent Med.* 2003;37(6):617–626

15. Fidler W, Lambert TW. A prescription for health: a primary care based intervention to maintain the non-smoking status of young people. *Tob Control.* 2001;10(1):23–26

16. Haggerty KP, Skinner ML, MacKenzie EP, Catalano RF. A randomized trial of parents who care: effects on key outcomes at 24-month follow-up. *Prevent Sci.* 2007;8(4):249–260

17. Hovell MF, Slymen DJ, Jones JA, et al. An adolescent tobacco-use prevention trial in orthodontic offices. *Am J Public Health.* 1996;86(12):1760–1766

18. Patnode CD, O'Connor E, Whitlock EP, et al. Primary care-relevant interventions for tobacco use prevention and cessation in children and adolescents: a systematic evidence review for the U.S. Preventive Services Task Force. *Ann Intern Med.* 2013;158(4):253–260

19. Jackson C, Dickinson D. Enabling parents who smoke to prevent their children from initiating smoking: results from a 3-year intervention evaluation. *Arch Pediatr Adolesc Med.* 2006;160(1):56–62

20. Pbert L, Druker S, DiFranza JR, et al. Effectiveness of a school nurse-delivered smoking-cessation intervention for adolescents. *Pediatrics.* 2011;128(5):926–936

21. Colby SM, Monti PM, Tevyaw TOL, et al. Brief motivational intervention for adolescent smokers in medical settings. *Addict Behav.* 2005;30(5):865–874

22. Colby SM, Nargiso J, Tevyaw TO, et al. Enhanced motivational interviewing versus brief advice for adolescent smoking cessation: results from a randomized clinical trial. *Addict Behav.* 2012;37(7):817–823

23. Killen JD, Robinson TN, Ammerman S, et al. Randomized clinical trial of the efficacy of bupro-pion combined with nicotine patch in the treatment of adolescent smokers. *J Consult Clin Psychol.* 2004;72(4):729–735

24. Muramoto ML, Leischow SJ, Sherrill D, Matthews E, Strayer LJ. Randomized, double-blind, placebo-controlled trial of 2 dosages of sustained-release bupropion for adolescent smoking cessation. *Arch Pediatr Adolesc Med.* 2007;161(11):1068–1074

25. US Food and Drug Administration. Overview of the family smoking prevention and tobacco con-trol act: consumer fact sheet. Available at: www.fda.gov/TobaccoProducts/GuidanceCompliance-RegulatoryInformation/ucm246129.htm. Published 2013. Accessed December 1, 2013

26. Husten CG, Deyton LR. Understanding the Tobacco Control Act: efforts by the US Food and Drug Administration to make tobacco-related morbidity and mortality part of the USA's past, not its future. *Lancet.* 2013;381(9877):1570–1580

27. US Food and Drug Administration. Section 901 of the Federal Food, Drug, and Cosmetic Act—FDA authority over tobacco products. Available at: www.fda.gov/TobaccoProducts/GuidanceComplianceRegulatoryInformation/ucm261879.htm#general. Published 2013. Accessed December 10, 2013

28. US Food and Drug Administration. Section 907 of the Federal Food, Drug, and Cosmetic Act—tobacco product standards. Available at: www.fda.gov/TobaccoProducts/GuidanceCompliance-RegulatoryInformation/ucm263053.htm. Published 2013. Accessed December 1, 2013

29. Alcohol and Tobacco Tax and Trade Bureau. Tax and fee rates. Available at: www.ttb.gov/tax_audit/atftaxes.shtml. Published 2013. Accessed November 26, 2013

30. The Legacy Foundation. Tobacco fact sheet: cigars, cigarillos and little cigars. Available at: www.legacyforhealth.org/content/download/642/7502/version/2/file/Fact_Sheet-Cigars_Cigarillos_LittleCigars.pdf. Published 2012. Accessed November 26, 2013

31. Delnevo CD, Hrywna M. "A whole 'nother smoke" or a cigarette in disguise: how RJ Reynolds reframed the image of little cigars. *Am J Public Health.* 2007;97(8):1368–1375

32. Kozlowski LT, Dollar KM, Giovino GA. Cigar/cigarillo surveillance. *Am J Prev Med.* 2008;34(5):424–426

33. Consumption of cigarettes and combustible tobacco—United States, 2000-2011. *MMWR Morb Mortal Wkly Rep.* 2012;61(30):565–569

34. National Cancer Institute. Smoking and Tobacco Control Monographs: Monograph 9: Cigars, Health Effects and Trends. Bethesda, MD: National Cancer Institute; 1998

35. Adkison SE, O'Connor RJ, Bansal-Travers M, et al. Electronic nicotine delivery systems: interna-tional tobacco control four-country survey. *Am J Prev Med.* 2013;44(3):207–215

36. Henningfield JE, Fant RV, Radzius A, Frost S. Nicotine concentration, smoke pH and whole tobacco aqueous pH of some cigar brands and types popular in the United States. *Nicotine Tob Res.* 1999;1(2):163–168

37. Boonn A. The Rise of Cigars and Cigar-Smoking Harms. Campaign for Tobacco-Free Kids. Avail-able at: www.tobaccofreekids.org/research/factsheets/pdf/0333.pdf. Published 2013. Accessed December 1, 2013

38. US Food and Drug Administration Tobacco Products Scientific Advisory Committee. Menthol ciga-rettes and public health: review of the scientific evidence and recommendations. Available at: www.fda.gov/downloads/AdvisoryCommittees/CommitteesMeetingMaterials/TobaccoProductsScienti-ficAdvisoryCommittee/UCM269697.pdf. Published 2011. Accessed December 3, 2013

39. Carpenter CM, Wayne GF, Pauly JL, Koh HK, Connolly GN. New cigarette brands with flavors that appeal to youth: tobacco marketing strategies. *Health Affairs.* 2005;24(6):1601–1610

40. Klein SM, Giovino GA, Barker DC, et al. Use of flavored cigarettes among older adolescent and adult smokers: United States, 2004-2005. *Nicotine Tob Res.* 2008;10(7):1209–1214

41. King BA, Tynan MA, Dube SR, Arrazola R. Flavored-little-cigar and flavored-cigarette use among US middle and high school students. *J Adolesc Health.* 2014;54(1):40–46

42. US Government Printing Office. Family Smoking Prevention and Tobacco Control Act. Public Law 111-31. Available at: www.gpo.gov/fdsys/pkg/PLAW-111publ31/content-detail.html. Pub-lished 2009. Accessed November 20, 2013

43. Galanti MR, Rosendahl I, Wickholm S. The development of tobacco use in adolescence among "snus starters" and "cigarette starters": an analysis of the Swedish "BROMS" cohort. *Nicotine Tob Res.* 2008;10(2):315–323

44. Mejia AB, Ling PM. Tobacco industry consumer research on smokeless tobacco users and product development. *Am J Public Health.* 2010;100(1):78–87

45. Popova L, Ling PM. Alternative tobacco product use and smoking cessation: a national study. *Am J Public Health.* 2013;103(5):923–930

46. Trinkets and Trash Artifacts of the Tobacco Epidemic. Marketing smokeless tobacco, moist snuff, snus and dissolvables. Available at: trinketsandtrash.org/tt-feature/pdf/currrent_feature.pdf. Published 2013. Accessed December 5, 2013

47. Agaku IT, Ayo-Yusuf OA, Vardavas CI, Alpert HR, Connolly GN. Use of conventional and novel smokeless tobacco products among US adolescents. *Pediatrics.* 2013;132(3):e578–e586

48. Substance Abuse and Mental Health Services Administration. *Results from the 2010 National Survey on Drug Use and Health: Summary of National Findings.* Rockville, MD: Substance Abuse and Mental Health Services Administration; 2011

49. Tomar SL, Giovino GA. Incidence and predictors of smokeless tobacco use among US youth. *Am J Public Health.* 1998;88(1):20–26

50. Tomar SL, Hatsukami DK. Perceived risk of harm from cigarettes or smokeless tobacco among U.S. high school seniors. *Nicotine Tob Res.* 2007;9(11):1191–1196

51. Boffetta P, Hecht S, Gray N, Gupta P, Straif K. Smokeless tobacco and cancer. *Lancet Oncol.* 2008;9(7):667–675

52. Smokeless tobacco and some tobacco-specific N-nitrosamines. *IARC Monogr Eval Carcinog Risks Hum.* 2007;89:1–592

53. Irina S, Joni J, Dorothy H, Stephen SH. New and traditional smokeless tobacco: comparison of toxicant and carcinogen levels. *Nicotine Tob Res.* 2008;10(12):1773–1782

54. Ashurst JV, Urquhart M, Cook MD. Carbon monoxide poisoning secondary to hookah smoking. *J Am Osteopath Assoc.* 2012;112(10):686–688

55. Jarrett T, Blosnich J, Tworek C, Horn K. Hookah use among U.S. college students: results from the National College Health Assessment II. *Nicotine Tob Res.* 2012;14(10):1145–1153

56. Elie AA, Mohammed J, Wai Yim L, et al. Motives, beliefs and attitudes towards waterpipe tobacco smoking: a systematic review. *Harm Reduct J.* 2013;10(1):12

57. Merlyn AG, Eric WF. Hookah smoking: behaviors and beliefs among young consumers in the United States. *Soc Work Public Health.* 2014;29(1):17–26

58. Primack BA, Sidani J, Agarwal AA, et al. Prevalence of and associations with waterpipe tobacco smoking among U.S. university students. *Ann Behav Med.* 2008;36(1):81–86

59. Cobb C, Ward KD, Maziak W, Shihadeh AL, Eissenberg T. Waterpipe tobacco smoking: an emerging health crisis in the United States. *Am J Health Behav.* 2010;34(3):275–285

60. Jamil H, Janisse J, Elsouhag D, et al. Do household smoking behaviors constitute a risk factor for hookah use? *Nicotine Tob Res.* 2011;13(5):384–388

61. Fielder RL, Carey KB, Carey MP. Predictors of initiation of hookah tobacco smoking: a one-year prospective study of first-year college women. *CORD Conf Proc.* 2012;26(4):963–968

62. Akl EA, Gaddam S, Gunukula SK, et al. The effects of waterpipe tobacco smoking on health outcomes: a systematic review. *Int J Epidemiol.* 2010;39(3):834–857

63. Notes from the field: electronic cigarette use among middle and high school students—United States, 2011-2012. *MMWR Morb Mortal Wkly Rep.* 2013;62(35):729–730

64. Shihadeh A, Saleh R. Polycyclic aromatic hydrocarbons, carbon monoxide, "tar", and nicotine in the mainstream smoke aerosol of the narghile water pipe. *Food Chem Toxicol.* 2005;43(5):655–661

65. Sepetdjian E, Shihadeh A, Saliba NA. Measurement of 16 polycyclic aromatic hydrocarbons in narghile waterpipe tobacco smoke. *Food Chem Toxicol.* 2008;46(5):1582–1590

66. Eissenberg T, Shihadeh A. Waterpipe tobacco and cigarette smoking: direct comparison of toxicant exposure. *Am J Prev Med.* 2009;37(6):518–523

67. Uyanik B, Arslan ED, Akay H, Ercelik E, Tez M. Narghile (hookah) smoking and carboxyhemoglobin levels. *J Emerg Med.* 2011;40(6):679

68. Barnett TE, Curbow BA, Soule EK, Tomar SL, Thombs DL. Carbon monoxide levels among patrons of hookah cafes. *Am J Prev Med.* 2011;40(3):324–328
69. Fiala SC, Morris DS, Pawlak RL. Measuring indoor air quality of hookah lounges. *Am J Public Health.* 2012;102(11):2043–2045
70. Daniel SM, Steven CF, Rebecca P. Opportunities for policy interventions to reduce youth hookah smoking in the United States. *Prev Chronic Dis.* 2012;9:E165–E165
71. Primack BA, Hopkins M, Hallett C, et al. US health policy related to hookah tobacco smoking. *Am J Public Health.* 2012;102(9):e47–e51
72. Caponnetto P, Campagna D, Cibella F, et al. EffiCiency and Safety of an eLectronic cigAreTte (ECLAT) as tobacco cigarettes substitute: a prospective 12-month randomized control design study. *PLoS One.* 2013;8(6):e66317
73. Etter J F, Zather E, Svensson S. Analysis of refill liquids for electronic cigarettes. *Addiction.* 2013;108:1671–1679
74. Cameron JM, Howell DN, White JR, et al. Variable and potentially fatal amounts of nicotine in e-cigarette nicotine solutions. *Tob Control.* 2014;23(1):77–78
75. Etter J-F, Bullen C. Saliva cotinine levels in users of electronic cigarettes. *Eur Respir J.* 2011;38(5):1219–1220
76. Flouris AD, Chorti MS, Konstantina PP, et al. Acute impact of active and passive electronic cigarette smoking on serum cotinine and lung function. *Inhal Toxicol.* 2013;25(2):91–101
77. Bullen C, McRobbie H, Thornley S, et al. Effect of an electronic nicotine delivery device (e cigarette) on desire to smoke and withdrawal, user preferences and nicotine delivery: randomised cross-over trial. *Tob Control.* 2010;19(2):98–103
78. Eissenberg T. Electronic nicotine delivery devices: ineffective nicotine delivery and craving suppression after acute administration. *Tob Control.* 2010;19(1):87–88
79. Vansickel AR, Cobb CO, Weaver MF, Eissenberg TE. A clinical laboratory model for evaluating the acute effects of electronic "cigarettes": nicotine delivery profile and cardiovascular and subjective effects. *Cancer Epidemiol Biomarkers Prev.* 2010;19(8):1945–1953
80. Richtel M. The E-cigarette industry, waiting to exhale. *New York Times.* October 27, 2013:BU1
81. Herzog B, Metrano B, Gerberi J. Tobacco talk survey— E-cigarettes a promising opportunity. Available at: www.stevevape.com/wp-content/uploads/2012/05/E-Cigs-A-Promising-Opportunity.pdf. Published 2012. Accessed August 2013
82. Pepper JK, Reiter PL, McRee AL, et al. Adolescent males' awareness of and willingness to try electronic cigarettes. *J Adolesc Health.* 2013;52(2):144–150
83. Camenga DR, Delmerico J, Kong G, et al. Trends in use of electronic nicotine delivery systems by adolescents. *Addict Behav.* 2013
84. Ayers JW, Ribisl KM, Brownstein JS. Tracking the rise in popularity of electronic nicotine delivery systems (electronic cigarettes) using search query surveillance. *Am J Prev Med.* 2011;40(4):448–453
85. Cahn Z, Siegel M. Electronic cigarettes as a harm reduction strategy for tobacco control: a step forward or a repeat of past mistakes? *J Public Health Policy.* 2011;32(1):16–31
86. McAuley TR, Hopke PK, Zhao J, Babaian S. Comparison of the effects of e-cigarette vapor and cigarette smoke on indoor air quality. *Inhal Toxicol.* 2012;24(12):850–857
87. Giorgio R, Elena A, Elena B, et al. Cytotoxicity evaluation of electronic cigarette vapor extract on cultured mammalian fibroblasts (ClearStream-LIFE): comparison with tobacco cigarette smoke extract. *Inhal Toxicol.* 2013;25(6):354–361
88. Konstantinos EF, Giorgio R, Elena A, et al. Comparison of the cytotoxic potential of cigarette smoke and electronic cigarette vapour extract on cultured myocardial cells. *Int J Environ Res Public Health.* 2013;10(10):5146–5162
89. Goniewicz ML, Knysak J, Gawron M, et al. Levels of selected carcinogens and toxicants in vapour from electronic cigarettes. *Tob Control.* 2013
90. Caponnetto P, Russo C, Bruno CM, et al. Electronic cigarette: a possible substitute for cigarette dependence. *Monaldi Arch Chest Dis.* 2013;79(1):12–19
91. Buchhalter AR, Acosta MC, Evans SE, Breland AB, Eissenberg T. Tobacco abstinence symptom suppression: the role played by the smoking-related stimuli that are delivered by denicotinized cigarettes. *Addiction.* 2005;100(4):550–559

92. Bullen C, Howe C, Laugesen M, et al. Electronic cigarettes for smoking cessation: a randomised controlled trial. *Lancet.* 2013;382(9905):1629–1637

93. KA Vickerman, KM Carpenter, T Altman, CM Nash, SM Zbikowski. Use of electronic cigarettes among state tobacco cessation quitline callers. *Nicotine Tob Res.* 2013;15(10):1787–1791

94. Etter J-F. Should electronic cigarettes be as freely available as tobacco? Yes. *BMJ.* 2013;346: f3845–f3845

95. US Food and Drug Administration. FDA warns of health risks posed by E-cigarettes. Available at: www.fda.gov/ForConsumers/ConsumerUpdates/ucm173401.htm. Published 2009. Accessed December 1, 2013

Adolesc Med 025 (2014) 50–69

Young People and Alcohol Use: Contextualizing and Responding to the Challenge of Problematic Drinking

Stewart Stubbs, BSS (Psych), MHS (Child & Adolescent Health)[a*]; David Bennett, MBBS[b]

[a]*Parenting Research Project Coordinator, NSW Centre for the Advancement of Adolescent Health, The Children's Hospital at Westmead, Sydney, Australia;* [b]*Clinical Professor in Adolescent Medicine, University of Sydney, Senior Staff Specialist, Department of Adolescent Medicine, The Children's Hospital at Westmead, Senior Clinical Adviser, Youth Health and Wellbeing, NSW Kids and Families, Sydney, Australia*

HEAVY SESSIONAL ALCOHOL CONSUMPTION

Underage drinking and heavy sessional consumption of alcohol (binge drinking, ie, having 5 or more drinks on 1 occasion) continues to be of concern in Australia and western developed countries, not only because of the detrimental physical health consequences that accrue but also because of the effect on social and psychological well-being.[1,2] Gathering reliable and comparative information about global adolescent alcohol use is hampered by inconsistent data collection and the lack of internationally agreed upon measurement instruments. Although recent surveys have provided mixed summaries of adolescent alcohol use (ie, in terms of age at initiation, gender differences, and amounts consumed), the overall trend, both within and between countries, is for adolescents to begin drinking alcohol at an earlier age and generally for binge drinking to increase throughout the adolescent years and into early adulthood.

The 2008 World Health Organization (WHO) Global Survey on Alcohol and Health reported on the 5-year trend in underage drinking.[3] Of the 73 responding countries, 71% indicated an increase in underage drinking, 4% a decrease, 8% a stable pattern, and 16% inconclusive results. This global trend in increase in alcohol consumption also extends into early adulthood. The 5-year trend in

*Corresponding author:
stewartstubbs@gmail.com

drinking among 18- to 25-year-olds from 82 responding countries showed 80% with an increase, 11% a decrease, and 6% stable.[3]

Data from the 2012 Monitoring the Future Survey (an annual North American survey of drug, alcohol, and cigarette use by 8th-, 10th-, and 12th-grade high school students) indicated a statistically significant rise in binge drinking from 22% to 24% among 12th-graders in the United States.[4] However, the overall trend in adolescent alcohol use has been declining across the United States since the 1990s (Figure 1). In contrast to their older adolescent peers, younger North American adolescents have continued to decrease their binge drinking.[4] Health researchers claim that the success of this reduction results not only from the higher perceived risk of binge drinking among younger cohorts but also from decreased access to alcohol by younger adolescents through the efforts of states, communities, and parents.

Like their American and Australian peers, Canadian high school students' most frequently used substance is alcohol.[5] Just over 50% of both female and male grade 10 Canadian students have engaged in binge drinking at least once in the past 12 months; however, the trend in regular weekly drinking of beer, wine, and spirits for the same cohort declined between 1990 and 2010 (Figure 1).

In Europe there are large differences between countries with regard to the amount of alcohol that adolescents consume and the relative incidence of ado-

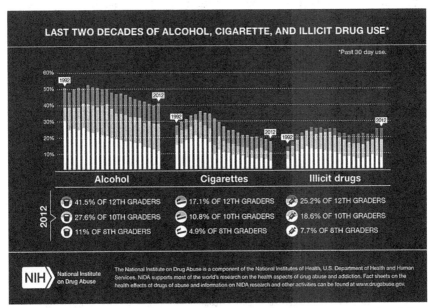

Fig 1. Alcohol, cigarette, and illicit drug use: monitoring the future 2012. (Reproduced from Johnston LD, O'Malley PM, Bachman JG, Schulenberg JE. *Monitoring the Future National Results on Drug Use: 2012 Overview, Key Findings on Adolescent Drug Use*. Ann Arbor, MI: Institute for Social Research, University of Michigan; 2013.)

lescent binge drinking. Data from the European School Project on Alcohol and Other Drugs (ESPAD), a large annual survey conducted with high school students, highlighted an overall downward trend in binge drinking between 2007 and 2011 among 15- to 16-year-olds.[6] Nevertheless, 2011 figures indicated that, on average, binge drinking was still the norm in 38% of female students and 43% of male students and that, in some European countries, the percentage of 15- to 16-year-olds who binge drank remained more than 50% (Table 1).[6]

Binge Drinking into Young Adulthood

In an Australian study that began in 1992, nearly 2000 Australian teenagers between 14 and 17 years of age were followed and assessed 9 times over 15 years.[7] Among the teenagers, 52% of boys and 34% of girls reported consuming 5 or more drinks on a single occasion within the past week. Most (90% of boys and 70% of girls) were highly likely to binge at the same or greater levels as young adults. The researchers also found that extremely risky binge drinking (defined as ≥20 drinks for males and ≥11 for females) was more common than thought. Almost half of the boys and one-third of the girls reported extreme binge drinking during either their adolescence or their 20s. Of these individuals, more than 40% first started heavy binge drinking when they were teenagers.[7]

A study analyzing health conditions, behaviors, and risks among young adults in the United States revealed that binge drinking and heavy alcohol use peaked in those between the ages of 21 to 25 years, with nearly 30% of people in that age group reporting binge drinking and 15% heavy alcohol use.[8] Although the young adults in this age group were 4 times more likely than adolescents to report past-

Table 1
Selected key variables by country for heavy episodic drinking* by 15- to 16-year-olds in the past 30 days

Country	Percentage
Croatia	54
Czech Republic	54
Denmark	56
Estonia	53
Malta	56
Slovenia	53
United Kingdom	52

*Having 5 or more drinks on 1 occasion. A "drink" is a glass/bottle/can of beer (~5 cL), a glass/bottle/can of cider (~50 cL), 2 glasses/bottles of alcopops (~50 cL), or a glass of wine (~5 cL) or mixed drink.
Data from Hibell B, Guttormsson U, Ahlström S, et al. *The 2011 ESPAD Report: Substance Use Among Students in 36 European Countries.* Stockholm, Sweden: Swedish Council for Information on Alcohol and Other Drugs (CAN); 2012.

month binge drinking, they also had the lowest perception of binge drinking risk, the greatest need for services, and the lowest access to services (Figure 2).

UNDERSTANDING DRINKING BEHAVIOR IN YOUNG PEOPLE

Early initiation, availability, and product types influence alcohol use. Since the late 20th century, the age of initiation to drinking alcohol in the west has become progressively younger. In Europe, students 13 years of age or younger have reported alcohol-related issues ranging from being drunk (12%) to performing poorly at school (13%) and having significant problems with family or friends (12% each).[9] Alcohol seems to be widely available and easily accessed by individuals, including older American adolescents.[4] European research suggests that consumption of beer and spirits by European adolescents predicts binge drinking.[9] In Australia, family and friends are the principal providers of alcohol, and adults are the primary supervisors of 64% of current drinkers younger than 18 years.[10]

The preferred types of alcoholic beverage by adolescents comes packaged as "ready to drink" in bottles or cans, premixed drinks, bottled spirits, and liqueurs.[2,10] In Australia, premixed spirits are becoming significantly more popular with underage male drinkers, whereas spirits, wine, and alcoholic sodas are more popular with underage female drinkers.[10] Interestingly, there has been a significant move away from consuming premixed spirits for Australian females and a move away from drinking straight spirits and beer for Australian males.[10] An Australian trend in both male and female underage drinkers is the consump-

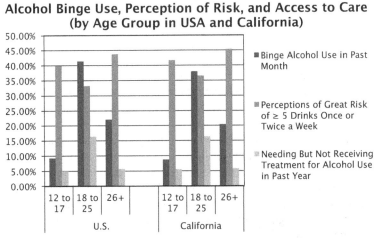

Fig 2. Binge drinking and heavy alcohol use by age, United States, 2010. (From Neinstein L. *The New Adolescents: An Analysis of Health Conditions, Behaviors, Risks, and Access to Services Among Emerging Young Adults*. Los Angeles, CA: University of Southern California; 2013. Copyright © Lawrence Neinstein. Reprinted with permission.)

tion of alcoholic cider. Although this alcoholic beverage has a small market share, it has seen a progressive and significant increase in use by 16- to 17-year-olds between 2005, 2008, and 2011.[10]

Reviewing quantitative data is a valuable way to map and understand the landscape of adolescent alcohol consumption, providing us with demonstrable trends and highlighting risks for drinking and correlated harms.[11] However, quantitative data do not generate insights into the nature of young people's decision-making about alcohol use or the effect of variables such as gender, leisure, and peer relationships, attitudes to alcohol, family influences, media promotion, and consumerism. Recent ethnographic research examining drinking behavior within the context of values that govern use and provide "its actions with meaning"[11] offers some explanation of young people's relationship to alcohol.

Attitudes Toward Drinking: Drinking to Get Drunk

Drinking to get drunk is another phenomenon associated with adolescent alcohol. The percentages of adolescents engaging in this behavior vary between countries.[6] Attitudes toward drinking influence both initiation and levels of consumption. In Australia, although most (66%) adolescents aged 12 to 17 describe themselves as nondrinkers, of those who drank in the past 7 days, 40% intentionally drank to get drunk *some of the time*, and approximately 36.5% drank to get drunk *most times* or *every time*. Younger female adolescents (12-15 years) and females aged 16 to 17 years outnumbered their male peers on intention to get drunk *some of the time*, whereas male adolescents across both age ranges outnumbered their female peers with intention to get drunk during *most occasions of current drinking* (38.5% and 34% respectively).[10] In Australia there seems to be a downward trend in the *total* number of 12- to 17-year-olds who are drinking. However, of those 12- to 17-year-olds who do drink, the number consuming more than 4 drinks on 1 occasion in the last 7 days increased during 2005 to 2011.[10]

> Female #1: *"I kind of stop drinking when I'm at a good drunkenness. Like when I'm happy and just feel like a bit tipsy but I don't feel like I'm going to vomit. Then I might have a little water and then I might have a little more...."*[11]

Australian research has shown that when young people discuss the desired outcome of consuming alcohol, they talk about a specifically sought-after state of mind. The difference between a desired state of mind and negative consequences (eg, vomiting) can influence the amount of alcohol individuals consume when they are trying to achieve a "good drunkenness" state. If the good time turns bad, then young people forgo their feeling of pleasure. Balancing on the tipping edge between a good time and a bad time is difficult, not only in terms of assessing the effect of alcohol as one continues drinking but also in preventing negative consequences such as having a hangover, experiencing social alienation, or not having an enjoyable night out.

Jonathan, 21: *"I'm one of those people that—I'll feel fine, fine, fine and then half a drink later and then I feel absolutely terrible and that's the end of it for me.*

... — you know you're in excess—until you just tip over the edge and then you realize that you're way over. And then that's the end of it and then you're not going to feel very good in the morning."[11]

What is viewed by health professionals as the irrationality of drinking to get drunk is highly valued by some young people because it provides social inclusion, belonging, and status within their peer groups. Instead of undermining the ideal state of mind (drunkenness), the intangibility of obtaining and keeping it adds to its value. Within drinking cultures, stigma may also be attached to remaining sober.

Male #1: *"I've been willing to take a risk (of) having a sh*t night."*
Female #1: *"just to have that good bit at least. That one good bit...."*
Male #1: *"have nothing and be completely sober."*
Female #1: *"Yeah."*[11]

Staying within the drunkenness state but not tipping over the edge into negative consequences can be viewed by young people as the ideal state and considered worthy of the investment. Having *"that one good bit..."* or *"hav[ing] nothing..."* for at least part of the "night out" seems to be a way for young people to rationalize decisions that place them at risk for short-term harm. Balancing on the edge without falling into negative territory may raise a person's status in peer groups and act as a behavioral reinforcer. In addition to gaining peer group status, success or otherwise balancing on the edge could mediate self-esteem; success may raise self-esteem while failure may decrease it.

Female: *"Everyone's having a good time and then that one person got really bad and ...messed it up for everyone else. Cause everyone else has to kind of leave and help them."*[11]
Laura, 17: *"People just miss out on the whole night. ...one of my friends ...he was passed out vomiting by 5 pm. ...And it's hard for his friends as well because they're kind of stuck like trying to make a decision ...."*[11]

Within a social context, drinking to get drunk acts as a social lubricant and is viewed as pleasurable, as long as individuals do not jeopardize their ability to remain contributors to the group. Taken too far, individuals risk missing out on group activities, and their relationship with other group members is threatened.

Function and Expectations of Alcohol Use

Early UK research with 16- to 21-year-olds whose substance use was above the national average highlighted the functionality of alcohol and other substance use in relation to motivating factors that affect young people's individual use decisions.[12] Examples include consuming alcohol to have a "good time" or to relax and increase one's confidence, whereas methamphetamine may be used to stay awake, to relieve the boredom of work, or to make one laugh.[12] Young people's (and adults') expectations about the effects of substance use, including alcohol, also influence decisions about use. For example, someone who wants to feel relaxed in a social situation and has previously experienced alcohol facilitating this feeling may consume alcohol with the expectation of feeling relaxed again. Alternatively, alcohol use and loss of control can act as motivators to set boundaries or limits. Australian research has found that adolescent expectations of alcohol interact across a diverse range of domains, such as increasing sociability, transgressing social conventions, adopting different personas or identities, and experiencing freedom.[11]

Motivational models of alcohol use have been applied to investigate drinking restraint (the ability to limit alcohol consumption), particularly in relation to binge drinking and alcohol dependence. Five factors have been suggested within the construct of drinking restraint to predict risk from alcohol use. One form of restraint—cognitive and emotional preoccupation (CEP)—is correlated to higher consumption of alcohol and related problems, whereas another form—cognitive and behavioral control (CBC)—measures attempts to control alcohol use.[13] Researchers on the Gold Coast in Queensland, Australia, investigated the relationship between drinking motives, drinking restraint, alcohol consumption, and alcohol problems with a sample of young adults aged 17 to 34 years to ascertain whether relationships between motivations to drink and drinking behavior were mediated by drinking restraint.[13] Whereas conforming to group norms was not related to alcohol consumption and problems, drinking to cope with negative affect and to enhance positive affect was. The researchers suggest that the counterintuitive finding on conformity may reflect a social change in attitudes toward pressuring others to drink while still engaging in personal consumption of alcohol at levels of risk. Social motives were found to be significantly related to consumption and problems. Data analyses also found that participants' anticipation of positive reinforcement of either a social nature or positive affect influenced the decision to consume alcohol.[13] New US data have shown the trend in lower-grade high school students to disapprove of and view binge drinking negatively in terms of perceived risk, with a corresponding downward trend in binge drinking rates in this cohort.[4]

Alcohol and Gender

In Australia today more young women are drinking at higher rates of "risky drinking for long-term harms" (risk of dependency and disease) than young men across early, middle, and late adolescence.[14] Similarly, young women are at higher risk for short-term monthly harm (ie, injury from accidents) compared to young men in the 12- to 19-year age range.[14] Comparing 12- to 15-year-old

Australians, fewer females than males abstain from alcohol consumption.[14] The gender divide between adolescent female and male drinking is narrowing.[11,15] In Australia, North America, and some European countries, the gender divide is virtually nonexistent, with a similar trend occurring in a number of developing countries (Table 2).[15]

Although Australian data from 2010 indicate that girls in early adolescence are drinking more than their male peers,[14] the global trend for young men to drink more frequently and heavily than young women across the adolescent years continues.[5-7,9,15,16] Twenty-three percent of Australian 18- to 19-year-old males drink at risk levels for short-term harm on a weekly basis compared to 11.5% of females of the same age.[13]

Australian research involving a young adult sample (17-34 years) indicated that women reached similar levels of intoxication and experienced similar alcohol-related problems as men.[13] For 17- to 23-year-old young women in Denmark and Finland, binge drinking has taken on an increasingly positive meaning, resulting in a corresponding rise in drunkenness.[17]

How are we to understand the narrowing gender divide in alcohol consumption? Traditionally, drinking by women occurred in the home or in the "Ladies Lounge." Drinking in public and drinking to excess has been the domain of men, with women banned from public bars and actively discouraged from "heavy" drinking. Historically, women who drank in public and to excess were considered "unfeminine, immoral, unrespectable and associated with uncontrolled sexual appetites."[18] However, the traditional male-dominated domain of drinking is changing, as evidenced earlier. In addition, women's roles are changing as well. The contemporary woman exists in a variety of public and private spheres, including study, work, professional life, leisure, and home. The social acceptance

Table 2
Differences in heavy episodic drinking among young people in selected countries by gender and age

Country	Year	Total (%)	Male (%)	Female (%)	Age group (y)
Australia	2001	10.7	9.6	11.8	14-19
Canada	2000-2001	15.3	26.3	5.2	15-19
Ireland	1999	31.0	32.0	32.0	15-16
Mexico	2000-2001	2.5	0.8	1.5	15-19
Nigeria	2000-2001	1.2	1.0	1.3	15-19
Norway	2003	15.0	17.0	14.0	15-16
United Kingdom	1999	30.0	33.0	27.0	15-16
United States	2002	10.7	11.4	9.9	12-17

Data from World Health Organization (WHO). *Global Status Report on Alcohol and Health.* Geneva, Switzerland: WHO; 2011.

of women's alcohol consumption is moderated by the cultural expectations of women, their growing emancipation (with young women themselves leading the change), and increasing gender equality. Although western society continues to place limitations and conditions on women's drinking,[18] young women have an expectation, like their male peers, that drinking is one way to experience pleasure within a fun and leisurely lifestyle.[11,19]

> Corinna, 24: "...I think it's fun to just relax especially after (a big few) weeks so alcohol's quite relaxing."[11]
> (P064): "If I have one I feel more relaxed. I feel more holiday mode. I feel work's finished. I've got a nice evening ahead of me...."[19]

Encapsulated in this construction of drinking for pleasure and leisure is an additional discourse about drinking as a reward for work, with women borrowing an accepted male theme of drinking at the end of a "hard working week."[19]

> (P037): "Just like the feeling of freedom, the feeling of, erm, you know, cause really I'm free to drink what I want without anybody you know raising their eyebrows or anything."[19]

Venturing into and existing within a previously male-dominated sphere confers rights, autonomy, and equality. In the preceding quote, the woman speaks about the freedom associated with drinking without retribution. Notwithstanding the sense of freedom alcohol can bring, the violation of alcohol use norms remains heavily criticized.[19] When women drink more than is culturally accepted or behave in ways that are constructed as deviant, such as being sexually assertive or "behaving like idiots,"[11] they can be ostracized by their peers and publicly humiliated.[18] Young women are perhaps at the cutting edge of challenging the traditional dichotomy of alcohol and gender: men can, women can't. In terms of sexual politics, alcohol may be the new frontier in attempts to challenge traditional male/female roles.

The gender shift in relation to alcohol use and the types of alcohol consumed also have been considered a reflection of a general trend toward feminization of drinking styles for both young men and women.[17] Qualitative research in Denmark and Finland suggests that young adult drinking culture is diversifying to a hybrid form, moving away from traditional masculine/feminine alcohol consumption to one that sees both genders engaged in a variety of drinking styles, including "heroic drinking" (traditional masculine drinking to get drunk) and "playful drinking." Playful drinking is characterized by self-representations, maintenance of some form of control, and social interactions that may lead to flirtation and romantic/sexual encounters. Playful drinking is considered to occur more frequently in public spaces (nightclubs, bars, parties) and to mediate levels of intoxication because of its "performative and controlled character."[17] Demant and Törrönen[17] challenge the view that young women are merely adopting a male drinking culture. They suggest that styles of alcohol consumption influence male and female drinking and that this is reflected in a modification toward playful drinking and a blurring of traditional alcohol-based gender roles.

ISSUES FOR VULNERABLE GROUPS

Gay, Lesbian, and Bisexual Young People

Evidence indicates that lesbian, gay, and bisexual young people report higher rates of substance use than their heterosexual peers.[20-22] It has been suggested that this disparity is mediated by environmental and cultural elements (eg, harassment, discrimination)[20,22] and that belonging to stigmatized and marginalized minority groups can result in psychosocial stress.[23] A longitudinal study found that young gay males' drinking was similar to that of heterosexual males but heavier than that of bisexual males.[24] Young lesbians, however, drank more heavily than female heterosexuals, and this disparity extended into later adolescence.[24] Young gay men and lesbians experiencing, for example, the transition of coming out, reported using alcohol to lessen the effect of internalized homophobia and to ease or cancel the stigma attached to their difference.[25]

Culturally and Linguistically Diverse Populations

Attention has been drawn to the vulnerabilities and susceptibilities of diverse cultural and ethnic young people to alcohol misuse and complex social influences on their health.[26,27] Challenges in delivery of drug and alcohol services to minority and newly emerging populations have been identified.[28] When young people migrate they leave behind cultural, language, community, social, and educational systems that are familiar to them. They face multiple adjustments as well as developmental changes experienced by all young people.[26] They may experience grief for the loss of their home country, stigma, discrimination, and difficulties with acculturation and navigating the social and cultural norms of their host country.[29]

Notwithstanding these challenges, Australian research indicates that substance use, including alcohol use, is lower among young people in culturally and linguistically diverse populations (CALD) than those in the general population.[26] The reasons for this difference are not fully understood, but prevailing cultural expectations, attitudes, and familial patterns of use may provide protection for some newly arrived young people and for those for whom English is not the first language spoken at home.[26,27] This is not to say that the stress of migration and adjusting to host countries such as Australia and Europe is without challenges. High levels of distress as a result of protracted asylum procedures and the psychological effects of torture, such as those experienced by asylum seekers and humanitarian migrants, are well documented.[30] Some people may use alcohol to cope with psychological symptoms, but the prevailing Australian evidence suggests that perceptions of excessive alcohol use by CALD young people is a myth.[26]

MEDIATING FACTORS

The Nuclear Family

Parents' personal alcohol consumption is positively correlated to adolescents' alcohol use. An Australian cross-sectional study found that primary school-aged children's *intention* to drink and *acceptance of* alcohol, unsurprisingly, are positively correlated to parental weekly alcohol use. Primary school-aged children from the same study identified as *occasional* or *more frequent* drinkers were significantly more likely to drink if a close friend or sibling drank.[10] In this study, intention to drink was mediated by parental alcohol use and drinking behavior by whether a friend or sibling drank. Parental attitudes to alcohol consumption have also been found to influence young people's beliefs about alcohol use. For example, a significant association has been found between parental drinking and parents giving permission to adolescents to take alcohol to parties.[10]

The relationship between *where* current drinkers consumed their last drink and how they *obtained* it also influenced alcohol consumption in high school students (Table 3). More "nondrinkers" and "occasional drinkers" obtained their alcohol from their parents and consumed it at home, whereas approximately

Table 3

Where current drinkers* who describe themselves as a nondrinker, occasional drinker, or party drinker consume alcohol and how they obtained it, Australia, 2011†

	Self-label					
	Nondrinker		Occasional drinker		Party drinker	
Age (y)	12-15	16-17	12-15	16-17	12-15	16-17
Alcohol obtained from:						
Parents	58.1	50.6	40.8	36.3	18.6	28.5
Friends	13.5	29.8	27.6	24.7	26.9	20.2
Someone else bought it for me	1.5	1.7	6.7	18.6	34.9	32.3
Where alcohol was consumed:						
Home	50.0	54.5	45.8	32.9	20.3	15.6
Party	16.2	12.3	20.7	31.6	48.6	48.5
Friend's place	7.8	16.2	14.3	21.1	14.9	18.1

Values are given as percentage unless otherwise indicated.
*Current drinkers are students who drank on any of the past 7 days.
†Percentages exclude responses from students who reported multiple drinking locations and multiple drinking sources.
Data from White V, Bariola E. *Australian Secondary School Students' Use of Tobacco, Alcohol, Over-The-Counter and Illicit Substance Use in 2011*. Melbourne, Australia: Centre for Behavioural Research in Cancer, The Cancer Council Victoria; 2012.

one-third of "party drinkers" obtained alcohol from "someone else" and close to 50% consumed their last drink at a party.[10]

Biologic links have been found between parental alcohol dependence and the propensity for adolescents to consume alcohol.[31] Furthermore, there is a significant correlation between parental alcohol dependency and alcohol-related behaviors in adolescents, hypothesized as the inability of these parents to maintain connection, involvement, and oversight of their adolescent.[31] However, controlled parental alcohol use has a protective effect when used within family rituals. Family structure also seems to influence adolescent alcohol use. For example, 2-parent families have been found to have fewer adolescent offspring engaged in problematic alcohol use compared to sole-parent households.[31]

Leisure Time and Peers

Young people are engaged in a variety of activities ranging from study and work to sport, recreation, and leisure. Involvement in these interests not only is mediated by the personal significance they hold for an individual or group but also is shaped by the young person's sociocultural environment.[32] Leisure time and the pursuit of enjoyment have been described as essential elements of youth culture. Integral to this leisure lifestyle is the consumption of alcohol as a mechanism to achieve group acceptance, identity, social bonding, and belonging.[11] The role of alcohol in the pursuit of a leisure lifestyle and the positive attributes derived from it compared to the spheres of work and study has a growing importance for today's young people.

As young people mature through adolescence, gain independence, and enter young adulthood, peers become increasingly influential and important. Groups may form and disband quickly because of the fluid nature of contemporary youth culture.[11] For example, individuals will mix with different friends to form groups in order to engage in specific shared activities. Interestingly, peer pressure (actual provocation and direct pressure) to consume alcohol has been discredited in recent UK research findings,[32] highlighting instead that friendship groups exert varying degrees of *peer influence* on each other through social mechanisms, group membership, and belonging compared to direct pressure to behave in certain ways. Perhaps not surprisingly, groups that aspire to moderate drinking have been found to be more accepting of individuals who do not drink.[32] However, young people who go out more frequently and spend less organized time with their friends (eg, hanging out) compared to those involved with structured sports or individual activities are more likely to drink and to do so heavily.[33] Additionally, going out at night, mixing with larger peer groups, having friends who are delinquent, and being a member of a gang are strongly associated with alcohol use.[33]

Media Promotion

Media plays a significant role in normalizing alcohol use. The alcohol industry has targeted young people for years through the promotion of sports, music events, and festivals. A number of studies have examined the effect of advertising on children and adolescents, and almost all showed advertising to be very effective in increasing young people's awareness of and emotional responses to alcohol, including recognition of brands, their desire to own or use the products, and their familiarity with the advertisement itself.[34] An analysis of 13 longitudinal studies found that alcohol advertising and promotion increases the likelihood that adolescents will start to use alcohol and to drink more if they already are using alcohol.[35] Alcohol advertisements frequently depict sexual and social stereotypes with fun-loving, seemingly successful young people enjoying themselves in large group parties or social activities.[34] Alcohol is marketed to young people with subtlety, reflecting their aspirations for success, freedom, fun, and independence. Marketers suggest that ads need to be "relevant, irreverent, mischievous and/or alternatively, as real as possible"[11] in order to connect to young people.

The alcohol industry invests large amounts of money in market research. Marketers ascertain what product appeals to young consumers, how they relate to it, and what makes it unique within a particular context (eg, a swimming pool party), and then they create an image of this ideal context and promote it back to the consumer.[11] For example, women's magazines connect alcoholic drinks with femininity, and magazines that target young adult women align drinking with professionalism, daring, and the public sphere, thus reinforcing changing gender roles.[18]

Studies have shown significant correlations between exposure to alcohol advertising and consumption.[34] The emotional association developed toward alcohol products also affects the likelihood of adolescents beginning to drink.[36] Those who binge drink tend to name a favorite and well-advertised brand.[37] Increased risk of drinking in early adolescence is correlated to frequent exposure to alcohol advertising.[38] Consumer choice and freedom are portrayed in the media as associated with alcohol use and young people. However, choice is limited by market provision and eroded by media campaigns that depict youth culture and fun as solely aligned to drinking cultures.[11] Thus choice is reduced to whether or not a person drinks alcohol in order to join social gatherings. Marketers and alcohol producers are in the business of promoting and selling product. Young people may be "savvy consumers"[11] of media, but the sophisticated techniques used by alcohol marketers and the portrayal of the rewards from a leisure lifestyle (eg, fun, freedom, social inclusion, relationships) take advantage of maturational processes and social aspirations to manipulate expectations through a lens of consumerism.[2]

RESPONDING TO THE CHALLENGE

There is increasing evidence that consumption of alcohol by young people can adversely affect brain development and lead to alcohol-related problems in later life. Governments have an obligation to act and have at their disposal a range of regulatory interventions. These include increasing the price of alcohol, restricting settings of use, and raising legal purchase age, all of which are effective in reducing alcohol use by young people and its related harms.[39] In integrating the findings of systematic reviews,[39] researchers have been able to summarize evidence for targeted strategies and other measures for preventing the onset of harmful patterns of drinking in settings, such as vulnerable families, schools, and communities, as well as universal strategies to reduce the attractiveness of substance use (eg, advertising and sponsorship bans). The optimal package for preventing alcohol-related harms comprises the following (in order of cost-effectiveness): volumetric taxation, advertising bans, increasing the minimum legal drinking age to 21 years, brief intervention by primary care practitioners, licensing controls, a drink-driving mass media campaign, and random breath testing.[40]

Restricting the Supply of Alcohol to Young People

Restricting young people's access to alcohol is an important supply reduction strategy for which there is substantial supporting evidence for efficacy. One such measure is raising the minimum age to 21 years at which it is legal to purchase and consume alcohol (in Australia and Europe it is legal to purchase and consume alcohol from the age of 18 years). Although Australian support for this legislative change rose from 40.7% in 2004 to 50.2% in 2010,[14] industry opposition related to potential lost revenue/patronage remains predictably strong. There are also "acceptability" issues for the public because the legal voting age is 18 years. Many believe that it simply wouldn't work. This debate has also raged in the United States.[41] In Australia it is reported that introduction of volumetric taxation (which would tax alcohol products based on alcohol volume) would be the most cost-effective intervention.[40]

Importance of a Comprehensive Response and Other Supporting Measures

Although the legal drinking age is important, it should not be viewed as the singular solution to the complex problem of alcohol use by underage young people. Cultural attitudes, parental and community norms, and public education also have been identified as important factors influencing youth behavior and behavioral change. An important consideration here, as noted earlier, is that parents/families themselves play a role in supplying alcohol to young people. The *Australian Secondary School Students' Use of Tobacco, Alcohol and Over-the-Counter and Illicit Substances* survey in 2011 found that 44.2% of current drinkers (students who drank on any of the past 7 days) aged 12 to 15 years and 38.3% of 16- to 17-years-olds nominated parents or siblings as the usual source of their alcohol.[10] Many parents (in some surveys, almost 50%) support underage drinking under parental supervision. Regardless of any legislative changes, therefore, educational campaigns that target parents and families are needed to provide information on the effect of alcohol on young people's development (especially on brain development) and to encourage parents to restrict supply and delay the initiation of consumption.

Unfortunately, little systematic research has been conducted on the needs of families of young people with problematic drug use. An Australian study noted that adolescents whose parents display a permissive attitude toward alcohol consumption tend to drink more.[42] They also found that sibling drug use may increase the likelihood of initial use by another child and that, once adolescents start experimenting with alcohol, increased parental monitoring is the most effective strategy for reducing the risk of excessive adolescent drinking. Schools, youth centers, and clubs are other important settings for education about alcohol-related harms.

Advertising and Sponsorship

Young people are exposed to alcohol marketing in more ways than ever before, not only through traditional media such as television, radio, newspapers and magazines, billboards, merchandise, and sponsorship, but also through the Internet, including social media sites such as Facebook, YouTube, and Twitter. At present, the only aspect of alcohol advertising that is government regulated in Australia is broadcasting times for alcohol advertising on television. Alcohol sponsorship of sporting and cultural events is prolific and highly visible in places where young people are present,[43] with the greatest exposure to alcohol advertising through televised sport events.[44] At least 29 countries have implemented bans on alcohol advertising in at least 1 medium. More countries have partial bans, most commonly on television, during times when young children are most likely to be watching. A few countries also have banned alcohol sponsorship at sporting events.[45]

Community Mobilization

Programs in the United States that have taken a whole community approach to addressing systemic issues affecting youth well-being have also been successful in reducing alcohol and other related harms.[46] These programs involve key agencies and stakeholders across communities in collaborating and working together to promote healthy social and personal development. Local data are collected and analyzed to identify behaviors that compromise health and gaps in the provision of services. Information is collected from youth surveys and the community and used to establish key prevention and intervention measures and health promotion targets. Plans are then implemented to select interventions that have been designed to address the local community's own identified priorities and objectives. Evaluation is a further step in ascertaining the intervention's effectiveness. Local communities are supported to strengthen their achievements through capacity building and to become self-sustaining in their efforts to address determinants of adolescent problems.[47] The United Kingdom, The Netherlands, and Australia have trialed similar programs and found them to be beneficial as an evidence-based approach to planning and delivering effective prevention initiatives to protect against social and health problems.[48]

The Australian-based community mobilization initiative "Hello Sunday Morning" (HSM) uses e-technology to provide a platform for individuals to reflect on their own drinking behavior.[49] HSM describes itself as "a movement towards a better drinking culture."[49] HSM is a blogging Web site where members can write blogs and post photos or videos about their experiences and the role that alcohol plays in their life while they are undertaking a period of sobriety.

HSMers elect to sign up to 3, 6, or 12 months of sobriety. The top 5 changes that HSMers identify as goals are the following:

1. Improving health (70.5%)
2. Improving well-being (51.9%)
3. Changing individual drinking behavior (26.9%)
4. Learning to socialize without needing alcohol (23.6%)
5. Saving money (23.3%)[48]

Qualitative analysis of the blog posts demonstrated that, over time, HSMers moved from being very self-focused to adopting a broader view of alcohol's role in society and helping others in their own goals.[49] Further analysis revealed that HSMers behavioral change is related to the individual's change in life outlook, well-being, cultural norms, life practices, and values.[49]

HSM takes a network approach to health promotion. HSMers communicate and network with each other as they attempt to change their drinking behavior and attitudes to alcohol.

> "...I look forward to clarity on my binge drinking, how it affects my life, and how not drinking like that anymore can change things for the better." (Days into HSM: 29, Post Count: 2, ID 45)[49]

Further research is needed to quantify any statistically significant effect of HSM as an initiative to measure changes in alcohol consumption and well-being data. Nevertheless, the research referred to here was able to identify how blogging and social networking creates a sense of community and a space where individuals can adapt another's language and experiences for their own purposes.[49] The blog posts become collective resources that provide support, guidance, and answerability to its community as members endeavor to change behavior.[49]

CONCLUSION

An examination of drinking patterns in young people is complicated by mixed data on adolescent alcohol use. Although some country and regional trends are on the decline in terms of overall consumption, problematic binge drinking seems to be on the rise. Early initiation, availability of alcohol, and a variety of ready-to-drink products influence consumption. In Australia, although most adolescents describe themselves as nondrinkers, of those who are current drinkers, approximately 38% intend to get drunk either some or every time they consume alcohol, and the number of 12- to 17-year-olds who binge drink increased between 2005 and 2011.

Young people's desired outcomes from alcohol consumption and the social context in which this occurs significantly affect the amount they drink. Seeking a balance between achieving an "ideal state of mind," obtaining pleasure, and risking negative consequences from excessive alcohol use are challenges faced by young people who drink to get drunk. An analysis of motivation reveals that attitudes toward drinking also influence levels of consumption. Personal reasons for alcohol use and expectations of the role that alcohol plays interact across a range of domains to mediate consumption patterns. Young people may consume alcohol for social reasons, as a rebellion, for experimentation with different identities, or as a demonstration of free will. Drinking to cope with negative affect and to enhance positive affect has been found to correlate with problematic alcohol use, whereas disapproval of and perceived risk from binge drinking tends to lessen alcohol consumption at this level.

Trends in problematic drinking are also associated with gender and sexuality. Australian data indicate that girls in early adolescence seem to drink more alcohol than their male peers. However, although a gender reversal occurs through adolescence, as women enter young adulthood some increase their drinking levels and experience alcohol-related problems similar to those of men. The changing role of women and the discourses about gender, the role of alcohol in the pursuit of a leisure lifestyle, and drinking styles all contribute to changes in gender-related alcohol use. The use of alcohol by gay, bisexual, and lesbian young people can be understood in the context of environmental influences on behavior and the self-medication theory, in which individuals use substances to reduce negative affect associated with psychological stress. Although leisure is an increasingly important factor in youth culture and alcohol use is correlated to group belonging, friendship groups are fluid, and group norms influence their members in a variety of ways. Spending structured time with friends and belonging to moderate drinking groups or groups that accept nondrinking peers are likely to protect against excessive drinking. Parental monitoring is a proven mechanism for reducing alcohol harms.

Within this complex and ever changing matrix of interrelated mitigating factors for problematic drinking, population health efforts have been struggling to keep pace. Those concerned with measures to protect young people from excessive harm recognize the compelling evidence about what works and want to implement a comprehensive package of prevention. However, obstacles to such interventions remain entrenched in most western societies. Alcohol manufacturers not only fight to maintain their market share (often presented as the primary reason for advertising alcohol) but also work assiduously to attract and build a youth market. Tax revenues present governments with an almost insurmountable conflict of interest, threatening political will to deal with the largely unregulated influence of the alcohol industry. Notwithstanding the many challenges involved, public health advocates must continue to find ways to address this foremost threat to the health and well-being of young people throughout the world.

ACKNOWLEDGMENT

We thank Emeritus Professor Ian Webster AO, School of Public Health and Community Medicine, University of New South Wales, for reading and commenting on the draft.

References

1. Boden JM, Fergusson DM. The short- and long-term consequences of adolescent alcohol use. In: Saunders JB, Rey JM eds. *Young People & Alcohol: Impact, Policy, Prevention, Treatment.* Chichester, West Sussex: Wiley-Blackwell; 2011
2. Roche AM, Bywood P, Borlagdan J, et al. *Young People and Alcohol: The Role of Cultural Influences.* Adelaide, Australia: National Centre for Education and Training on Addiction; 2008
3. World Health Organization. *Global Survey on Alcohol and Health.* Geneva, Switzerland: WHO; 2008
4. Johnston LD, O'Malley PM, Bachman JG, Schulenberg JE. *Monitoring the Future National Results on Drug Use: 2012 Overview, Key Findings on Adolescent Drug Use.* Ann Arbor, MI: Institute for Social Research, University of Michigan; 2013
5. Freeman JG, King M, Pickett, W. *The Health of Canada's Young People: A Mental Health Focus.* Ottawa, Canada: Public Health Agency of Canada; 2011
6. Hibell B, Guttormsson U, Ahlström S, et al. *The 2011 ESPAD Report: Substance Use Among Students in 36 European Countries.* Stockholm, Sweden: Swedish Council for Information on Alcohol and Other Drugs (CAN); 2012
7. Degenhardt L, O'Loughlin C, Swift W, et al. The persistence of adolescent binge drinking into adulthood: findings from a 15-year prospective cohort study. *BMJ Open.* 2013;3:e003015
8. Neinstein L. *The New Adolescents: An Analysis of Health Conditions, Behaviors, Risks, and Access to Services Among Emerging Young Adults.* Los Angeles, CA: University of Southern California; 2013
9. Kuntsche P, Rehm J, Gmel G. Characteristics of binge drinkers in Europe. *Soc Sci Med.* 2004;59: 113–127
10. White V, Bariola E. *Australian Secondary School Students' Use of Tobacco, Alcohol, Over-The-Counter and Illicit Substance Use in 2011.* Melbourne, Australia: Centre for Behavioural Research in Cancer, The Cancer Council Victoria; 2012
11. Borlagdan J, Freeman T, Duvnjak A, et al. *From Ideal to Reality: Cultural Contradictions and Young People's Drinking.* Adelaide, Australia: National Centre for Education and Training on Addiction; 2010
12. Boys A, Marsden J, Fountain J, et al. What influences young people's use of drugs? A qualitative study of decision-making. *Drugs Educ Prev Policy.* 1999;6:373–387
13. Lyvers M, Hasking P, Hani R, Rhodes M, Trew E. Drinking motives, drinking restraint and drinking behaviour among young adults. *Addict Behav.* 2010;35:116–122
14. *2010 National Drug Strategy Household Survey.* Canberra, Australia: Australian Institute of Health and Welfare; 2011
15. World Health Organization (WHO). *Global Status Report on Alcohol and Health.* Geneva, Switzerland: WHO; 2011
16. Isidore S, Room R. *Alcohol, Gender and Drinking Problems: Perspectives from Low and Middle Income Countries.* Geneva, Switzerland: World Health Organization; 2005

17. Demant J, Törrönen J. Changing drinking styles in Denmark and Finland. Fragmentation of male and female drinking among young adults. *Subst Use Misuse.* 2011;46:1244-1255
18. Plant MA. The role of alcohol in women's lives: a review of issues and responses. *J Subst Use.* 2008;13(3);155-191
19. Rolfe A, Orford J, Dalton S. Women, alcohol and femininity: a discourse analysis of women heavy drinkers' accounts. *J Health Psychol.* 2009;14:326-335
20. Marshal MP, Friedman MS, Stall R, Thompson AL. Individual trajectories of substance use in lesbian, gay and bisexual youth and heterosexual youth. *Addiction.* 2009;104(6):974-981
21. Marshal MP, Friedman MS, Stall R, et al. Sexual orientation and adolescent substance use: a meta-analysis and methodological review. *Addiction.* 2008;103:546-556
22. Austin EL, Bozick R. Sexual orientation, partnership formation, and substance use in the transition to adulthood. *J Youth Adolesc.* 2012;41:167-178
23. Hughes TL. Alcohol use and alcohol-related problems among lesbians and gay men. *Annu Rev Nurs Res.* 2005;23:283-325
24. Corliss H, Rosario M, Wypij D, et al. Sexual orientation disparities in longitudinal alcohol use patterns among adolescents: findings from the Growing Up Today Study. *Arch Pediatr Adolesc Med.* 2008;162(11):1071-1078
25. Peralta L. "Alcohol allows you to be yourself": toward a structured understanding of alcohol use and gender difference among gay, lesbian and heterosexual youth. *J Drug Issues.* 2008;389(2):373-399
26. Manderson L. Alcohol and other drug prevention in culturally and linguistically diverse communities: responding to the challenges. *Drug Info.* 2010;8(4):1-16
27. Bryan B, Batch JA. An Australian perspective: the complexities of ethnic adolescent health. *Youth Studies Aust.* 2002;21(1):24-33
28. Nguyen P. *Challenges for CALD Drug & Alcohol Service Delivery.* Carlton, Australia: Ethnic Communities' Council of Victoria; 2007:1-15
29. Transcultural Mental Health Centre. Personal communication from Michele Sapucci. March 3, 2013
30. Heeren M, Mueller J, Ehlert U, et al. Mental health of asylum seekers: a cross-sectional study of psychiatric disorders. *BMC Psychiatry.* 2012;12:114
31. Australian Institute of Family Studies (AIFS). *Family and Environmental Factors–Adolescent Alcohol Use. Research Report No. 10.* Melbourne: AIFS; 2004
32. Townshend TG. Youth, alcohol and place-based leisure behaviours: a study of two locations in England. *Soc Sci Med.* 2013;1:153-161
33. Steketee M, Aussems C, van den Toorn J, Jonkman H. *Leisure Time, Peers and Their Influence on Alcohol and Drug Consumption Amongst the Youth.* Utrecht, The Netherlands: Verwey-Jonker Institute; 2012:1-17
34. Borzekowski DLG, Strasburger VC. Tobacco, alcohol, and drug exposure. In: Calvert S, Wilson BJ, eds. *Handbook of Children and the Media.* Boston: Blackwell; 2008: 432-452
35. Anderson P, de Bruijn A, Angus K, Gordon R, Hastings G. Impact of alcohol advertising and media exposure on adolescent alcohol use: a systematic review of longitudinal studies. *Alcohol Alcohol.* 2009;44:229-243
36. McClure AC, Stoolmiller M, Tanski SE, Worth KA, Sargent JD. Alcohol-branded merchandise and its association with drinking attitudes and outcomes in US adolescents. *Arch Pediatr Adolesc Med.* 2009;163:211-217
37. Tanski SE, McClure AC, Jernigan DH, Sargent JD. Alcohol brand preference and binge drinking among adolescents. *Arch Pediatr Adolesc Med.* 2011;165:675-676
38. Morgenstern M, Isensee B, Sargent JD, Hanewinkel, R. Exposure to alcohol advertising and teen drinking. *Prev Med.* 2011;52:146-151
39. Toumbourou JW, Stockwell T, Neighbors C, et al. Interventions to reduce harm associated with adolescent substance use: an international review. *Lancet Adolesc Health Series,* 2007;4:41-45
40. Doran CM, Hall WD, Shakeshaft AP, Vos T, Cobiac LJ. Alcohol policy reform in Australia: what can we learn from the evidence? *Med J Aust.* 2010;192(8):468-470

41. Toomey TL, Nelson TF, Lenk KMK. The age-21 minimum legal drinking age: a case study linking past and current debates. *Addiction*. 2009;104(12):1958–1965

42. Fry S, Dawe S, Harnett P, Kowalenko S, Harlen, M. *Supporting the Families of Young People with Problematic Drug Use: Investigating Support Options. ANCD Research Paper No. 15.* Canberra, Australia: Australian National Council on Drugs; 2008

43. Callinan S, Wilkinson C, Livingston M. *Australian Attitudes Toward Alcohol Policy: 1995-2010.* Deakin, NSW, Australia: Foundation for Alcohol Research & Education and Centre for Alcohol Policy Research; 2013

44. Winter MV, Donovan RJ, Fielder LJ. Exposure of children and adolescents to alcohol advertising on television in Australia. *J Studies Alcohol Drugs*. 2008;69:676–683

45. Nicholson M, Hoye R. Reducing adolescents' exposure to alcohol advertising and promotion during televised sports. *J Am Med Assoc*. 2009;301:1479–1482

46. Hawkins JD, Oesterie S, Brown EC, et al. Results of a type 2 transactional research trial to prevent adolescent drug use and delinquency: a test of Communities That Care. *Arch Pediatr Adolesc Med*. 2009;163:789–798

47. The Royal Children's Hospital Melbourne. Communities That Care: Introduction. Available at: www.rch.org.au/ctc. Accessed November 3, 2013

48. Carlon C. Investing in Our Youth: Implementing Communities That Care in Western Australia. Unpublished paper. 2002;1–12

49. Hamley B, Carah N. *One Sunday At A Time: Evaluating Hello Sunday Morning.* Deakin, NSW, Australia: Foundation for Alcohol Research & Education; 2012

Adolesc Med 025 (2014) 70–88

Marijuana

Seth Ammerman, MD

Clinical Professor, Division of Adolescent Medicine, Department of Pediatrics, Stanford University, Lucile Packard Children's Hospital, Stanford, California

DEFINITIONS

Marijuana/Cannabis

Marijuana refers to the cannabis plant of which there are numerous species and subspecies. Buds and leaves of the plant are smoked, vaporized, cooked for eating, and liquefied for drinking for both their pleasurable psychoactive and medicinal effects. The 2 most common species used for medicinal purposes are *Cannabis sativa* and *Cannabis indica*. Psychotropically, *C sativa* typically causes increased alertness and an energetic sense, whereas *C indica* is reported to cause more of a sense of relaxation and, in some cases, lethargy. However, both species have been hybridized repeatedly, and a typical medical marijuana plant will have varying amounts of both *C sativa* and *C indica*.[1]

Cannabinoids

Regardless of the species, the cannabis plant contains a large number of biologically active molecules called *cannabinoids*. Marijuana is a complex mixture of cannabinoids (more than 200 have been identified) and other molecules, and the risk-benefit ratio of this mixture has not been well defined. Over the past several decades, selective breeding of marijuana species has resulted in higher concentrations of cannabinoids in the plant oil, resulting in a more potent psychotropic effect as well as possible increased risk of adverse effects.

The main active ingredients responsible for the desired medicinal effects are the 2 exogenous cannabinoids delta-9-tetrahydrocannabinol (THC), a psychoactive cannabinoid, and cannabidiol (CBD), a nonpsychoactive cannabinoid. A third cannabinoid, arachidonoylethanolamide (anadamide), is an endogenous ligand

---

*Corresponding author:
seth.ammerman@stanford.edu

that is involved in binding THC and CBD to endocannabinoid receptors. The 2 major endocannabinoid receptors are CB1, found in the brain and nervous system, and CB2, found in the immune system. Both naturally occurring and synthetic cannabinoid molecules can bind the human endocannabinoid receptors and have biologic activity. Cannabinoids have a number of regulatory functions in the human body, although currently cannabinoid biology is poorly understood.

Cannabinoids and marijuana have been used for a wide variety of pathologic states and diseases, including chronic pain, nausea, anorexia, cancer, autoimmune and rheumatic diseases, inflammatory bowel disease, attention-deficit/hyperactivity disorder, multiple sclerosis and spasticity, depression, anxiety, and posttraumatic stress disorder. No US Food and Drug Administration (FDA) safety or efficacy data concerning marijuana for medical use are available. There are 2 FDA-approved cannabinoid pharmaceutical products (see later for further discussion). Two recent articles have reviewed, respectively, current and emerging research on the physiologic mechanisms of cannabinoids and their applications in managing chronic pain, muscle spasticity, cachexia, and other debilitating problems, and the efficacy of marijuana for treatment of chemotherapy-induced nausea and vomiting.[2,3] Research has demonstrated that cannabinoids may be useful in treating anorexia associated with cancer, nausea and vomiting associated with chemotherapy, chronic pain, multiple sclerosis, and seizures.[4-12] A recently published study also demonstrated that current marijuana use was associated with lower levels of fasting insulin levels, lower homeostasis model assessment-estimated insulin resistance (HOMA-IR), and smaller waist circumference.[13] No studies on the use of cannabinoids or marijuana for treatment of health conditions in children or adolescents have been published.

Two legal synthetic forms of cannabinoids are available in the United States and approved by the FDA; a third is available in the United Kingdom and Canada. The first form, dronabinol (Marinol), is a schedule III oral medication approved by the FDA for treatment of wasting related to acquired immunodeficiency syndrome (AIDS) and for chemotherapy-induced nausea and vomiting.[14] Dronabinol is a capsule that must be taken whole orally, which may prove problematic in cases of nausea or vomiting. Additionally, the onset to symptom relief with dronabinol is significantly longer versus that with smoked marijuana. The second form, nabilone (Cesamet), is an oral capsule with properties similar to dronabinol but is a schedule II medication because of its possibly higher abuse potential. Nabilone is also prescribed for spasticity secondary to spinal cord injury.[15]

A third form is known as Sativex, a fast-acting nonsynthetic cannabinoid-based oral-mucosal spray.[16] Sativex is currently approved in Canada and the United Kingdom for symptomatic relief of neuropathic pain in multiple sclerosis. In Canada it also is approved as an adjunctive analgesic treatment for patients with cancer pain. Sativex is currently undergoing late-stage clinical testing in Europe and the United States for similar indications. Sativex contains equal amounts of THC and CBD. Sativex is rapidly absorbed and easy to titrate, which may make it a more effective and easy-to-use medication than dronabinol. Onset of desired effects typically occurs within minutes. However, in addition to the desired responses, adverse side effects can occur, ranging from relatively benign (eg, tachycardia and palpitations) to serious (eg, disorders in mood, anxiety, and thought).[17] Controlled studies have found that pharmaceutical preparations that combine cannabinoids with varying affinities for the CB1 and CB2 receptors seem to be able to deliver therapeutic effects while protecting against adverse effects.

THC

THC, also known as delta-9-tetrahydrocannibinol or tetrahydrocannabinol, is the primary psychoactive cannabinoid in the marijuana plant. The amount of THC in a given plant varies widely depending on the species and subspecies of marijuana used in breeding the plant.

Hemp

Hemp, a low-THC strain of *C sativa,* is not used for psychoactive effects. Rather, hemp is used to make a variety of consumer products, including paper, textiles, clothing, health food, and biofuel. Commercially available hemp products (eg, hemp milk) are devoid of cannabinoids. Hemp is legally grown in a number of countries, including Spain, China, Japan, Korea, France, and Ireland.

EPIDEMIOLOGY OF MARIJUANA USE AMONG YOUTH

Three major US national databases track substance use, including marijuana, over time: Monitoring the Future (MTF),[18] which is sponsored by the University of Michigan and the National Institute of Drug Abuse; the Youth Risk Behavior Survey (YRBS),[19] which is sponsored by the Centers for Disease Control and Prevention; and the National Survey on Drug Use and Health (NSDUH),[20] which is sponsored by the Substance Abuse and Mental Health Services Administration. Although the methodologies used differ with each database, all track substance use on a longitudinal basis. MTF annually surveys approximately 50,000 middle and high school students (12th-graders since 1975, and 8th- and 10th-graders since 1991). The data from MTF 2012 found that 6.5% of 8th-graders, 17.0% of 10th-graders, and 22.9% of 12th-graders had used marijuana at least once in the past 30 days (current use). Current-use rates peaked in 1996 for 8th-graders at 11.3%, and in 1997 for 10th-graders (20.5%) and 12th-graders (23.7%). Current-use rates have decreased for 8th-graders during the past 2 years, remained stable for 10th-graders in 2012 after increasing 3 years in a row; and increased for 12th-graders the past 6 years. All current rates remain lower than the peak rates in the 1990s. Daily-use rates for 8th-, 10th-, and 12th-graders in 2012 were 1.1%, 3.5%, and 6.5%, respectively. Note too that in 2011, The Partnership Attitude Tracking Study, sponsored by the MetLife Foundation and the Partnership at DrugFree.org, found that in a school-based sample of teens in grades 9 to 12, 9% reported smoking marijuana heavily (at least 20 times) in the past month. Overall, past-month heavy marijuana use is up 80% among US teens since 2008 in this same survey.[21] Based on NSDUH 2011 data, peak current use rates were 8.2% in 2002, 6.7% in 2006 and 2007, 7.3% in 2009, and 7.9% in 2011 for 12- to 17-year-olds. Marijuana use rates have also increased for 18- to 25-year-olds each year between 2008 and 2011, from 16.5%, 18.1%, 18.5%, and 19.0%, respectively. Note that approximately 100 million adult Americans have ever used marijuana, with a current use rate of 17.4 million.[22]

Specific state data are available in many states through their use of YRBSs or their equivalent. Table 1 compares these national data with youth use rates in

Table 1
Change in overall adolescent marijuana use by oldest high school grade surveyed, pre- and post-legalization of medical marijuana

State	Percent use pre-legalization and most recent data
California	11th grade: 25.9[1] to 24.2[2]
Alaska	12th grade: 30.9 to 22.2[3]
Oregon	11th grade: 21.0 to 20.9[4]
Washington	12th grade: 28.7[5] to 26.7[6]
Maine	12th grade: 33.1 to 27.3[7]
Hawaii	12th grade: 27.2 to 25.4[8]
Nevada	12th grade: 27.5 to 22.7[9]
Montana	12th grade: 29.1 to 27.2[10]
Vermont	12th grade: 37.2 to 31.5[11]
Rhode Island	12th grade: 34.3 to 34.0[12]
New Mexico	12th grade: 25.4 to 26.8[13]
Michigan	12th grade: 19.0 to 21.1[14]
Arizona	12th grade: 28.2 to 27.1[15]
New Jersey	12th grade: 31.0 to 33.4[16]
Washington, DC; Delaware; Connecticut; Massachusetts; Illinois; New Hampshire	N/A (no post-legalization data available yet)

[1] The 6th biennial California Student Survey (CSS) 1995-1996.
[2] The 13th biennial California Student Survey (CSS) 2009-2010, Table 2.14.
[3] Alaska YRBS, 1995 and 2011, respectively.
[4] 1998 Oregon Public Schools Drug Use Survey and the Oregon Healthy Teens 2013, Table 134.
[5] The 1998 Washington State Survey of Adolescent Health Behaviors, p. 35.
[6] Washington State Department of Health, "Healthy Youth Survey 2012, question 29.
[7] Maine YRBS, 1997 and 2011, respectively.
[8] Hawaii YRBS, 1999 and 2011, respectively.
[9] Nevada YRBS, 1999 and 2009, respectively.
[10] Montana YRBS, 2003 and 2011, respectively.
[11] Vermont YRBS, 2003 and 2011, respectively.
[12] Rhode Island YRBS, 2005 and 2011, respectively.
[13] New Mexico YRBS, 2007 and 2011, respectively.
[14] Michigan YRBS, 2007 and 2011, respectively.
[15] Arizona YRBS, 2009 and 2011, respectively.
[16] New Jersey YRBS, 2009 and 2011, respectively.

states with medical marijuana laws (MMLs). Use rates are variably higher or lower than the MTF and NSDUH data, but notably, youth use rates have not significantly increased or decreased in all states with MMLs for which data are available post-MML enactment. The one exception is Alaska, where there has been a significant decrease in youth use rates. A number of factors may affect youth use rates in the future, including perceived harm of marijuana use, locations and numbers of medical marijuana dispensaries in a given locale, and outright legalization of marijuana for nonmedical purposes.

SIDE EFFECTS OF MARIJUANA USE

The most consistent physical side effects are a mild increase in heart rate and systolic blood pressure. These effects tend to be dose related. Other possible side effects are conjunctival injection, dry mouth, orthostatic hypotension, increased appetite, increased thirst, drowsiness, insomnia, anxiety, short-term memory loss, hallucinations, and ataxia.[23,24] In a larger overdose, severe anxiety or a panic reaction can occur; treatment with a benzodiazepine may be helpful.[23] Ingestion of marijuana by children can result in a variety of symptoms, including drowsiness, ataxia, nystagmus, hypothermia, and hypotonia. Respiratory depression or coma, primarily in toddlers, has rarely been reported.[25] There is no specific antidote for an overdose of medical marijuana, and no fatalities have ever been reported solely as a result of a marijuana overdose. However, a number of cases of toddlers presenting to emergency rooms with toxic reactions, including lethargy, ataxia, and respiratory insufficiency after unintentional ingestion of marijuana, have been reported.[26]

EFFECT OF MARIJUANA USE ON ADOLESCENT BRAIN DEVELOPMENT

New research on adolescent brain development has found that brain maturation, particularly in the areas of the prefrontal cortex, continues into the mid-20s (see "Neurobiology of Adolescent Substance Use and Addictive Behaviors: Treatment Implications" in this issue). This maturation includes substantial changes in specialization and efficiency that occur through myelination and synaptic pruning. Synaptic pruning or refining consists of a reduction in gray matter primarily in the prefrontal and temporal cortex areas as well as in subcortical structures through the elimination of neural connections that are unnecessary.[27-31] Increased myelination also occurs, which allows for increased neural connectivity and efficiency and better integrity of white matter fiber tracts.[32,33] The prefrontal lobes are the last areas of the adolescent brain to undergo these neuromaturational changes, which when complete allow smoother communication between the higher-order regions areas of the brain and the lower-order sensorimotor areas; this allows for better "top-down" cognitive control.[34,35]

It has been postulated that the developing adolescent brain is particularly at risk for the development of substance use disorders, although a number of factors are involved, including genetic predisposition, epigenetic factors, environmental stressors, and untreated comorbid disorders. The younger the adolescent is when he or she initiates substance use, the more likely a substance use disorder, such as dependence or addiction, will occur.[36-40] Now, with newer techniques for studying both brain structure and function, emerging data suggest that use of marijuana may alter the developing brain, paralleling what has been found in studies on adolescent neurocognitive functioning. For example, studies have shown that adolescents who report regular marijuana use perform more poorly on tests of working memory, visual scanning, cognitive flexibility, and learning.[39] Furthermore, the number of episodes of lifetime marijuana use reported by subjects has been correlated with overall lower cognitive functioning,[41,42] although these findings are controversial.[43]

Recently, studies looking at brain structure have found effects of marijuana use on hippocampal, prefrontal cortex, and white matter volume. Specifically, heavy marijuana users have been found to have larger gray matter volume, particularly in the left hippocampal area, suggesting interference with the synaptic pruning that results in smaller volume.[44-46] Furthermore, heavy marijuana use that was correlated with increased gray matter volumes also was correlated with poorer verbal and attention performance.[47] In terms of brain functioning, functional magnetic resonance imaging studies looking at neural activity in abstinent marijuana users have found abnormalities in activation during cognitive tasks, which is postulated to be correlated with marijuana-related changes seen in cognition and attention such as deficits in spatial working memory, verbal encoding, and inhibition.[47]

Additionally, use of substances may alter the developing brain itself in ways that are not yet fully understood but are different than usual brain development; further studies using multimodal neuroimaging approaches are needed.[48] It is probable that there are critical periods during adolescence when there is heightened vulnerability to substances, and whether these changes can be reversed with abstinence or reduced use is not known.[48] A number of models have been proposed to explain the adolescent's heightened vulnerability to substance use disorders as occurs with marijuana, and emerging research should elucidate this more fully. However, the documented effects on cognition and the data that correlate them with detrimental effects on brain structure and function should serve as cautionary evidence to discourage any recreational marijuana use in adolescents.

MEDICAL AND RECREATIONAL MARIJUANA

As of December 2013, medical marijuana (cannabis) is legal for adults in 20 states and the District of Columbia (Table 2). Cannabis is illegal by federal law and is a schedule I drug under the federal Drug Enforcement Agency (no legitimate medical use). California was the first state to legalize medical marijuana in 1996. Efforts

Table 2

States with medical marijuana laws, by year

State	Year medical marijuana legalized
California	1996
Alaska	1998
Oregon	1998
Washington	1998
Maine	1999
Colorado	2000
Hawaii	2000
Nevada	2000
Montana	2004
Vermont	2004
Rhode Island	2006
New Mexico	2007
Michigan	2008
Arizona	2010
New Jersey	2010
Washington, DC	2010
Delaware	2011
Connecticut	2012
Massachusetts	2012
New Hampshire	2013
Illinois	2013

are underway in a number of nonmedical marijuana states to legalize the use of medical marijuana. Specifics of the MMLs vary state by state,[49] but all allow adults to use marijuana for medical purposes, usually for certain specified conditions, if recommended by a physician, although general categories also often include "pain." Minors are able to obtain medical marijuana with parents' written permission (and in some cases other restrictions) in most medical marijuana states.

As of December 2013, 2 states, Colorado and Washington, have legalized the recreational use of marijuana for adults ages 21 years and older. Although the specific rules and regulations on legalization are still being determined, they likely will be modeled after similar laws governing alcohol use, including driving under the influence.

MARIJUANA DELIVERY METHODS

Medical marijuana dispensaries provide marijuana in forms that can be either smoked through combustion or vaporization or ingested to produce the desired medical effects. Smoking marijuana results in rapid onset (minutes) of desired effects, whereas ingestion results in a more gradual and delayed onset (30 minutes to hours). Vaporization is considered less harmful because the marijuana is slowly heated to its vaporization point, releasing THC and water vapor, rather than burning the marijuana to its combustion point to release THC (as well as tar and other potentially harmful products in smoke). Most medical marijuana dispensaries sell vaporizers for their patients; vaporizers are also widely available for purchase online. The dose of THC is the same whether the marijuana is vaporized or burned.[50-52]

It should be noted that use of a water pipe to smoke marijuana does not eliminate any of the harmful products in the smoke.

MEDICAL MARIJUANA AND POTENTIAL EFFECT ON ADOLESCENT USE OF RECREATIONAL MARIJUANA

One concern of parents and pediatricians is whether the legalization of medical marijuana will result in increased use of recreational marijuana by adolescents. This concern is multipronged: that legitimizing marijuana as a medication may lead adolescents to believe that marijuana is a safe drug whether or not it is prescribed; that access to marijuana will be more widespread; and that marketing will be targeted to youths. As an example, the abuse of prescription drugs such as pain relievers, sedatives, tranquilizers, and stimulants for nonmedical purposes has increased among adolescents and young adults with the increased prescribing of these substances.[53] Table 1 shows specific state-level changes in teen marijuana use rates comparing pre- and post-legalization of medical marijuana for all states with these laws, using YRBS or equivalent data. When all high school grade data are combined for each medical marijuana state in which data are available pre- and post-medical marijuana legalization (13 states to date), no medical marijuana state has shown a statistically significant increase in adolescent recreational marijuana use. Only one state (Alaska) has shown a significant decrease in adolescent recreational marijuana use. One recent study found that states with MMLs on average reported higher rates of marijuana use in 12- to 17-year-olds over the time period from 2002 to 2008 compared with the average rate reported by the same age group in all of the states without such laws: 8.68% (85% confidence interval [CI], 7.95-9.42) versus 6.94% (95% CI 6.60-7.28).[54] These MML states also reported lower rates of perception of riskiness of marijuana than did non-MML states. However, this study was not able to determine the changes within each individual state with MMLs before the passage of the laws compared to after passage of the laws. In fact, in the 8 states that passed MMLs within the time period studied (since 2004), the baseline rate already was higher than in states without MMLs, but no data were provided comparing those individual states' differences pre- and post-passage of the MML.[54] To date, data have shown that state-specific legalization of medical marijuana has not led to an increase in recreational use of marijuana by adolescents. This relationship is complex, and further research and epidemiologic surveillance need to continue.

COMPARISONS BETWEEN MARIJUANA, ALCOHOL, AND TOBACCO

Those who support the legalization of marijuana argue that alcohol and tobacco use causes more harm to society, in terms of financial and health costs, than marijuana. Part of their argument is based on their belief that current restrictions and criminalization of the use, possession, and sale of marijuana are inconsistent with policies that permit the legal use of substances such as alcohol and tobacco. Few would argue that the use of tobacco and the underage or abusive use of alcohol are not harmful. However, opponents argue that marijuana is not a benign substance and that legalizing yet another psychoactive addictive substance has no merit. Proponents also claim that marijuana legalization would facilitate tighter control of its use through regulation, such as requiring a license for selling, restricting sale to those 21 years of age or older, and taxation, similar to that done for alcohol and tobacco.[55] However, often lax enforcement of such laws for alcohol and tobacco and the push of advertisers to market these products to adolescents, despite legal sanctions, both suggest that it will be difficult to enforce similar limits of legal sale and advertising of marijuana to youth.

The high rates of underage alcohol and tobacco use, despite state laws barring the sale of alcohol to those younger than 21 years and tobacco to those younger than 18 years, support this concern. In fact, recent data from NSDUH from 2011 have shown that the declines in use of illicit substances, tobacco, and alcohol seen throughout the 2000s not only have reached a plateau but have reversed from 2008 to 2010.[56] An additional concern is that over the past decade, adolescents' perception of the risks of heavy drinking, tobacco use, and marijuana use have declined, with significantly fewer youth now reporting that there is great risk associated with routine or heavy use of these substances. Researchers cite these changes in perception of risk as contributors to this reversal of rates among youth. Of note, these perceptions have changed despite the emergence of societal norms reducing the acceptance of tobacco use in public[57] and media coverage about excessive alcohol use and driving.[58,59]

SOCIAL JUSTICE

Ongoing criminal prosecution solely for marijuana possession has led to serious and often permanent legal problems for adolescents arrested for these acts. Since 1991, marijuana arrests have nearly doubled,[60,61] whereas levels of marijuana use have not increased to a similar extent.[19] Marijuana arrests disproportionately affect young males and particularly young blacks. In 2009, there were 858,408 arrests for marijuana, of which 755,399 were for possession (88% of the total). Of the marijuana possession arrests, 52% were in adolescents and young adults. Males aged 15 to 19 years accounted for 28% of all possession arrests, and those ages 20 to 24 years accounted for another 24%. Thus, approximately 392,807 adolescents and young adults were arrested for marijuana possession in 2009. With regard to race, although blacks account for 12% of the population and only 15% of current marijuana users, they also account for 31% of marijuana possession arrests.[60,61]

Currently the criminal penalties for marijuana possession and use by teens and young adults adversely affect almost 400,000 youth per year in the United

States. Imprisonment represents direct removal of individuals from needed roles in society: adults away from jobs, parents away from young children, and adolescents from school and their families. Furthermore, these individuals are placed in environments where they are likely to have close contact with individuals who have committed serious violent offenses or are career criminals.

Seventeen states currently offer legal alternatives to incarceration, and possible felony conviction, for marijuana possession.[62] Advocates of decriminalization cite the importance, particularly for youth, of ensuring that criminal offenses are limited to misdemeanors, petty offenses, or even noncriminal civil violations. These reduced violations do not carry the requirement for short-term prison time or probation, or the longer-term stigma of a felony drug conviction,[62] which may result in the individual's inability to obtain student loans or attend school, ineligibility for certain housing, and difficulties with future employment. For example, students applying to college may be denied federal financial aid because of a drug conviction, including marijuana possession (part of the Higher Education Act Aid Elimination Penalty passed by the US Congress in 1998). Penalties for marijuana possession of 1 ounce or less range widely from state to state; maximum penalties range from a fine of $100 to $5000 and 5 years in prison. Possession of more than 1 ounce of marijuana usually results in larger maximum fines and jail time.[63]

Detention facilities are ill equipped to deal with issues that may be related to an individual's substance abuse problem, and many adolescents will not receive any treatment.[64] Likewise, for many youth, treatment programs that deal with abuse and dependence are seldom available as an alternative to incarceration. The criminal justice system typically has punishment as a primary goal. Treatment and diversion programs for drug use are not a usual focus of the criminal justice system, although some jurisdictions require drug education or community service for minors convicted of drug possession. Juvenile drug courts have also been used for drug education and for treatment of minors convicted of drug possession,[65] as mentioned in "Assessment and Treatment of Substance Abuse in the Juvenile Justice Population" in this issue of AM:STARS.

The main argument against decriminalization is that it will lead to increased rates of marijuana use, and of illicit substances in general, and that this in turn will lead to increases in criminal activity in terms of selling and distribution. However, it also has been argued that adolescents are frequent buyers of small amounts of marijuana because of the fear of being caught with larger quantities and that this is a major impetus for local drug sellers, often other teens. For example, 15.9% of 12- to 17-year-olds bought marijuana from someone they had just met or did not know.[66] Opponents also argue that it sends the wrong message to young people when the penalties for use are reduced to minor infractions that may carry little incentive to change behaviors.

DRIVING UNDER THE INFLUENCE

The issue of driving while intoxicated may need specific treatment. Cannabis is the most prevalent illicit drug detected in fatally injured drivers and motor vehicle crash victims.[67] However, currently there are no accepted lower levels of blood concentration for THC or standards on serum thresholds indicating intoxication.[68] Furthermore, because THC is lipid soluble, a positive serum level is possible several weeks after abstinence in the chronic user.[68] Individual drivers can vary widely in their sensitivity to THC-induced impairment, as evinced by weak correlations between THC in serum and magnitude of performance impairment.[68] Plasma of drivers showing substantial impairment contained both high and low THC concentrations; and drivers with high plasma concentrations showed substantial, but also no, impairment, and some even showed some improvement.[69] Additionally, although blood alcohol content can be accurately measured and correlated with behavioral impairment, this may not be the case with cannabis, in part because alcohol is water soluble whereas cannabis is stored in the fat and is metabolized differently, making a direct correlation with behavior difficult to measure.[70] Because marijuana use may cause impaired driving, driving under the influence of marijuana should be actively discouraged.

ADOLESCENT USE OF MEDICAL MARIJUANA

There are anecdotal reports of the successful use of marijuana by adolescents for treatment of a variety of health conditions, ranging from attention-deficit/hyperactivity disorder to anxiety and depression to autism, anorexia, chronic pain, and post-chemotherapy nausea and vomiting. There are no data on the rates of adolescent use of medical marijuana obtained through licensed dispensaries. There also are no published studies on the use of marijuana in the pediatric or adolescent patient populations, with the exception of 1 study that evaluated the source of marijuana used by adolescents receiving care in a substance abuse treatment facility.[71] This study found that diverted medical marijuana had been used by 74% of the adolescents in the treatment facility.[71]

In 2008, the American College of Physicians (ACP) issued a position paper emphasizing the importance of sound scientific study to evaluate the role of marijuana in modern medical therapy.[72] The ACP paper stressed that marijuana was neither devoid of potentially harmful effects nor universally effective.

In 2010, the California Society for Addiction Medicine issued a statement on the medical aspects of marijuana legalization that addressed the following 7 points[73]:

1. The importance of developing effective regulations to minimize access to marijuana for anyone younger than 21 years.
2. Treatment for adolescent marijuana abusers, rather than punishment, should be made universally available.

3. Revenues from fees and taxes on marijuana sales should go specifically to treatment programs.
4. The need for warning labels placed on smokable products.
5. The need for strict regulation of marketing (advertising), distribution, and sales of marijuana.
6. The need for comprehensive evaluation components to document the effect of legalization.
7. Technical difficulties documenting driving under the influence should be further addressed and clarified. Three other concerns were expressed concerning medical marijuana: administering any medication via drawing hot smoke into the lungs is inherently unhealthy; although use of vaporizers, sprays, and tinctures solves problems inherent in smoking, treatment of illness without standardized dose or content of the medication remain a safety issue; and if the public wants to legalize marijuana, there is no reason to force physicians to be gatekeepers in a manner that enables liberal access to marijuana but generally fails to uphold accepted standards of practice for recommending a potentially addicting medication/drug.

Current research has demonstrated that cannabinoids may be helpful for adults with certain health care conditions as noted earlier. However, medical marijuana currently is problematic for the following reasons: it is not regulated by the FDA; neither its purity nor its THC or other cannabinoid content can be consistently verified; and the risk-benefit ratio is poorly described. Available data have shown that medical marijuana has not led to a significant increase in the use of recreational marijuana by adolescents. Pediatricians may legally recommend or prescribe medical marijuana in some states. Without any peer-reviewed studies on the use of medical marijuana in pediatric populations, recommendation of its use would be based only on limited scientific evidence in adult populations and anecdotal case reports.

PARENTAL GUIDANCE

Parents may turn to their child's and adolescent's physician for questions concerning the potential benefits and risks of marijuana use, whether for recreational or medical use, by their child or adolescent. Parents may request that the physician recommend medical marijuana for their child and adolescent for a myriad of issues, including anxiety, depression, attention-deficit/hyperactivity disorder, chronic pain, autism, and seizures, especially when the patient has not responded to the usual medical treatment. Many parents themselves have used or currently use marijuana for these purposes; the most recent data reveal that 100 million adults in the United States have ever used marijuana, and approximately 1 million adults have recommendations for the use of medical marijuana.[74] Parents often want guidance as well on how much information to share with their adolescent about their own past or current marijuana use.

A useful approach to counseling parents includes the following recommendation:

- Nonmedical use of marijuana is to be discouraged in children and adolescents, except in compassionate care or end-of-life care situations as deemed necessary, and on a case-by-case basis as deemed appropriate when standard treatments have failed. As noted earlier, marijuana may affect the developing brain in ways that are poorly understood, and serious side effects have occurred in adolescent users, including debilitating mental health disorders such as addiction, depression, and psychosis.
- Medical use of marijuana may have benefits for adults in helping treat certain diseases, as noted previously, but no studies on any use of medical marijuana in children or adolescents have been reported to date. Issues regarding dosing, effects, and side effects all are unknowns in the pediatric and adolescent populations. When usual medical treatments fail, it is understandable that parents will look for alternative therapies to try to help their child or adolescent, but no current data provide specific recommendations for the use of medical marijuana. This does not mean that certain cannabinoids may not have therapeutic benefit for a variety of diseases, only that no pediatric or adolescent data are available to help guide decision-making along these lines.
- Parents are role models for their children and adolescents, and actions usually speak louder than words. Use of nonmedical marijuana by parents may lead to a higher likelihood that their child or adolescent will use marijuana. Parents need to assess their own use, including intensity and frequency of use, to be sure there are no problems associated with use. For medical marijuana use, making sure the adolescent understands that use is for a specific purpose for a specific diagnosis and that all medications have risks and benefits associated with use.
- Generally it has been shown that sharing information about past drug use, including marijuana, in general terms with an adolescent will not promote use in the adolescent. For example, saying "I smoked marijuana when I was in college, and it was OK, but I found that I couldn't remember any of the conversation I had had the night before, so that seemed stupid" is preferable to "I smoked marijuana when I was in college, we used to party a lot, every weekend, it was a lot of fun, and I still do it when I'm on vacation" because the latter statement is more likely to be appealing to an adolescent to consider trying it. Parents should not feel that because they used marijuana as a teen or young adult themselves that it is not appropriate for them to advise their own adolescent against use.
- Any product that requires smoking to release the desired effects cannot be recommended by physicians because smoke contains tar and other harmful chemicals.

COUNSELING THE ADOLESCENT PATIENT

A number of useful counseling approaches for the adolescent include the following:

- Ask the adolescent how much and how often he or she uses marijuana. Also ask about the circumstances of use: is it social (ie, uses with others), or does he or she use it while alone? What does the adolescent think are the benefits of using marijuana? Can he or she think of any risks to using?
- Ask the adolescent, "Are you in control?" Does the adolescent have control over where and when he or she uses, or does the drug have control over the adolescent? If the adolescent is using regularly and does not think there is a problem, offer a little test to see if that is the case. Ask the adolescent to try not to use it under the usual circumstances for a brief period of time and see what happens. If the adolescent can't *not* use, that can be helpful in showing that he or she may have a problem. On the other hand, if the adolescent can stop use, then perhaps he or she can stop for a longer period of time. Discuss triggers and alternate methods of getting the same perceived benefits from marijuana use.
- For medical marijuana, state that marijuana does have certain specific indications in adults but that we do not know about use in adolescents. Also, a medication may be safe overall for a specific indication, but that does not mean that the medication is safe, period.
- All medications may have side effects, including possible serious ones.
- Never drive under the influence of marijuana or drive with someone who is under the influence of marijuana. Fatal car accidents are the number one cause of death in adolescents, and 80% of these accidents result because the driver is under the influence of alcohol or of alcohol and a drug such as marijuana.
- Marijuana can be addictive. Do you know that 1 in 10 adolescents who use marijuana are addicted to it?

INTERVENTION AND REFERRAL

The psychiatric diagnoses of cannabis abuse and cannabis dependence in the *DSM-IV-TR* have been changed to 1 diagnosis, cannabis use disorder, in the *DSM-5*.[75] *DSM-5* diagnostic criteria for a cannabis use disorder are as follows: "A problematic pattern of cannabis use leading to clinically significant impairment or distress, as manifested by 2 or more of the following within a 12-month period":

1. Cannabis is often taken in larger amounts or over a longer period than was intended
2. Persistent desire or unsuccessful efforts to cut down or control cannabis use
3. A great deal of time is spent in activities necessary to obtain cannabis, use cannabis, or recover from its effects
4. Craving, or a strong desire or urge to use cannabis
5. Recurrent cannabis use resulting in a failure to fulfill major role obligations at work, school, or home
6. Continued cannabis use despite having persistent or recurrent social or interpersonal problems caused or exacerbated by the effects of cannabis

7. Important social, occupational, or recreational activities are given up or reduced because of cannabis use
8. Recurrent cannabis use in situations in which it is physically hazardous
9. Continued cannabis use despite knowledge of having a persistent or recurrent physical or psychological problem that is likely to have been caused or exacerbated by cannabis
10. Tolerance
11. Withdrawal

The severity of a cannabis use disorder is based on the number of *DSM-5* symptoms present and is defined as mild (2-3 symptoms), moderate (4-5 symptoms), or severe (≥6 symptoms).

Diagnostic criteria for cannabis withdrawal in the *DSM-5* are as follows (note that cannabis withdrawal is not a life-threatening condition):

- Cessation of cannabis use that has been heavy and prolonged (ie, usually daily or almost daily over a period of at least a few months)
- Three or more of the following signs and symptoms develop within approximately 1 week after the cannabis cessation:
  - Irritability, anger, or aggression
  - Nervousness or anxiety
  - Sleep difficulty (eg, insomnia, disturbing dreams)
  - Decreased appetite or weight loss
  - Restlessness
  - Depressed mood
- At least one of the following physical symptoms causing significant discomfort: abdominal pain, shakiness/tremors, sweating, fever, chills, or headache
- The signs or symptoms cause clinically significant distress or impairment in social, occupational, or other important areas of functioning
- The signs or symptoms are not attributable to another medical condition and are not better explained by another mental disorder, including intoxication or withdrawal from another substance

Patients diagnosed with a cannabis use disorder or cannabis withdrawal should receive brief intervention or referral to a substance abuse specialist or program for further evaluation and treatment (see "Screening and Brief Intervention for Alcohol and Other Abuse" in this issue of AM:STARS).

SUMMARY

Marijuana use in pediatric populations remains an ongoing concern, and marijuana use by adolescents has known medical, psychological, and cognitive side effects. Marijuana alters brain development and has detrimental effects on brain structure and function in ways that are incompletely understood at this point in time. Furthermore, marijuana smoke contains tar and other harmful chemicals, so marijuana cannot be recommended by physicians. At this time, no studies suggest a benefit of marijuana use by children and adolescents. In the context of limited but clear evidence showing harm or potential harm from marijuana use by adolescents, any recommendations for medical marijuana use by adolescents are based on research studies with adults and on anecdotal evidence.

Criminal prosecution for marijuana possession adversely affects hundreds of thousands of youth yearly in the United States, particularly minority youth. Current evidence does not support a focus on punishment for youth who use marijuana. Rather, drug education and treatment programs should be encouraged to better help youth who are experimenting with or are dependent on marijuana. Decriminalization of recreational use of marijuana by adults has not led to an increase in youth use rates of recreational marijuana. Thus, decriminalization may be a reasonable alternative to outright criminalization, as long as it is coupled with drug education and treatment programs. The effect of outright legalization of adult recreational use of marijuana on youth use is unknown.

RESOURCES

National Institute on Drug Abuse: www.drugabuse.gov
Office of National Drug Control Policy: www.whitehouse.gov/ondcp
Marijuana Policy Project: www.mpp.org
Drug Policy Alliance: www.drugpolicy.org
Substance Abuse and Mental Health Services Administration: www.samhsa.gov

References

1. Holland J, ed. *The Pot Book: A Complete Guide to Cannabis: Its Role in Medicine, Politics, Science, and Culture.* Rochester, VT: Park Street Press; 2010
2. Aggarwal SK, Carter GT, Sullivan MD, et al. Medicinal use of cannabis in the United States: historical perspectives, current trends, and future directions. *J Opoid Manag.* 2009;5(3):153–168
3. Cotter J. Efficacy of crude marijuana and synthetic delta-9-tetrahydrocannabinol as treatment for chemotherapy-induced nausea and vomiting: a systematic literature review. *Oncol Nursing Forum.* 2009;36(3):345–352
4. Scotter EL, Abood ME, Glass M. The endocannabinoid system as a target for the treatment of neurodegenerative disease. *Br J Pharmacol.* 2010;160(3):480–498
5. Rahn EJ, Hohmann AG. Cannabinoids as pharmacotherapies for neuropathic pain: from the bench to the bedside. *Neurotherapeutics.* 2009;6(4):713–737
6. Lynch ME, Campbell F. Cannabinoids for treatment of chronic non-cancer pain: a systemic review of randomized trials. *Br J Clin Pharmacol.* 2011;72(5):735–744
7. Peat S. Using cannabinoids in pain and palliative care. *Int J Palliat Nurs.* 2010;16(10):481–485
8. Nevalainen T. Recent development of CB2 selective and peripheral CB1/CB2 cannabinoid receptor ligands. *Curr Med Chem.* 2014;21(2):187–203
9. Pertwee RG. Targeting the endocannabinoid system with cannabinoid receptor agonists: pharmacological strategies and therapeutic possibilities. *Philos Trans R Soc Lond B Biol Sci.* 2012;367(1607): 3353–363

10. Gloss D, Vickrey B. Cannabinoids for epilepsy. *Cochrane Database Syst Rev.* 2012;6:CD009270
11. Jones NA, Glyn SE, Akiyama S, et al. Cannabidiol exerts anti-convulsant effects in animal models of temporal lobe and partial seizures. *Seizure.* 2012;21(5):344–552
12. Jones NA, Hill AJ, Smith I, et al. Cannabidiol displays antiepileptiform and antiseizure properties in vitro and in vivo. *J Pharmacol Exp Ther.* 2010;332(2):569–577
13. Penner E, Buettner H, Mittleman MA. The impact of marijuana use on glucose, insulin, and insulin resistance among US adults. *Am J Med.* 2013;126(7):583–589
14. Navari RM. Antiemetic control: toward a new standard of care for emetogenic chemotherapy. *Expert Opin Pharmacother.* 2009;10(4):629–644
15. Pooyania S, Ethans K, Szturm T, et al. A randomized, double-blinded, crossover pilot study assessing the effect of nabilone on spasticity in persons with spinal cord injury. *Arch Phys Med Rehabil.* 2010;91(5):703–77
16. Sastre-Garriga J, Vila C, Clissol S, et al. THC and CBD oromucosal spray (Sativex) in the management of spasticity associated with multiple sclerosis. *Expert Rev Neurother.* 2011;11(5):627–637
17. Wang T, Collet JP, Shapiro S, et al. Adverse effects of medical cannabinoids: a systematic review. *CMAJ.* 2008;178:1669–1678
18. Monitoring The Future. 2010 Data Tables, Table 3. National Institute on Drug Abuse & The Institute for Social Research, University of Michigan. Available at: www.monitoringthefuture.org/data/10data/pr10t3.pdf. Accessed November 30, 2013
19. Centers for Disease Control and Prevention. Youth risk behavior surveillance system. 2012. Available at: www.cdc.gov/HealthyYouth/yrbs. Accessed November 30, 2013
20. National Survey on Drug Use and Health. Substance abuse and mental health services administration, Research Triangle Institute. Available at: nsduhweb.rti.org. Accessed November 30, 2013
21. The Partnership Attitude Tracking Study, MetLife Foundation & The Partnership at Drugfree.org, 2011. Parents and teens full report, released May 2, 2012. Available at: www.metlife.com/assets/cao/foundation/PATSFULL-ReportFINAL-May.pdf. Accessed November 30, 2013
22. US Department of Health and Human Services, Substance Abuse and Mental Health Services Administration, Center for Behavioral Health Statistics and Quality. Results of the 2010 national survey of drug use and health: Summary of national findings. Available at: oas.samhsa.gov/NSDUH/2k10NSDUH/2k10Results.htm#1.1. Accessed November 30, 2013
23. Borgelt LM, Franson KL, Nussbaum AM, Wang GS. The pharmacologic and clinical effects of medical cannabis. *Pharmacotherapy.* 2013;33(2):195–209
24. Wang T, Collet JP, Shapiro S, et al. Adverse effects of medical cannabinoids: a systematic review. *CMAJ.* 2008;178:1669–78
25. Appelboam A, Oades PJ. Coma due to Cannabis toxicity in an infant. *Eur J Emerg Med.* 2006;13(3):177–179
26. Wang GS, Roosevelt G, Heard K. Pediatric marijuana exposures in a medical marijuana state. *JAMA Pediatr.* 2013;167(7):630–633
27. Yakovlev PI, Lecours AR. The myelogenetic cycles of regional maturation of the brain. In: Minkowski A, ed. *Regional Development of the Brain in Early Life.* Boston, MA: Blackwell Scientific; 1967:3–70
28. Sowell ER, Thompson PM, Welcome SE, Kan E, Toga AW. Longitudinal mapping of cortical thickness and brain growth in normal children. *J Neurosci.* 2004;24(38):8223–8231
29. Giedd JN. Structural magnetic resonance imaging of the adolescent brain. *Ann N Y Acad Sci.* 2004;1021:77–85
30. Sowell ER, Thompson PM, Holmes CJ, Jernigan TL, Toga AW. In vivo evidence for post-adolescent brain maturation in frontal and striatal regions. *Nat Neurosci.* 1999;2(10):859–861
31. Hüppi PS, Dubois J. Diffusion tensor imaging of brain development. *Semin Fetal Neonatal Med.* 2006;11:489–497
32. Gogtay N, Giedd JN, Lusk L, et al. Dynamic mapping of human cortical development during childhood through early adulthood. *Proc Natl Acad Sci U S A.* 2004;101:8174–8179
33. Luna B, Sweeney JA. The emergence of collaborative brain function: fMRI studies of the development of response inhibition. *Ann N Y Acad Sci.* 2004;1021:296–309
34. Schepis TS, Adinoff B, Rao U. Neurobiological processes in adolescent addictive disorders. *Am J Addict.* 2008;17(1):6–23

35. Casey BJ, Getz S, Galvan A. The adolescent brain. *Dev Rev.* 2008;28(1):62–77
36. Winters KC, Lee C-Y. Likelihood of developing an alcohol and cannabis use disorder during youth: association with recent use and age. *Drug Alcohol Depend.* 2008; 92:239–247
37. Casey BJ, Jones RM. Neurobiology of the adolescent brain and behavior: implications for substance use disorders. *J Am Acad Child Adolesc Psychiatry.* 2010;49(12):1189–201; quiz 1285
38. Perkonigg A, Goodwin RD, Fiedler A, et al. The natural course of cannabis use, abuse, and dependence during the first decades of life. *Addiction.* 2008;103(3):439–449
39. Von Sydow K, Lieb R, Pfister H, et al. The natural course of cannabis use, abuse, and dependence over four years: a longitudinal community study of adolescents and young adults. *Drug Alcohol Depend.* 2001;64(3):347–361
40. Medina KL, Hanson K, Schweinsburg AD, et al. Neuopsychological functioning in adolescent marijuana users: subtle deficits detectable after 30 days of abstinence. *J Int Neuropsychol Soc.* 2007;13(5):207–220
41. Gonzalez R, Swanson JM. Long-term effects of adolescent-onset and persistent use of cannabis. *Proc Natl Acad Sci U S A.* 2012;109(40):15970–15971
42. Meier MH, Caspi A, Ambler A, et al. Persistent cannabis users show neuropsychological decline from childhood to midlife. *Proc Natl Acad Sci U S A.* 2012;109(40):E2657–E2664
43. Rogeberg O. Correlations between cannabis use and IQ change in the Dunedin cohort are consistent with confounding from socioeconomic status. *Proc Natl Acad Sci U S A.* 2013;110(11):42514242
44. Medina KL, Schweinsburg AD, Cohen-Zion M, Nagel BJ, Tapert SF. Effects of alcohol and combined marijuana and alcohol use during adolescence on hippocampal volume and asymmetry. *Neurotoxicol Teratol.* 2007;29:141–152
45. Nagel BJ, Schweinsburg AD, Phan V, Tapert SF. Reduced hippocampal volume among adolescents with alcohol use disorders without psychiatric comorbidity. *Psychiatry Res.* 2005;139:181–190
46. Medina KL, McQueeny T, Nagel BJ, Hanson KL, Schweinsburg AD, Tapert SF. Prefrontal cortex volumes in adolescents with alcohol use disorders: unique gender effects. *Alcohol Clin Exp Res.* 2008;32(3):386–394
47. Schweinsburg AD, Nagel BJ, Schweinsburg BC, et al. Abstinent adolescent marijuana users show altered fMRI response during spatial working memory. *Psychiatry Res.* 2008;163:40–51
48. Squeglia LM, Jacobus J, Tapert SF. The influence of substance use on adolescent brain development. *Clin EEG Neurosci.* 2009;40(1):31–38
49. ProCon.org. 20 Legal Medical Marijuana States and D.C. Laws, Fees, and Possession Limits. Summary. Available at: medicalmarijuana.procon.org/view.resource.php?resourceID=000881. Accessed November 30, 2013
50. Hazekamp A, Ruhaak R, van Gerven J, et al. Evaluation of a vaporizing device (Volcano) for the pulmonary administration of tetrahydrocannabinol. *J Pharm Sci.* 2006;95:1308–1317
51. Abrams VI, Vizoszo HP, Shade SB, et al. Vaporization as a smokeless cannabis delivery system: a pilot study. *Clin Pharmacol Ther.* 2007;82(5):572–578
52. Fischedick J, Van Der Kooy F, Verpoorte R. Cannabinoid receptor 1 binding activity and quantitative analysis of Cannabis sativa L smoke and vapor. *Chem Pharm Bull.* 2010;58(2):201–207
53. Substance Abuse and Mental Health Services Administration. Results from the 2010 National Survey on Drug Use and Health: Summary of National Findings. NSDUH Series H-41, HHS Publication No. (SMA) 11-4658. Rockville, MD: Substance Abuse and Mental Health Services Administration; 2011
54. Wall MM, Poh E, Cerdá M, Keyes KM, Galea S, Hasin DS. Adolescent marijuana use from 2002 to 2008: higher in states with medical marijuana laws, cause still unclear. *Ann Epidemiol.* 2011;21(9):714–716
55. Marijuana Policy Project. Marijuana: decriminalization vs. tax & regulate. Available at: www.mpp.org/legislation/approaches.html. Accessed November 30, 2013
56. US Department of Health and Human Services, Substance Abuse and Mental Health Services Administration, Center for Behavioral Health Statistics and Quality. Results of the 2011 national survey of drug use and health: Summary of national nindings. Available at: www.samhsa.gov/data/nsduh/2k11results/nsduhresults2011.htm. Accessed November 30, 2013
57. Levy DT, Boyle RG, Abrams DB. The role of public policies in reducing smoking: the Minnesota SimSmoke tobacco policy model. *Am J Prev Med.* 2012;43(5 Suppl 3):S179–S186

58. Clapp JD, Johnson M, Voas RB, Lange JE, Shillington A, Russell C. Reducing DUI among US college students: results of an environmental prevention trial. *Addiction.* 2005;100(3):327–334

59. Perkins HW, Linkenbach JW, Lewis MA, Neighbors C. Effectiveness of social norms media marketing in reducing drinking and driving: a statewide campaign. *Addict Behav.* 2010;35(10):866–874

60. Drugscience.org. Marijuana, science, and public policy. Marijuana arrests in the United States, (2007). A special report in the November, 2009 edition of the Bulletin of Cannabis reform. Available at: www.drugscience.org. Accessed November 30, 2013

61. US Census Bureau. Annual county resident population estimates by age, sex, race, and Hispanic origin. 2010. Available at: 2010.census.gov/2010census/data/index.php. Accessed November 30, 2013

62. National Organization for the Reform of Marijuana Laws. States That Have Decriminalized Marijuana Laws. Available at: norml.org/aboutmarijuana/item/states-that-have-decriminalized. Accessed November 30, 2013

63. Get Smart About Drugs: A Drug Enforcement Agency Resource for Parents. What are the penalties for possession of marijuana. Available at: mobile.getsmartaboutdrugs.com/identify/what_are_the_penalties_for_possession_or_marijuana.html Accessed November 30, 2013

64. The National Survey on Drug Use and Health. The NSDUH Report. Published February 27, 2004. Available at: www.samhsa.gov/data/2k4/DetainedYouth/detainedYouth.pdf. Accessed November 30, 2013

65. US Department of Justice, Office of Justice Programs, Bureau of Justice Assistance. Juvenile drug courts: strategies in practice monograph. March 2003. Available at: www.ncjrs.gov/pdffiles1/bja/197866.pdf. Accessed November 30, 2013

66. The National Survey on Drug Use and Health. The NSDUH Report. Published March 12, 2004. Available at: www.samhsa.gov/data/2k4/MJsource/MJsource.pdf. Accessed November 30, 2013

67. US Department of Transportation, National Highway Traffic Safety Administration. State of knowledge of drugged driving: final report. September 2003. Available at: www.nhtsa.gov/people/injury/research/stateofknwlegedrugs/stateofknwlegedrugs/. Accessed November 30, 2013

68. Ramaekers JG, Berghaus G. Dose related risk of motor vehicle crashes after cannabis use: an update. In: Verster JC, Pandi-Perumal SR, Ramaekers JG, de Gier JJ, eds. *Drugs, Driving, and Traffic Safety.* Geneva, Switzerland, World Health Organization, 2009:477–499

69. US Department of Transportation, National Highway Traffic Safety Administration. Marijuana and actual driving performance: final report. 1993. Available at: ntl.bts.gov/lib/25000/25800/25867/DOT-HS-808-078.pdf. November 1993. Accessed November 30, 2013

70. Elliott M, Smith A, La Cava C.Marijuana DUI Workgroup: recommendation to the Drug Policy Task Force and Colorado Commission on Criminal and Juvenile Justice. September 1, 2011. Available at: norml.org/pdf_files/MMIG_Workgroup_Recommendation_9-6-11.pdf. Accessed November 30, 2013

71. Salomensen-Sautel S, Sakai JT, Thurstone C, et al. Medical marijuana use in adolescents in substance abuse treatment. *J Am Acad Child Adolesc Psychiatry.* 2012;51(7):694–702

72. American College of Physicians. Supporting research into the therapeutic role of marijuana. Philadelphia: American College of Physicians; 2008: Position Paper. (Available from American College of Physicians, 190 N. Independence Mall West, Philadelphia, PA 19106). Available at: www.acponline.org/acp_policy/policies/supporting_medmarijuana_2008.pdf Accessed November 30, 2013

73. California Society of Addiction Medicine (CSAM). CSAM statement on the medical aspects of marijuana legalization. Adopted by the CSAM Executive Council April 2010 Available at: www.csam-asam.org/sites/default/files/pdf/misc/Legalization.pdf. April 2010. Accessed November 30, 2013

74. Procon.org. Medical marijuana. how many people in the United States use medical marijuana? Available at: medicalmarijuana.procon.org/view.answers.php?questionID=001199. Accessed November 30, 2013

75. American Psychiatric Association. *Diagnostic and Statistical Manual of Mental Disorders,* Fifth Edition. Arlington, VA: American Psychiatric Association; 2013

Adolesc Med 025 (2014) 89–103

Nonmedical Use of Prescription Stimulants by Adolescents

Alain Joffe, MD, MPH*

*Director, Student Health and Wellness Center, Johns Hopkins University,
Associate Professor of Pediatrics, Johns Hopkins University School of Medicine, Baltimore, Maryland*

INTRODUCTION

Prescribed and used correctly, stimulant medications such as methylphenidate and various forms of amphetamines can be an important component of treatment of attention-deficit/hyperactivity disorder (ADHD). Over the past decade, concern has arisen about adolescents' use of these medications without a doctor's prescription. A 2012 article in the *New York Times* characterized these drugs as the "good-grade pill" and suggested that their use by adolescents who did not have a doctor's prescription was widespread, especially at academically competitive high schools.[1]

PREVALENCE

Use of amphetamines by adolescents is not a new phenomenon. According to the Monitoring the Future (MTF) survey, an annual in-school survey of a nationally representative sample of approximately 50,000 8th-, 10th-, and 12th-graders, adolescents reported use of amphetamines for many decades. In 1991, for example, 6% of 8th-graders and 8% of 10th- and 12th-graders each reported past-year use of amphetamines (www.monitoringthefuture.org//pubs/monographs/mtf-vol1_2012.pdf, accessed November 23, 2013). However, as prescriptions for ADHD medications have increased (a 6.5% annual increase among adolescents from 1996 to 2008[2] and a 26% rise in prescriptions written for 10- to 19-year-olds since 2007 alone[1]), greater attention has focused specifically on ADHD medications and their nonmedical use by adolescents. As a marker of the potential problems with nonmedical use, data from the Drug Abuse Warning Network indicate that visits in 2010 by 12- to 17-year-olds to the emergency department, secondary to medical misuse of stimulants, greatly outnumbered visits for medication side effects (1830

---

*Corresponding author:
ajoffe@jhu.edu

vs. 685 visits).[3] Also, from 1998 to 2005, calls related to adolescent (age 13-19 years) prescription ADHD abuse rose 76%, which was greater than calls related to adolescent substance abuse in general.[4]

Defining the extent of the problem of nonmedical use of stimulant medications is challenging. First, there is a certain degree of imprecision in the term *nonmedical use*.[5] The MTF survey defines nonmedical use as the use of a specified medication not under a doctor's orders ("On how many occasions [if any] have you ever used [NAME OR CLASS OF DRUG] on your own—that is without a doctor telling you to take them"). In the National Survey on Drug Use and Health (NSDUH; www. samhsa.gov/data/NSDUH.aspx, accessed November 23, 2013), an in-home survey of a representative sample of the noninstitutionalized population of the United States, nonmedical use of a prescription drug is defined as "use without a prescription of the individual's own or simply for the experience or feeling the drugs caused" ("Have you ever, even once, used [NAME OF DRUG], that was not prescribed for you or that you took only for the experience or feeling it caused?"). Under this definition, nonmedical use includes both individuals who use a prescription medication not prescribed for them as well as individuals who use their own prescription medication for purposes other than that for which the medication was prescribed (eg, getting high). Some investigators draw a distinction between the 2, separating individuals who use prescription medications without having prescriptions for those medications (nonmedical use) from those who misuse their own prescription medications (too much, too little, or for a purpose other than for which it was prescribed). Still others refer to excessive use of prescription medications. Hence, when comparing statistics across surveys, it is important to understand how the investigators are defining the pattern of use they are studying. For example, a student who takes extra doses of a prescribed stimulant to get high would answer yes to the NSDUH question but might say no to the parallel item in the MTF.

Another limitation is that some surveys group together prescribed stimulants with methamphetamine. Furthermore, stimulant medications include so-called diet-pills, which are more likely to be used by girls; hence, gender differences may be masked or exaggerated, depending on whether the dataset or the investigators distinguish between or group together nonmedical use of prescription medications typically used to treat ADHD and diet pills.

Because the MTF survey is administered in school, students who are absent on the day of the survey or who have dropped out of school are excluded. Students who are chronically absent and youth who are out of school may have higher rates of misuse. In contrast, the NSDUH surveys are administered at home, and despite attempts to reassure adolescents that their answers will be kept confidential from parents, respondents still may underreport their misuse of the drug in question.

Table 1 summarizes nonmedical use rates of stimulants according to the MTF. Before 2001, the MTF grouped together a wide variety of stimulant medications

Table 1
Nonmedical use of prescription stimulants by adolescents based on Monitoring the Future data

	Past-year use (%)										
	1992	1998	2001	2004	2006	2007	2008	2009	2010	2011	2012
Amphetamines											
8th grade	6.2	7.2	6.7	4.9	4.7	4.2	4.5	4.1	3.9	3.5	2.9
10th grade	8.2	10.7	11.7	8.5	7.9	8.0	6.4	7.1	7.6	6.6	6.5
12th grade	8.2	10.1	10.9	10.0	8.1	7.5	6.8	6.6	7.4	8.2	7.9
Ritalin											
8th grade			2.9*	2.5	2.6	2.1	1.6	1.8	1.5	1.3	0.7
10th grade			4.8	3.4	3.6	2.8	2.9	3.6	2.7	2.6	1.9
12th grade			5.1	5.1	4.4	3.8	3.4	2.1	2.7	2.6	2.6
Adderall											
8th grade								2.0†	2.3	1.7	1.7
10th grade								5.7	5.3	4.6	4.5
12th grade								5.4	6.5	6.5	7.6

*Ritalin use was first surveyed in 2001.
†Adderall use was first surveyed in 2009.
Data from Johnston LD, O'Malley PM, Bachman JG, Schulenberg JE. Monitoring the Future: National Survey Results on Drug Use 1975–2012. Secondary School Students. Ann Arbor, MI: Institute for Social Research, The University of Michigan; 2012

under a single heading. In 2001, in response to increasing concerns about misuse of ADHD medications in particular, the principal investigators for the MTF survey added a question specifically about misuse of Ritalin (methylphenidate). In 2009, they added an additional question about Adderall.

A number of authors have reported on the extent of misuse of prescription stimulants by adolescents using NSDUH data. Kroutil et al[6] provided adolescent data from the 2002 NSDUH. In that study, 2.6% of 12- to 17-year-olds reported nonmedical use of any stimulant in the past year, but only 0.9% reported past-year use of ADHD stimulants only. Wu et al[7] reported that in 2003, 5.4% of 16- to 17-year-old males and 5.5% of 16- to 17-year-old females had used prescription stimulants (thereby excluding methamphetamine) in their lifetime. Comparable figures for past-year misuse were 2.5 and 3.1%, respectively. Gender differences are notable in that study: 78% of males who reported lifetime use of a stimulant used methylphenidate, and almost 14% used diet pills or amphetamines. For females, 58.4% used methylphenidate and almost 38% reported lifetime use of diet pills or other amphetamines.

The study by Kroutil et al[6] also showed that stimulant misuse was as common, if not more common, among youth living in nonmetropolitan areas compared to youth living in urban or suburban areas. Levine and Coupey[8] and Havens et al[9] also noted significant risk among rural youth. In the study by Levine and Coupey, 34% of the 849 rural Vermont high school students surveyed reported lifetime nonmedical use of prescription medications, and 20% reported current use. Ritalin was the fourth most popular drug used, following Tylenol with codeine, Valium, and Percocet. The study by Havens et al used data on almost 18,000 adolescents from the 2008 NSDUH. Rural adolescents were 26% more likely than urban adolescents to use prescription drugs nonmedically, even after controlling for race, health, and other drug and alcohol use. However, that difference seemed to be driven by greater nonmedical use of prescription pain relievers. Only 2.6% of rural youth used prescription stimulants compared to 3% of suburban and 2.3% of urban youth. The most recent data from the 2011 and 2012 NSDUH surveys are listed in Table 2.

The Partnership at Drugfree.org also tracks prescription stimulant misuse by adolescents. In their most recent (2012) survey of almost 3900 adolescents (www.drugfree.org/wp-content/uploads/2013/04/PATS-2012-KEY-FINDINGS. pdf, accessed November 12, 2013), the Partnership reports that 9% of teenagers (up from 6% in 2008) had misused Adderall or Ritalin in the past year, and of these teenagers, 6% (up from 4% in 2008) did so in the past month.

Wilens et al[10] performed a systematic review of stimulant misuse and diversion among adolescents. Based on 21 studies, they found that 5% to 9% of youths of grade school and high school age had misused stimulants of any kind in the past year. Poulin[11] studied nonmedical use of prescription stimulants (amphetamine

Table 2

Lifetime, past-year, and past-month nonmedical use of prescription stimulants (% using) based on National Survey on Drug Use and Health 2011-2012 data

Age (y)/drug	Lifetime		Past year		Past month	
	2011	2012	2011	2012	2011	2012
12-13						
Stimulants	0.9	0.4	0.5	0.2	0.2	0.1
Methamphetamines	0.4	0.1	0.2	0.1	0.0	0.0
14-15						
Stimulants	1.7	1.7	1.2	1.2	0.4	0.4
Methamphetamines	0.5	0.5	0.4	0.3	0.2	0.2
16-17						
Stimulants	3.4	3.7	1.9	2.4	0.6	0.9
Methamphetamines	1.2	1.0	0.7	0.6	0.2	0.2

Data from Substance Abuse and Mental Health Services Administration. Results from the 2012 National Survey on Drug Use and Health: Summary of National Findings and Detailed Tables. Available at: www.samhsa.gov/data/NSDUH/2012SummNatFindDetTables/Index.aspx. Accessed March 13, 2014

and methylphenidate) among 12,000 students (mean age 12.6 years) in the Atlantic provinces of Canada from 2002 to 2003. She found that 6.2% of students reported nonmedical use of those 2 stimulants in the 6 months before the survey.

Finally, McCabe et al performed 2 web-based surveys of a racially diverse sample of Detroit-area public school children in 2005 (1086 students, grades 7-12)[12] and in 2009 to 2010 (2744 students, mean age 14.8 years)[13] to assess medical and nonmedical use of prescription drugs. In the 2005 survey, 1.2% of students were classified as nonmedical users of stimulant medications, and another 1.2% of students were classified as both medical and nonmedical users.[12] Of the 2597 out of 2744 students in the 2009 to 2010 study who completed all survey items, 91 (3.5%) reported receiving a prescription for stimulant medications from a physician. Of these, 20 (22%) reported some misuse, 20 reported taking too much, and 10 reported using their medication to get high or to increase the effects of alcohol or other drugs.[13]

CHARACTERISTICS OF ADOLESCENTS WHO MISUSE PRESCRIPTION STIMULANTS

Most adolescents, including those with a prescription for stimulant medication, do not misuse prescription stimulants. What distinguishes those who do not from those who do? A number of studies have addressed this question. In a 2004 study of more than 1500 midwestern schoolchildren in grades 6 to 12, McCabe et al[14] divided study participants into 4 groups: those who did not use stimulants, those who did so only with a doctor's prescription, those who had a prescription for stimulants but also used stimulants not in accordance with a physician's recommendations, and those who only used stimulants illicitly (no prescription).

Compared to the first 2 groups, the latter 2 had significantly higher rates of tobacco, alcohol (including binge drinking), marijuana, and ecstasy use. Students in the latter 2 groups also were more likely to ride with someone who had consumed any alcohol and consumed 5 or more drinks in the two weeks prior to the survey. In fact, the substance abuse and risk behavior profiles of the latter 2 groups were quite similar.

Additional analyses of data from the 1086 7th- to 12th-grade students surveyed in 2005 found that, compared to nonusers of stimulants, those with a prescription for stimulant use (but no nonmedical use) were 6 times more likely to score positive on the Drug Abuse Screening Test (DAST) and 3.5 times more likely to report past-year use of illicit drugs other than marijuana; they were not more likely to report past-year marijuana use. However, medical/nonmedical users and nonmedical-only users were 31 and 44 times more likely to score positive on the DAST, 52 and 12 times more likely to use marijuana in the past year, and 36 and 22 times more likely to report past-year use of illicit drugs other than marijuana than the nonuser group.[12] Whereas those who had a prescription for stimulants (presumably to treat ADHD) had an increased risk for substance abuse, clearly those who misused stimulants had a much greater risk.

Data from this same study also detail why adolescents use stimulants nonmedically.[15] Students cited the following reasons for using these medications nonmedically. The drugs (1) help them with concentration, alertness, and ability to study; (2) help them to lose weight; (3) give them a high; (4) counteract the effects of other drugs; and (5) are safer than other drugs. The students also use the drugs (6) for experimentation and (7) because they are addicted to them.

Schepis and Krishnan-Sarin[16] used data from the 2005 NSDUH to examine differences between adolescents who reported misuse of stimulant medications from those who did not. Black and Asian youth were approximately 70% less likely than white youth to misuse stimulants, and Hispanic youth were about 15% less likely to do so. Factors that increased the odds of reporting past-year stimulant misuse were being female, being 15 years or older, having grades of D or worse, reporting a past-year major depressive disorder or mental health treatment, and having a history of juvenile justice involvement and past-year alcohol, tobacco, or other drug use. Adolescents who reported greater pleasure in taking risks were almost 5 times as likely to misuse prescription stimulants as those who reported lower levels of risk-taking. Adolescents who reported purchasing their stimulants had the worst risk profile; they were at greater risk for daily cigarette smoking, monthly marijuana use, and past-year use of cocaine.

Using data from the 2002 NSDUH, Herman-Stahl et al[17] found that high levels of sensation-seeking behavior, past mental health treatment, and past-year marijuana and other illegal drug use all increased the risk for past-year nonmedical use of prescription stimulants. However, being female, being black, or past-month binge drinking neither increased risk nor was protective. Youth reporting high conflict with parents were almost 1.6 times as likely to misuse prescription stimulants compared to those with lower levels of conflict.

A report from the 2005 and 2006 NSDUH surveys combined also demonstrated distinct drug use and risk behavior profiles between youth aged 12 to 17 years who used stimulants nonmedically and those who did not.[18] Those who reported non-medical use of stimulant medications were much more likely to use a wide variety of other illicit drugs and to engage in a variety of risky behaviors such as stealing, fighting, selling drugs, and carrying a handgun than were those who did not report such use (Figures 1 and 2). Furthermore, 22.8% of youth who endorsed past-year nonmedical use of stimulants reported an episode of major depression compared to just 8.1% of those who did not use stimulants nonmedically.

In her study, Poulin[11] examined characteristics of nonmedical users of prescription stimulants (methylphenidate and amphetamine) in the Atlantic provinces of Canada. Almost 13,000 students participated in the survey, which included a standardized screening test for ADHD (6-item Ontario Child Health Study Hyperactivity Scale) and 1 for depression (short version of the Center for Epidemiological Studies-Depression Scale [CES-D]). Students were also asked whether they had received a prescription for stimulant medications, whether they had ever used stimulants nonmedically, and whether they had ever diverted their medications. In a logistic regression model, students who reported nonmedical use of methylphenidate were more likely to be male and to report heavy

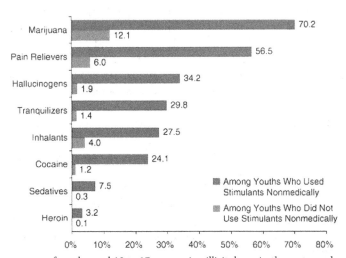

Fig 1. Percentages of youths aged 12 to 17 years using illicit drugs in the past year by past-year nonmedical stimulant use from 2005 to 2006. (From Substance Abuse and Mental Health Services Administration, Office of Applied Studies. The NSDUH Report, February 28, 2008. Nonmedical stimulant use, other drug use, delinquent behaviors, and depression among adolescents. Available at: www.oas.samhsa.gov/2k8/stimulants/depression.pdf. Accessed December 13, 2013.)

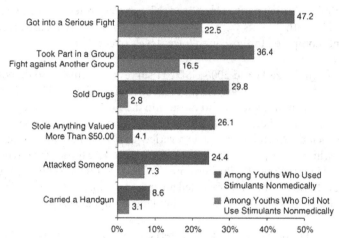

Fig 2. Percentages of youths aged 12 to 17 engaging in delinquent behaviors in the past year, by past year nonmedical stimulant use: 2005 and 2006. Youths aged 12 to 17 were asked how many times in the past 12 months they had participated in each delinquent behavior. The response options were (a) 0 times, (b) 1 or 2 times, (c) 3 to 5 times, (d) 6 to 9 times, and (e) 10 or more times. For this report, youths were counted as engaging in the behavior if they reported participating one or more times. Youths with unknown or missing data of delinquent behavior were excluded from this analysis. (From Substance Abuse and Mental Health Services Administration, Office of Applied Studies. The NSDUH Report, February 28, 2008. Nonmedical stimulant use, other drug use, delinquent behaviors, and depression among adolescents. Available at: www.oas. samhsa.gov/2k8/stimulants/depression.pdf. Accessed December 13, 2013.)

alcohol use, cigarette smoking, and cannabis use. Of particular note is that nonmedical use was also associated with depressive symptoms (adjusted odds ratio [AOR] 1.49 for a somewhat elevated CES-D score and AOR 1.56 for a very elevated score) and a positive ADHD screening test score (AOR 2.59 compared to students who screened negative). Nonmedical use also was associated with being in a classroom where 1 or more students diverted their medication.

In a parallel model for nonmedical use of amphetamines, the relationship with alcohol and cannabis use as well as cigarette smoking was confirmed. Similarly, the links between nonmedical amphetamine use and depressive symptoms (AOR 1.56 for somewhat elevated and 2.03 for very elevated CES-D scores) as well as a positive ADHD screen (AOR 2.0) were noted. Although cross-sectional in nature, taken together the NSDUH study and the study by Poulin suggest that adolescents who use prescription stimulants nonmedically may, in part, be self-medicating their undiagnosed depression and ADHD with stimulants as well as other drugs.

Using data from the 2003 NSDUH, Simoni-Wastila et al[19] found that having moved in the past year significantly increased the risk for past-year nonmedical prescription stimulant misuse. Their analyses also confirmed that, compared to youth of "other race/ethnicity," whites (AOR 5.36) had higher rates of misuse, followed by Hispanics (AOR 3.89) and blacks (AOR 2.42).

Attitudes about illicit drugs are related to levels of use among adolescents. For example, data from the MTF surveys show that as adolescents perceive less risk in using a drug, they are more likely to use it. Whether a similar relationship exists with nonmedical use of prescription drugs, including stimulants, is unknown. However, it is worth noting that in the 2012 Partnership Attitude Tracking Study (PATS):

- 33% of adolescents indicated "it's okay to use prescription drugs that were not prescribed to them to deal with an injury, illness or physical pain";
- 23% said "their parents don't care as much if they are caught using Rx drugs without a doctor's prescription, compared to getting caught with illegal drugs";
- 27% believed "that misusing and abusing prescription drugs is safer than using street drugs" and
- 26% believed "that prescription drugs can be used as a study aid."

From a parental perspective, PATS also reports that 29% of parents agreed that "ADHD medication can improve a child's academic or testing performance, even if the teen does not have ADHD." Adolescents also report that although 80% of their parents have discussed alcohol and marijuana use with them and 30% have discussed use of cocaine or crack, only 14% have discussed misuse of prescription medications.

SOURCES OF MEDICATION

How are adolescents without a prescription for stimulant medications able to access these drugs? Are the sources for these medications the same as for other illicit drugs such as marijuana?

The National Monitoring of Adolescent Prescription Stimulants Study (N-MAPSS) was launched to detect current levels of nonmedical use of prescription stimulants among preteens and teens.[20] In this sample of more than 11,000 youths aged 10 to 18 years recruited from entertainment venues (shopping malls, parks, movie theaters, food courts, etc.), 3% of respondents reported selling a prescription stimulant, 4.6% gave a prescription stimulant away, 2.4% traded prescription stimulants, and 1.6% reported their stimulants being stolen. Additionally, 2.1% of the sample reported stealing a stimulant, 7% obtained a prescription stimulant without cost, and 4.2% borrowed a prescription stimulant. Across age groups (10-12, 13-15, 16-18 years), there was a trend for diversion to increase with age, and suburban youth were more likely than urban or rural youth to be involved in diverting (either incoming or outgoing) medications (Table 3).

Table 3
Diversion of prescription (Rx) stimulants by residential area and age (% of respondents) based on National Monitoring of Adolescent Prescription Stimulants Study data

| | Rural | | | Suburban | | | Urban | | | Total |
| | Age (y) | | | | | | | | | |
	10-12	13-15	16-18	10-12	13-15	16-18	10-12	13-15	16-18	
No. of respondents in each category	211	633	836	553	1635	1935	642	2126	2488	11,048
Approached to divert Rx	1.0	10.7	18.4	7.6	9.4	16.9	3.8	8.2	14.1	11.7
Asked to sell Rx	0.5	6.3	10.3	5.6	4.9	10.6	2.5	4.7	7.3	6.7
Asked to give Rx	1.0	8.6	14.5	5.3	6.7	12.6	3.2	5.3	11.1	8.8
Asked to trade Rx	1.0	4.5	7.6	4.0	2.8	6.8	1.6	2.6	6.2	4.6
Sold Rx	0	2.6	5.9	0.9	1.6	4.9	0.6	1.5	4.1	3.0
Gave Rx	0.5	4.1	7.4	2.7	2.6	7.1	1.6	2.9	6.0	4.6
Traded Rx	0.0	2.3	5.4	1.1	1.3	4.1	0.3	0.9	3.1	2.4
Had Rx stolen	0.5	2.8	2.9	2.0	1.1	2.0	0.8	1.0	1.7	1.6

Adapted from Cottler LB, Striley CW, Lasopa SO. Assessing prescription stimulant use, misuse, and diversion among youth 10 to 18 years of age. Curr Opin Psychiatry. 2013;26:511–519, with permission from Wolters Kluwer.

Schepis and Krishnan-Sarin[21] analyzed data from the 2005 and 2006 NSDUH to identify sources of prescriptions for misuse among adolescents. They found that 49.7% of misusers obtained stimulants for free from a friend or relative, followed by purchasing stimulants from a friend/relative (11.8%), drug dealer/stranger (7.1%), or the Internet (1.6%); from 1 (10.8%) or multiple (1.5%) physicians; and through theft or faking a prescription (10.9% stole from a friend/relative, 0.8% stole from a medical source, and 0.5% faked a prescription). There were no differences in source by gender, but there were differences by race/ethnicity. White youth were most likely to get medications from a friend/relative (52.1%), through purchase (21.9%), or from a physician (10.9%). Black youth were most likely to get medications from theft/fake prescriptions (51.5%), from a friend/relative (25.9%), or from a physician (13%). Hispanic/Latino youth listed friend/relative (46.7%), physicians (19.6%), purchase (15%), and theft/fake prescription (13%) as their major sources. These findings could represent differences in access to medical care, which vary by race/ethnicity for both the students and their friends.

In their study of 2744 secondary school students from 2 southeastern Michigan school districts during 2009 to 2010, McCabe et al[22] found that of the approximately 141 students with a prescription for stimulant medication, 24.1% had been approached to divert their medication, 9.6% had sold their medication, 13.7% had given or loaned their medication to others, and 7.5% had traded their medication. In her study of Canadian youth, Poulin[11] reported that 3% of youth had been forced to give up some of their medication.

WHO DIVERTS MEDICATION?

As indicated earlier, most adolescents who misuse stimulants report getting medications from a friend or relative, and a small but significant percentage of students give away, sell, or trade their stimulant medications to others. Are there characteristics that define those who divert their medications from those who do not?

McCabe et al[22] analyzed the characteristics of 2744 adolescents from grades 7 to 12 who diverted any one or more of 4 classes of prescribed medications (pain, stimulants, antianxiety, and sleeping). In this sample, 33% of students reported having a prescription for at least 1 of these medications, and of these students, 13.8% reported ever selling, trading, loaning, or giving away their medications. Of students with prescriptions, 16.4% of those with stimulant prescriptions diverted their medications versus 14% for pain, 11.1% for antianxiety, and 9.6% for sleep.

In a multivariate analysis for any diversion (not limited to stimulants), those who diverted (compared to those who did not and those without a prescription) were significantly more likely to smoke cigarettes, report binge drinking, score positive on 2 measures of substance abuse (the CRAFFT and DAST screens), and report past-year use of marijuana, other illicit drugs, and nonmedical use of a prescription medication. Those with a prescription who did not divert were no more likely than those without a prescription to score positive on the CRAFFT or DAST or to engage in any of the other risk behaviors.

PREVENTION

Almost no data are available on how to prevent prescription stimulant misuse by adolescents. Prevention is critical because *each year* beyond age 13 that non-medical use of prescriptions medications (not just stimulants) can be delayed results in a 2% decrease in the risk of lifetime prescription drug dependence.[23] Although misuse of prescription stimulants has increased somewhat during the same period with the more widespread prescribing of stimulant medications for ADHD, a direct cause-and-effect relationship cannot be drawn. Furthermore, it is essential that adolescents with appropriately diagnosed ADHD have access to stimulant medications if needed as part of a comprehensive treatment strategy. Nonetheless, to minimize any potential fabrication of symptoms by adolescents (or their parents) with the goal of obtaining prescription stimulants purely to enhance cognitive abilities absent ADHD or to divert the drugs, physicians should perform careful evaluations according to accepted guidelines.[24]

Given the potential link between undiagnosed ADHD and mood disorders and misuse of prescription stimulants (as well as other prescription medications), it is important that adolescents with symptoms suggestive of ADHD be evaluated for other comorbidities. The United States Preventive Services Task Forces recommends routine screening of 12- to 18-year-olds for major depressive disorder when systems are in place to ensure accurate diagnosis, psychotherapy (cognitive-behavioral or interpersonal), and follow-up (www.uspreventiveservicestask-force.org/uspstf09/depression/chdeprrs.htm, accessed November 23, 2013). If some adolescents with undiagnosed ADHD or depression are self-medicating by misusing prescription medications, better recognition and treatment of those youths could decrease the number misusing these medications. Assessment for a co-occurring substance abuse disorder is essential because it likely will affect the choice of medications if they are to be prescribed.

Physicians who prescribe ADHD medications should carefully monitor requests for refills and regularly assess the adolescent's symptom control. Just as an adolescent's repeated requests for an albuterol inhaler can signal that his or her asthma is poorly controlled, so too can requests for stimulant refills at less than the indicated interval, regardless of the reason, signal that an adolescent is diverting the medication or that he or she is using extra doses because the symptoms of ADHD are not well controlled. Given the overlap between substance abuse problems and misuse of prescription stimulants, it is important that physicians perform a careful drug and alcohol assessment before prescribing stimulant medications.

Physicians can discuss with adolescents and their parents where the medications will be kept and who will administer them. In a recent study, 74% of adolescents with prescriptions for pain medications, stimulants, and anxiety/sedative medications reported that they had unsupervised access to these medications.[25] Sizeable numbers of parents and adolescents believe that prescription medications are safer if abused than illicit drugs, so it is worthwhile for physicians to review with them that this statement is true only if these medications are taken within the context of a careful evaluation by a physician. Adolescents should be cautioned never to give or share their medications with others.

Whether preferentially choosing long-acting over shorter-acting stimulants reduces the risk of diversion and abuse is unknown, especially if the goal of the diversion is to provide or obtain a study aid. In general, however, these formulations are less likely to be used for the purposes of getting high.[26] Although drugs such as guanfacine, atomoxetine, and bupropion might be preferred treatment for an adolescent with ADHD and a substance use disorder, these medications may not otherwise be as effective for first-line treatment of ADHD in individuals without a substance abuse disorder. An individualized and tailored treatment plan is essential for each adolescent with ADHD.

Community-based universal prevention interventions hold promise for reducing prescription drug misuse. Spoth et al[27] reported on 3 separate studies using the Iowa Strengthening Families Program (later renamed the Strengthening Families Program) conducted in rural communities or small towns with populations of less than 50,000 in Iowa and in communities in Pennsylvania. The programs were school based, and each included a parent component. Subjects were between 11 and 13 years of age at baseline; they were followed to age 25 years in studies 1 and 2 and to the 12th grade in study 3. Nonmedical use of prescription stimulants was not measured separately. Rather, students were assessed on misuse of prescription opioids in particular and on misuse of 4 prescription drugs grouped together (barbiturates, tranquilizers, amphetamines, and narcotics). In study 1, lifetime prescription drug abuse in the intervention groups was reduced by two-thirds in comparison to the control group at age 25. In study 2, lifetime use was significantly reduced to age 22, with continued significant reductions to age 25 among the higher-risk group that had initiated some illicit drug use at the time of the baseline evaluation. In study 3, there were significant reductions in misuse at grade 12 in the intervention versus control students.

Statewide or nationwide prescription monitoring programs theoretically could reduce misuse of prescription stimulants by allowing physicians to determine if patients are receiving stimulants from multiple sources. However, the limited evidence to date suggests that relatively few adolescents obtain prescriptions from multiple physicians.[21]

One final aspect of prevention merits consideration. To the extent that adolescents' misuse of prescription stimulants is driven largely by the belief that use of such medications enhances learning or compensates for inadequate or last-minute preparation, it is critical to gain a better understanding of whether these medications enhance learning and academic performance when taken by individuals without ADHD. A recent review demonstrates that the evidence supporting claims of enhanced cognition is mixed.[28] However, none of these studies involved adolescents, although a number involved young adults aged 18 to 25. Research regarding the effect of prescription stimulants on the academic performance of adolescents without ADHD would face many ethical and regulatory challenges. Even if stimulants were shown to have a positive effect, any potential benefit would need to be weighed against the potential effect on the still developing adolescent brain, along with a myriad of ethical, legal, and social justice issues.[29]

References

1. Schwarz A. Risky rise of the good-grade pill. New York Times. June 9, 2012. Available at: www. nytimes.com/2012/06/10/education/seeking-academic-edge-teenagers-abuse-stimulants.html?_r=0. Accessed November 23, 2013

2. Zuvekas SH, Vitiello B. Stimulant medication use in children: a 12-year perspective. Am J Psychiatry. 2012;169:160–166

3. Substance Abuse and Mental Health Services Administration, Center for Behavioral Health Statistics and Quality. The DAWN Report, January 24, 2013. Emergency department visits involving attention deficit/hyperactivity disorder stimulant medications. Available at: www.samhsa.gov/data/2k13/DAWN073/sr073-ADD-ADHD-medications.htm. Accessed November 23, 2013

4. Setlik J, Bond GR, Ho M. Adolescent prescription ADHD medication abuse is rising along with prescriptions for these medications. Pediatrics. 2009;124:875–880

5. Boyd CJ, McCabe SE. Coming to terms with the non-medical use of prescription medications. Subst Abuse Treat Prev Policy. 2008;3:22–24

6. Kroutil LA, Van Brunt DL, Herman-Stahl MA, et al. Non-medical use of prescription stimulants in the United States. Drug Alcohol Depend. 2006;84:135–143

7. Wu LT, Pilowsky DJ, Schlenger WE, Galvin DM. Misuse of methamphetamine and prescription stimulants among youths and young adults in the community. Drug Alcohol Depend. 2007;89:195–205

8. Levine SB, Coupey SM. Nonmedical use of prescription medications: an emerging risk behavior among rural adolescents. J Adolesc Health. 2009;44:407–409

9. Haven JR, Young AM, Haven CE. Nonmedical prescription drug us in a nationally representative sample of adolescents. Arch Pediatr Adolesc Med. 2011;165:250–255

10. Wilens TE, Adler LA, Adams J, et al. Misuse and diversion of stimulants prescribed for ADHD: a systematic review of the literature. J Am Acad Child Adolesc Psychiatry. 2008;47:21–31

11. Poulin C. From attention-deficit/hyperactivity disorder to medical stimulant use to the diversion of prescribed stimulants to non-medical stimulant use: connecting the dots. Addiction. 2007;102:740–751

12. McCabe SE, Boyd CJ, Young A. Medical and non-medical use of prescription drugs among secondary school students. J Adolesc Health. 2007;40:76–83

13. McCabe SE, West BT, Cranford JA, et al. Medical misuse of controlled medications among adolescents. Arch Pediatr Adolesc Med. 2011;165:729–735

14. McCabe SE, Teter CJ, Boyd CJ. The use, misuse and diversion of prescription stimulants among middle and high school students. Subst Use Misuse. 2004;39:1095–116

15. Boyd CJ, McCabe SE, Cranford JA, Young A. Adolescents' motivations to abuse prescription medications. Pediatrics. 2006;118:2472–2480

16. Schepis TS, Krishnan-Sarin S. Characterizing adolescent prescription misusers: a population based study. J Am Acad Child Adolesc Psych. 2008;47:745–754

17. Herman-Stahl MA, Krebs CP, Kroutil LA, Heller DC. Risk and protective factors for nonmedical use of prescription stimulants and methamphetamine among adolescents. *J Adolesc Health.* 2006;39:374–380

18. Substance Abuse and Mental Health Services Administration, Office of Applied Studies. The NSDUH Report, February 28, 2008. Nonmedical stimulant use, other drug use, delinquent behaviors, and depression among adolescents. Available at: www.oas.samhsa.gov/2k8/stimulants/depression.pdf. Accessed November 23, 2013

19. Simoni-Wastila L, Yang HWK, Lawler J. Correlates of prescription drug nonmedical use and problem use by adolescents. *J Addict Med.* 2008;2:31–39

20. Cottler LB, Striley CW, Lasopa SO. Assessing prescription stimulant use, misuse, and diversion among youth 10-18 years of age. *Curr Opin Psychiatry.* 2013;26:511–519

21. Schepis TS, Krishnan-Sarin S. Sources of prescriptions for misuse by adolescents: differences in sex, ethnicity, and severity of misuse in a population-based study. *J Am Acad Child Adolesc Psy.* 2009;48:828–836

22. McCabe SE, West BT, Teter CJ, Ross-Durow P. Characteristics associated with the diversion of controlled medications among adolescents. *Drug Alcohol Depend.* 2011;118:452–458

23. McCabe SE, West BT, Morales M, Cranford JA, Boyd CJ. Does early onset of non-medical use of prescription drugs predict subsequent prescription drug abuse and dependence? Results from a national study. *Addiction.* 2007;102:1920–1930

24. Wolraich M, Brown L, Brown RT, et al. ADHD: clinical practice guideline for the diagnosis, evaluation, and treatment of attention-deficit/hyperactivity disorder in children and adolescents. *Pediatrics.* 2011;128:1007–1022

25. Ross-Durow PL. McCabe SE, Boyd CJ. Adolescents' access to their own prescription medications in the home. *J Adolesc Health.* 2013;53:260–264

26. Croft HA. Physician handling of prescription stimulants. *Pediatric Ann.* 2006;35:557–562

27. Spoth R, Trudeau L, Shin C, et al. Longitudinal effects of universal preventive intervention on prescription drug misuse: three randomized controlled trials with late adolescents and young adults. *Am J Public Health.* 2013;103:665–672

28. Smith ME, Farah MJ. Are prescription stimulants "smart pills"? *Psychol Bull.* 2011;137:717–741

29. Graf WD, Nagel SK, Epstein LG, et al. Pediatric neuroenhancement: ethical, legal, social, and neurodevelopmental implications. *Neurology.* 2013;80:1251–1260

Adolesc Med 025 (2014) 104–112

Responding to the Prescription Opioid Epidemic: Practical Information for Pediatricians

Martha J. Wunsch, MD[a*]; Pamela K. Gonzalez, MD, MS[b]

[a]Medical Director, Addiction Medicine, Kaiser Permanente–GSAA,
Chemical Dependency Recovery Program, Union City, California; [b]Adjunct Assistant Professor,
Department of Psychiatry, University of Minnesota, St. Paul, Minnesota

EPIDEMIOLOGY

Nonmedical or illicit use of psychoactive prescription medications without one's own legal prescription, outside of a doctor's guidance, by a modality other than orally, or only for the effect or feeling caused by the medication has emerged as a public health problem in the United States since 1995. The National Survey on Drug Use and Health (NSDUH), a nationwide confidential health survey, uses the National Institute on Drug Abuse definition of nonmedical use, which is "taking a psychoactive medication either without a legitimate prescription or for the experience or feeling the medications cause."[1] The NSDUH reports nonmedical use of stimulants, sedatives, tranquilizers, and opioids for individuals aged 12 years and older during the last 30 days and in the individuals' lifetime. Prescription opioids are the psychoactive medications most commonly used nonmedically.[2] Increased nonmedical use has been accompanied by a 5-fold increase in admissions for opioid abuse and addiction in the first decade of the 21st century (8000 admissions in 2000 vs. 150,000 in 2010).[3]

In the 2012 NSDUH survey, the prevalence of youth aged 12 to 17 years who used psychotherapeutic medications illicitly in the last 30 days was 2.8%, a slight decrease from 4% in 2002. Among young adults aged 18 to 24 years, the prevalence of nonmedical use of psychoactive medications in the last 30 days was 5.3%, a small decrease from a peak of 6.5% in 2006. In addition, although youth aged 12 to 17 years report cannabis as the first substance used, prescription opi-

---

*Corresponding author:
Martha.J.Wunsch@kp.org

oids have risen to be the second most commonly used drug at initiation of drug use. According to NSDUH, the peak age for initiation of nonmedical use of pain relievers is 16 years (4.3%), although the age at initiation in some is as early as 12 to 13 years (1.3%).[2]

Whereas NSDUH surveys individuals aged 12 years and older, 2 epidemiologic surveys focus solely on youth behavior. The Youth Risk Behavior Surveillance System (YRBSS) is a national school-based survey of 150,000 young people conducted by the Centers for Disease Control and Prevention (CDC); state, territorial, and local education and health agencies; and tribal governments. YRBSS asks about 6 high-risk health behaviors, including drug and alcohol use, among 9th- to 12th-graders. With regard to prescription medications, youth are asked about "taking a prescription medication without a doctor's prescription one or more times during their lifetime." The medications asked about include Oxy-Contin, Percocet, Vicodin, codeine, Adderall, Ritalin, and Xanax. For youth nationwide, one-fifth (20.7%) endorsed nonmedical use of 1 of these 7 medications. Among high school seniors, 25.6% reported taking a medication without a doctor's prescription 1 or more times. In contrast, 2.9% of youth nationwide had ever used heroin. Unfortunately, when pills become unavailable or too costly, youngsters may shift use from prescription opioids to snorted or smoked heroin and eventually escalate to intravenous forms.[4,5] Heroin use among non-medical users of opioid pain relievers increased between 2002 and 2004 and between 2008 and 2010. Most individuals reported nonmedical use of opioid pain relievers before initiating heroin.[6]

Monitoring the Future (MTF), the other youth-focused project, surveys 8th-, 10th-, and 12th-graders every other year. MTF defines prescription drug *misuse* as use "on your own—that is, without a doctor telling you to take them." In 2012, 8% of 12th-graders reported use of opioid narcotics other than heroin in the last 12 months.[7] Half of these high school seniors reported that getting access to narcotics other than heroin was "fairly or very easy." MTF asks specifically about use of Oxy-Contin and Vicodin. Among 12th-graders, 4% had used OxyContin and 8% had used Vicodin, both in the past 12 months. Use was less but present among 8th- and 10th-graders. Of note, both MTF and NSDUH have documented decreases in past-month use rates of alcohol and tobacco over the past decade.

SOURCE OF MEDICATIONS

According to NSDUH, the source for nonmedical use rarely includes the Internet, strangers, or drug dealers but instead is as close as the family medicine cabinet. In the 2012 survey, most individuals (54%) who initiated nonmedical use cited the primary source of pills as "Free from Friend/Relative," and in 16.6% of cases medication was taken or bought, again from friends or family (Figure 1).[8] Between 1994 and 2007, opioid prescribing increased from 6.2% to 10.6% among 15- to 19-year-olds, and from 8.3% to 15.9% among young adults (20-29 years of

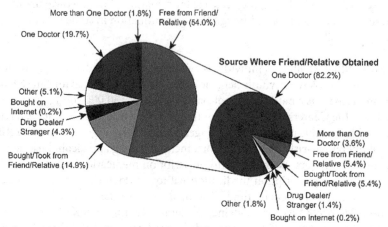

Fig 1. Source where pain relievers were obtained for most recent nonmedical use among past-year users aged 12 years or older: 2011 to 2012. (From Substance Abuse and Mental Health Services Administration. *Results from the 2011 National Survey on Drug Use and Health: Summary of National Findings.* NSDUH Series H-44, HHS Publication No. [SMA] 12-4713. Rockville, MD: Substance Abuse and Mental Health Services Administration, 2012.)

age).[9] Another important opportunity for nonmedical use is prescription left-overs. McCabe et al[10] analyzed the 2007 to 2010 cohorts of high school seniors and found that more than one-third (36.9%) of past-year nonmedical users endorsed using leftovers from their own prescriptions. On entry to treatment, teens reported that they have been prescribed opioids on multiple occasions.[11] The most common prescribers for the 10- to 19-year-old age group are family physicians/general practitioners, followed by dentists, emergency room physicians, orthopedic surgeons, and pediatricians.[12]

EFFECT OF NONMEDICAL USE

The National Epidemiologic Survey of Alcohol and Related Conditions (NESARC) described an increased risk of addiction when abuse of psychoactive drugs, including alcohol, begins in adolescence.[13] Similarly, the earlier nonmedical use of medications is initiated, the more likely an individual will be diagnosed with prescription drug dependence as an adult.[14] The estimated prevalence of prescription medication use disorder for a youngster who initiates nonmedical use by age 13 years is 25%, whereas the prevalence for an individual who begins first nonmedical use at age 21 years is estimated to be less than 10% (Figure 2).

Nonmedical prescription use often is associated with use of other substances, including alcohol, tobacco, marijuana, and other illicit drugs. Specifically,

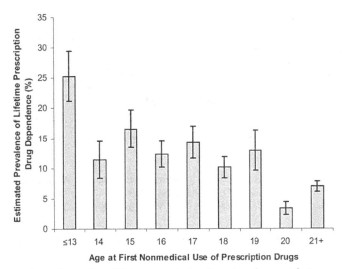

Fig 2. Estimated prevalence of any lifetime prescription drug abuse by age at first nonmedical use of any prescription drugs, 2001 to 2002. Error bars indicate ±1 standard error. (From McCabe SE, West BT, Morales M, Cranford JA, Boyd CJ. Does early onset of non-medical use of prescription drugs predict subsequent prescription drug abuse and dependence? Results from a national study. *Addiction.* 2007;102(12):1920–1930. Reprinted with permission.)

youth who are nonmedical opioid users who also coingested other drugs were more likely to report intranasal administration, recreational motives, and a greater subjective "high."[15] A study not specifically focused on youth reported that, in rural Appalachia, if the first illicit drug used was illicit methadone, oxycodone, or OxyContin, there is an increased hazard for transitioning to injection drug use.[16]

The most devastating consequences of nonmedical use are overdose deaths and drug poisonings. For the United States in general, drug-poisoning deaths in which prescription opioids are identified now outpace deaths attributed to heroin and cocaine.[17] Deaths in which prescription opioids are identified on toxicology tests have steadily increased over the same time period as increased nonmedical use of these medications. Among the 15- to 24-year-old age group, such deaths have more than doubled from 3.2:100,000 in 1999 to 8.2:100,000 in 2008 (Figure 3).

MOTIVATIONS FOR USE

Similar to the general population, adolescents and young adults endorse many different reasons for nonmedical use of prescription medications. A midwestern survey of 10- to 18-year-olds reported motivations varying from experimentation and seeking euphoria, "to getting high" and "because I'm addicted," to treatment of symptoms for which the medication usually is prescribed. These young people

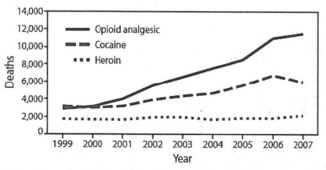

Fig 3. Unintentional drug overdose deaths involving opioid analgesics, cocaine, and heroin in the United States from 1999 to 2007. (From Paulozzi L, Baldwin G. CDC grand rounds: prescription drug overdoses—a U.S. epidemic. *MMWR Morb Mortal Wkly Rep.* 2012;61(01):10–13.)

endorsed using stimulants to study, focus, and lose weight; pain medication to relieve pain; and tranquilizers and sedative-hypnotics to treat anxiety or as sleep aids.[18,19] Among undergraduates, young adults who endorsed reasons other than self-treatment for nonmedical use, such as experimentation to seek feelings of novel intoxication or euphoria, were significantly more likely to have substance abuse problems as indicated by high scores on the Drug Abuse Screening Test-10.[20] Given the possibility of combining prescription medications with alcohol and other drugs, the potential for accidental unintended overdose is a significant concern.

ANTICIPATORY GUIDANCE: THE DANGER OF THE FAMILY MEDICINE CABINET

As prescribers, the most important message to give to patients and families is that *any sharing of medication is diversion* and, in the case of controlled substances, is illegal. Prescribers and support staff can remind patients and families that all medications should be taken as directed and only by the person for whom they are prescribed, with no changes in dose or dosage interval made without discussion with the prescriber. They also should be informed that medications should never be combined with alcohol or other psychoactive substances.

Point out to families that medications are labeled "controlled" by the Drug Enforcement Administration (DEA) and thus can only be prescribed with great care because of the potential for abuse and addiction. Like heroin, prescription opioids can cause respiratory depression, are metabolized by the body to similar compounds, and, when taken incorrectly, can have adverse consequences, including inadvertent overdose that may lead to a fatality. As noted earlier, most people procure pills for nonmedical use from friends or family. Parents and other caregivers should be encouraged to include nonmedical use of prescription medications in discussions with their children about the dangers of alcohol, tobacco, and other psychoactive drugs.

The American Academy of Pediatrics Committee on Substance Abuse suggests that the following may be important anticipatory information to give to patients and their families in order to prevent diversion or nonmedical use of controlled substances:

1. Actively discourage parents and caretakers from sharing their own medications with their children.
2. Actively discourage patients from sharing their medications with *anyone,* including family members and friends.
3. Prevent "accidental sharing" by advising parents, caretakers, and patients to keep medications secured under lock and key.
4. Determine who in the family will secure and administer medication.
5. Consider the risk for diversion or nonmedical use in the household.

Ask if there is anyone in the household, including the patient, who may be placed at risk by having controlled medications in the home. Has there been problematic use of any psychoactive substance, including prescription medications? If there is risk of diversion or nonmedical use, suggest that the parent or caretaker control and administer doses.

Physicians should specifically discourage stockpiling of unused prescription medications. Instruct caretakers and patients to destroy rather than stockpile any unused medications because leftover pills are often the source of initial nonmedical use by youth. Instructions for proper disposal of medications are available online (www.fda.gov/ForConsumers/ConsumerUpdates/ucm101653.htm). In addition, local police departments may sponsor, in concert with the DEA, community locations and times when consumers can drop off any unused medications for disposal.

PRESCRIBER AWARENESS

Physicians, researchers, and the World Health Organization have established guidelines for the treatment of pain in infants, children, and adolescents.[21-25] These guidelines are helpful for pediatricians faced with the assessment, diagnosis, management, and treatment of acute and chronic pain. In addition, when prescribing controlled medications, consider the following questions:

1. Is the medication appropriate for the indication?
2. Are the potential risks worth the anticipated benefits?
3. How long do I anticipate the condition to last, and how many doses does the patient need?
4. What are my expectations for follow-up?
5. At what point do I need to stop prescribing the medication because I need specialty input?

OFFICE POLICIES: MINIMIZING NONMEDICAL USE

Patients and families should be familiar with office procedures that physicians establish and universally apply when controlled substances are prescribed. Before prescribing a medication, having a discussion of anticipatory guidance and office policies that discourage nonmedical use will minimize conflicts over prescribing practices. All physicians should store paper prescription pads under lock and key. If printing controlled prescriptions, use a secure printer with limited staff access, prescribe only the necessary number of pills, minimize or do not allow refills, and inquire about current or past patient prescriptions from the state prescription monitoring databases before prescribing any controlled substance. In addition, prescribers should be aware of the parent or patient who does not keep scheduled appointments and requests refills without face-to-face visits. Urine drug tests for substances of abuse, including cannabis and other prescribed controlled substances, may be requested at the time of initial prescription. A "random unscheduled" urine drug test may be helpful when concerns emerge about patient or family behavior. Asking for early refills, losing prescriptions, or appearing intoxicated at a visit may trigger a random urine drug test.[26] If the adolescent already shows evidence of a substance use disorder, the physicians may choose to use nonopioid medications to control pain and refer the patient to an addiction specialist for further evaluation.

SCREENING FOR NONMEDICAL USE

There is no specific screening tool for nonmedical use; however, some evidence supports the good sensitivity of the CRAFFT screening tool.[27] In addition to using an appropriate screening tool (eg, CRAFFT), the physician may ask additional questions to enhance the detection of nonmedical use, such as "Have you ever taken a prescription pill that wasn't yours?" or, for youth who are currently prescribed psychoactive medications, "Have you ever taken your medication not as prescribed (eg, extra dose, increased dose on your own)?"

Many nonmedical users of prescription drugs have significant psychiatric comorbidities, so follow existing guidelines for mental health screening assessment at every pediatric encounter, including those when controlled medications are being prescribed.

TREATMENT

The Drug Abuse Treatment Act (DATA 2000) authorized the use of medication to treat opioid addiction in a medical office (ie, office-based opioid treatment [OBOT]). Buprenorphine, a partial agonist-antagonist, is combined with naloxone in a sublingual formulation. This is a powerful pharmaceutical that stabilizes the physiologic problems resulting from opioid withdrawal and can be prescribed as maintenance during addiction treatment. Pediatricians who are interested in the treatment of adolescent opioid addiction, both pharmaceutical and illicit, can complete 8 hours of focused training in addiction medicine to qualify for a specific DEA number that allows them to prescribe buprenorphine/naloxone. Online training to qualify as a DATA 2000 waiver physician is offered through the American Psychiatric Association, American Society of Addiction Medicine, American Academy of Addiction Psychiatry, and American Academy of Osteopathic Addiction Medicine (buprenorphine.samhsa.gov. Accessed January 19, 2014).

CONCLUSION

The definition of nonmedical use of psychoactive prescriptions varies; however, it is generally defined as use of a psychoactive medication without the supervision of a physician or use for the experience or feeling that results from taking the medication. Types of psychoactive medications used include prescription opioids, stimulants, and sedative-hypnotics. Initiation of nonmedical use occurs as early as ages 12 to 13 years, the peak age of initiation is 16 years, and opioid medications are most commonly used. In most cases, the source of medications for nonmedical use is friends or family and is free, although youth may use their own leftover medications. The increased rates of nonmedical opioid use is of great concern, especially for early adolescents, because early initiation of nonmedical use of medications is associated with higher occurrence of prescription drug dependence in adulthood and often co-occurs with use of alcohol and other drugs. Deaths from overdose of nonmedical use of opioids have more than doubled since 1999. Families should be reminded that prescription medications, if used inappropriately, can be as dangerous as alcohol and illegal drugs. Important prevention messages to give to patients and their families are that any sharing of controlled medication is diversion, family and friends are major sources of medications for nonmedical use, all medications should be stored securely, stockpiling is dangerous, and medications should be disposed of according to federal guidelines.

References

1. Compton WM, Volkow ND. Abuse of prescription drugs and the risk of addiction. *Drug Alcohol Depend*. 2006;83(Suppl 1):S4–S7
2. Substance Abuse and Mental Health Services Administration. *Results from the 2012 National Survey on Drug Use and Health: Summary of National Findings*. NSDUH Series H-46, HHS Publication No. (SMA) 13-4795. Rockville, MD: Substance Abuse and Mental Health Services Administration; 2013
3. Substance Abuse and Mental Health Services Administration, Center for Behavioral Health Statistics and Quality. *Treatment Episode Data Set (TEDS): 2000-2010. State Admissions to Substance Abuse Treatment Services*. DASIS Series S-63, HHS Publication No. (SMA) 12-4729. Rockville, MD: Substance Abuse and Mental Health Services Administration; 2012
4. Mars SG, Bourgois P, Karandinos G, Montero F, Ciccarone D. "Every 'never' I ever said came true": transitions from opioid pills to heroin injecting. *Int J Drug Policy*. 2013;13:167–169
5. Pollini RA, Banta-Green CJ, Cuevas-Mota J, et al. Problematic use of prescription-type opioids prior to heroin use among young heroin injectors. *Subst Abuse Rehabil*. 2011;2(1):173–180

6. Jones CM. Heroin use and heroin use risk behaviors among nonmedical users of prescription opioid pain relievers–United States, 2002-2004 and 2008-2010. *Drug Alcohol Depend.* 2013;132(1–2):95–100

7. Johnston LD, O'Malley PM, Bachman JG, Schulenberg JE. *Monitoring the Future National Results on Adolescent Drug Use: Overview of Key Findings, 2012.* Ann Arbor, MI: Institute for Social Research, The University of Michigan; 2013

8. Substance Abuse and Mental Health Services Administration. *Results from the 2011 National Survey on Drug Use and Health: Summary of National Findings.* NSDUH Series H-44, HHS Publication No. (SMA) 12-4713. Rockville, MD: Substance Abuse and Mental Health Services Administration, 2012

9. Fortuna RJ, Robbins BW, Caiola E, Joynt M, Halterman JS. Prescribing of controlled medications to adolescents and young adults in the United States. *Pediatrics.* 2010;126(6):1108–1116

10. McCabe SE, West BT, Boyd CJ. Leftover prescription opioids and nonmedical use among high school seniors: a multi-cohort national study. *J Adolesc Health.* 2013;52(4):480–485

11. Matson SC, Bentley C, Dughman VH, Bonny AE. Receipt of prescribed controlled substances by adolescents and young adults prior to presenting for opiate dependence treatment. *J Addict.* Volume 2013. Available at: www.hindawi.com/journals/jad/2013/680705/. Accessed March 13, 2014

12. Volkow ND, McLellan TA, Cotto JH, Karithanom M, Weiss SR. Characteristics of opioid prescriptions in 2009. *JAMA.* 2011;305(13):1299–1301

13. Hermos J, Winter M, Heeren T, Hingson R. Alcohol-related problems among younger drinkers who misuse prescription drugs: results from the national epidemiologic survey of alcohol and related conditions (NESARC). *Subst Abus.* 2009;30(2):118–126

14. McCabe SE, West BT, Morales M, Cranford JA, Boyd CJ. Does early onset of non-medical use of prescription drugs predict subsequent prescription drug abuse and dependence? Results from a national study. *Addiction.* 2007;102(12):1920–1930

15. McCabe SE, West BT, Teter CJ, Boyd CJ. Co-ingestion of prescription opioids and other drugs among high school seniors: results from a national study. *Drug Alcohol Depend.* 2012;126(1–2):65–70

16. Young AM, Havens JR. Transition from first illicit drug use to first injection drug use among rural Appalachian drug users: a cross-sectional comparison and retrospective survival analysis. *Addiction.* 2012;107(3):587–596

17. Paulozzi L, Baldwin G. CDC grand rounds: prescription drug overdoses—a U.S. epidemic. *MMWR Morb Mortal Wkly Rep.* 2012;61(01):10–13

18. McCabe SE, Boyd CJ. Sources of prescription drugs for illicit use. *Addict Behav.* 2005;30(7):1342–1350

19. Boyd CJ, McCabe SE, Cranford JA, Young A. Adolescents' motivations to abuse prescription medications. *Pediatrics.* 2006;118(6):2472–2480

20. McCabe SE, Boyd CJ, Cranford JA, Morales M, Slayden J. A modified version of the Drug Abuse Screening Test among undergraduate students. *J Subst Abuse Treat.* 2006;31(3):297–303

21. American Academy of Pediatrics Committee on Psychosocial Aspects of Child and Family Health; Task Force on Pain in Infants, Children, and Adolescents. The assessment and management of acute pain in infants, children, and adolescents. *Pediatrics.* 2001;108(3):793–797

22. Zempsky WT, Cravero JP. Relief of pain and anxiety in pediatric patients in emergency medical systems. *Pediatrics.* 2004;114(5):1348–1356

23. Kost-Byerly S. Management of chronic pain in children. In: McInerny TK, Adam HM, Campbell D, Kamat DK, Kelleher KJ, eds. *Textbook of Pediatric Care.* Elk Grove Village, IL: American Academy of Pediatrics; 2008

24. World Health Organization. WHO guidelines on the pharmacological treatment of persisting pain in children with medical illnesses. Available at: whqlibdoc.who.int/publications/2012/9789241548120_Guidelines.pdf. Accessed December 28, 2013

25. Lewis DW, Ashwal S, Dahl G, et al. Quality Standards Subcommittee of the American Academy of Neurology; Practice Committee of the Child Neurology Society. Practice parameter: evaluation of children and adolescents with recurrent headaches. *Neurology.* 2002;59(4):490–498

26. Weaver M, Heit H, Savage S, Gourlay D. Clinical case discussion: chronic pain management. *J Addict Med.* 2007;1(1):11–14

27. McCabe SE, West BT, Teter CJ, et al. Adolescent nonmedical users of prescription opioids: brief screening and substance use disorders. *Addict Behav.* 2012;37:651–656

Adolesc Med 025 (2014) 113–125

Performance-Enhancing Substances

Cora Collette Breuner, MD, MPH*

Professor Adolescent Medicine Section, Department of Pediatrics, Adjunct Professor Orthopedics and Sports Medicine, Seattle Childrens Hospital University of Washington, Seattle, Washington

INTRODUCTION

"If I could give you a pill that would make you an Olympic champion—and also kill you in a year—would you take it?" Mirkin asked this Faustian question of elite competitive runners in advance of a Washington, DC, road race in 1967. Half of the athletes responded, and more than 50% stated "Yes."[1] In a separate survey, Goldman and Klatz[2] asked aspiring Olympians 2 questions. Question 1: "If you were offered a banned performance-enhancing substance that guaranteed that you would win an Olympic medal and you could not be caught, would you take it?" Not astonishingly, 195 of 198 athletes said "Yes." Question 2: "Would you take a banned performance-enhancing drug with a guarantee that you will not be caught, you will win every competition for the next 5 years, but will then die from adverse effects of the substance?" Fifty percent of the athletes said "Yes."

Where are we now, years after these oft quoted and overscrutinized surveys? With more than 57% of high school and middle school students (>30 million children and adolescents) playing on formal sports teams, the growing use of performance-enhancing substances is a significant health concern. The increased use most likely is fueled by the rise in popularity of team/competitive sports, easy and affordable availability of performance-enhancing substances via the Internet and social media chat groups, hyped media focus on thinness or muscular bodies, parental and coach pressure, and a propensity for adolescents to engage in quick-fix risk-taking behaviors. The inherent and natural desire to win is countered by the ethical dilemma of obtaining a victory by cheating. Is the only issue getting caught? Or are there health risks?[3]

---

*Corresponding author:
cora.breuner@seattlechildrens.org

In this article, performance-enhancing substances available to adolescents are discussed, including steroids, steroid precursors, growth hormone, supplements, stimulants, and beta-blockers.

WHAT ARE PERFORMANCE-ENHANCING SUBSTANCES?

A performance-enhancing substance is any substance used by a person to perform better on the playing field, on the stage, or in the classroom. Historians have reported that Greek Olympians used material such as figs, mushrooms, and strychnine, and Mayans chewed on cocoa leaves to improve their competitive edge.[4]

THERE ARE SEVERAL DISTINCT CLASSES OF SUBSTANCES (TABLE 1):

1. *Lean mass builders* amplify the growth of muscle and lean body mass and may reduce recovery time from an injury. This class of drugs includes anabolic steroids, hormone precursors, and human growth hormone (hGH).
2. *Stimulants* promote optimal body and mind performance by enhancing focus, energy, and aggression. Examples include caffeine, amphetamine, and methamphetamine.

Table 1
Classes of Commonly Used Performance-Enhancing Drugs

Anabolic Agents
Anabolic steroids
Testosterone
Steroid precursors
   Dehydroepiandosterone
   Androstenedione

Nutritional Supplements
Creatine
Protein/amino acids
β-hydroxy β-methylbutryic acid

Stimulants
Ephedrine
Caffeine/Guarana

Other
Human growth hormone
Erythropoietin
Blood doping
Diuretics
Actovegin (calf blood extract)

From Calfee R, Fadale P. Popular ergogenic drugs and supplements in young athletes. *Pediatrics.* 2006;117(3):e577–e589.

3. *Analgesics* may mask pain, allowing performers to compete and perform beyond their usual pain thresholds. These substances range from common over-the-counter medicines such as nonsteroidal anti-inflammatory drugs (eg, ibuprofen) to powerful prescription narcotics.
4. *Sedatives* and *beta-blockers* have been used by athletes in sports such as archery and golf, which require steady hands and accurate aim, and by athletes or stage performers attempting to overcome excessive nervousness or discomfort. Alcohol, diazepam, propranolol, and marijuana are examples.
5. *Diuretics* are often used by athletes such as wrestlers, who need to meet weight restrictions. Importantly, stimulants can have secondary diuretic effects.
6. *Erythropoietin* (EPO) can increase the oxygen-carrying capacity of blood and is used in endurance sports such as cycling and Nordic skiing.
7. *Drug Masking* can be used to mask the detection of other classes of drugs. An example is epitestosterone, a drug with no performance-enhancing effects, which restores the testosterone/epitestosterone ratio (a common criterion in steroid testing) to normal levels after anabolic steroid supplementation.
8. *Supplements* such as vitamins, proteins, and creatine, which are easily obtained with a proper diet, are considered by some to enhance athletes' performance.

ANABOLIC ADRENAL STEROIDS

History

In 1889, the prominent physiologist and Harvard Professor Charles-Edouard Brown-Sequard, MD was studying the effects of dog and guinea pig testicular extracts in hopes of finding a means to prolong life and preserve youth. Brown-Sequard probably is most famous for his self-injection of testicular substances (extracted from guinea pigs and dogs), the results of which were published in 1889.[5] He described an invigorating effect, manifested as increased strength, mental abilities, and appetite. His reports and the provision of free samples to physicians prompted further investigations, which unfortunately were of poor quality and in many instances were ethically unsound. However, his theories and study of adrenal glands, testes, thyroid, pancreas, liver, spleen, and kidneys later promoted the development of the field of endocrinology.[6]

The use of synthetic testosterone rose dramatically after publication of the book *The Male Hormone* by Paul de Kruif in 1945, with reports that testosterone increased libido and enhanced performance. Beginning in the late 1940s and early 1950s, testosterone was used by bodybuilders and weight lifters in the United States to increase muscle mass. The US Food and Drug Administration (FDA) approved methandrostenolone in 1958. In the 1950s, Soviet Union and East German Olympic athletes used anabolic steroids, as did many other Olympic competitors.

Beginning in the 1950s, testosterone was modified into derivatives that possessed more anabolic qualities. In the 1970s, the oral testosterone undecenoate was synthesized but did not fare well in the oral form because of poor hepatic clearance, hepatotoxicity, and ineffective bioavailability. The only active forms of testosterone are injectable or transdermal or buccal gels.

The US Congress placed anabolic adrenal steroids (AAS) in the schedule III category of the Controlled Substance Act (CSA) in the Anabolic Steroid Control Act of 1990. This act included testosterone and all related chemical or pharmacologic substances that promoted muscle growth. Later, the Anabolic Steroid Act of 1994 was passed as an amendment to the CSA, where anabolic steroids as well as their precursors were placed on the controlled substance list. Possession and use of the drugs without a prescription became a federal crime. The decision of pharmaceutical companies to stop producing anabolic steroids in the 1990s prompted a huge surge in black market sales.

Steroids bind to androgen receptors within the cell cytoplasm and then are transported into the nucleus before they bind DNA and increase mRNA transcription, enhancing contractile and structural protein synthesis. The beneficial effects of steroids are improved positive muscle nitrogen balance, anticatabolic/antiaging effects, and significant emotional outcomes such as increased aggression and drive to compete.[7,8]

Current Use

The National Youth Risk Behavior Surveillance System, which is conducted every 2 years, surveys 16,500 9th- through 12th-graders in private and public schools on priority health risk behaviors. One survey question asks if the teenager "ever took steroid pills or shots without a doctor's prescription one or more times during their life." From 1991 to 2003, reported rates of lifetime use increased 2.7% to 6.1% and then decreased to 3.3% in 2009. Males (4.4%) were more likely than females (2.2%) to have used steroids at least once.[9]

Monitoring the Future is an annual long-term study of 50,000 8th-, 10th-, and 12th-grade adolescents and adults based at the University of Michigan Institute for Social Research. The 2010 survey demonstrated annual male adolescent prevalence rates for steroid use of 0.7% for 8th-graders, 1.3% for 10th-graders, and 2.5% for 12th-graders. The annual female adolescent prevalence was 0.3% for 8th-graders, 0.5% for 10th-graders, and 0.3% for 12th-graders.[10]

In an interesting study published in 2014, sexual minority adolescent boys were more likely to report a lifetime use of anabolic steroids than their heterosexual counterparts (21% versus 4%).[11]

From the National Longitudinal Study of Adolescent Health, 15,000 adolescents in grades 7 to 12 were assessed in order to determine the relationship between high school sports participation and the subsequent use of anabolic steroids and legal performance-enhancing dietary supplements. Males had a higher tendency than females to use anabolic steroids and legal supplements, with a positive association between anabolic steroid and supplement use. High school sports participation was associated with use of supplements in young adulthood.[12]

Steroids can be injected, taken orally, or absorbed transdermally. Injectable forms of steroids are more potent and longer lasting. Anabolic steroids often are "stacked," when multiple steroids are taken at the same time and also in 4- to 12-week cycles. The doses often are in a pyramid sequence, with the largest dose at the middle of the cycle. These doses often are 50 to 100 times what would be needed to maintain the normal physiologic level of testosterone. A large black market has developed that creates designer steroids, which are modified to evade detection.

Testing for exogenous testosterone can be accomplished by determining the urinary ratio of testosterone glucuronide to epitestosterone glucuronide. The ratio is normally 1:1 up to 3:1. When a person is taking anabolic steroids, endogenous testosterone glucuronide and epitestosterone glucuronide are suppressed, leaving just the exogenous testosterone. A testosterone to epitestosterone ratio of more than 4:1 is considered positive. Another method of monitoring exogenous testosterone is determination of urine testosterone and luteinizing hormone (LH) levels. Because exogenous testosterone suppresses LH, the ratio of testosterone to LH is high (>30) in those taking anabolic steroids.

There are many adverse effects of anabolic steroids, and some can be serious and long term. Table 2 highlights the major adverse effects.[13] Other adverse effects include hepatotoxicity (jaundice, cancer, and cystic lesions called peliosis hepaticus), hypercoagulability, hypertension, left ventricular hypertrophy, acne, hypercholesterolemia with increased low-density lipoprotein and decreased high-density lipoprotein levels, and increased risk for cerebrovascular accident and acute myocardial infarction. Other risks include those associated with sharing needles, such as hepatitis B and C, human immunodeficiency virus (HIV)/acquired immunodeficiency syndrome (AIDS), endocarditis, local pain, and abscess formation. Steroid abuse among adolescents also can lead to precocious puberty and stunted adult height secondary to premature epiphyseal closure.[14] In men, side effects include dysuria, baldness, gynecomastia, testicular atrophy, decreased sperm production, and even infertility. In women, side effects include masculinization, decreased body fat and breast size, hair loss, and clitoral enlargement. Numerous studies have linked aggression and violence to high-dose steroid abuse with associated increase in fighting, rage, and committing criminal acts.[15] Anabolic steroid withdrawal can lead to restlessness, insomnia, decreased libido, headaches, arthralgias, myalgias, fatigue, decreased appetite, depression, and even suicide.

Table 2

Adverse Effects of Androgenic-Anabolic Steroids and Steroid Precursors

Musculoskeletal
Acne
Muscle hypertrophy
Epiphyseal closure
Increased rate of tendon strains and rupture

Reproductive
Boys/Girls
   Altered libido
Girls
   Deepening of voice due to thickening of vocal cords
   Hypertrophy of the clitoris*
   Hirsutism
   Amenorrhea
   Uterine atrophy
   Breast atrophy
Boys
   Testicular atrophy
   Oligospermia
   Abnormal sperm morphology
   Prostate hypertrophy
   Prostate cancer
   Impotence
   Gynecomastia*

Endocrine
Increased glucose tolerance

Skin
Striae
Hirsutism
Edema
Male pattern baldness

Cardiovascular
Elevated cholesterol
Decreased high-density lipoproteins
Increased blood pressure
Thrombosis

Urinary
Wilms tumor

Immunologic
Decreased immune globulin A

Psychologic
Aggression
Psychosis
Depression
Emotional instability
Addiction
Withdrawal and dependency

Gastrointestinal
Liver tumor-benign hepatoadenoma
Hepatic carcinoma
Peliosis hepatitis
Cholestasis
Gastrointestinal irritation

Infectious
Local wound infection at injection site
Septic arthritis
Hepatitis B or C
HIV infection

---

*Irreversible and permanent
From Dandoy C, Gereige RS. Performance-Enhancing Drugs. *Pediatr Rev.* 2012;33(6):265–271

Steroid Precursors

In the late 1990s and early part of 2000, the use of steroid precursors increased dramatically. These steroid precursors included, but were not limited to, andro-stenedione (also known as "andro"), androstenediol, nor-androstenedione, nor-androstenediol, and dehydroepiandrosterone (DHEA). The efficacy and safety of these prohormones are not well established, but they are promoted as having the same androgenic effects on muscle mass and strength as anabolic-androgenic steroids. Studies[16–19] referenced below demonstrated consistently that acute and long-term administration of these oral testosterone precursors does not effectively increase serum testosterone levels and fails to produce any significant changes in lean body mass, muscle strength, or performance improvement compared with placebo.

DHEA is secreted from the adrenal cortex and then converted to androstenedi-one and androstenediol; this latter substance is then converted to testosterone. Steroid precursors were thought to increase free testosterone, but they have not been shown to do so. Most studies in athletes and in the elderly have revealed that DHEA increases androstenedione and estradiol levels but results in little to no increase in serum testosterone levels[16] or muscle mass and does not lead to improved athletic performance or memory function.[17–19]

Although these AAS precursors have minimal desired effects, they still have many of the negative effects of anabolic steroids (Table 2). In female athletes these substances have an androgenizing influence, including general virilization and male pattern baldness. Males can experience gynecomastia, acne, and testicular atrophy. In both genders, decreased levels of high-density lipoproteins, increased levels of undesirable lipids, and stunted growth can result. Finally, these substances can downregulate endogenous testosterone over time.

In 2005, androstenedione was classified as a schedule III controlled substance. DHEA continues to remain an over-the-counter nutritional supplement. The Dietary Supplement Health and Education Act of 1994 (DSHEA) allows many steroid precursors to be sold over the counter with minimal regulation.[20,21]

Growth Hormone

Human growth hormone has been used by sports competitors for performance enhancement since the 1970s. Human growth hormone is an endogenous hormone produced in the pituitary gland. It is used medically to treat growth hormone deficiency and short stature. Growth hormone may increase lean body mass and decreases fat mass, yet it has limited effect on strength and athletic performance. Adverse effects such as diabetes, cardiomyopathy, hepatitis, and renal failure have occurred with the use of high-dose growth hormone. Currently, hGH is on the World Anti-Doping Agency banned substance list.

There are 2 methods of detection of hGH in the blood. The markers method looks for alterations in the ratios of serum proteins as a result of exogenous hGH. The isoform method looks for alterations in the growth hormone structure.[22-24]

Supplements

Use of nutritional supplements has become increasingly popular among adolescents in the past 18 years.[25] Based on DSHEA legislation, dietary supplements are in a special category under the general umbrella of foods, not drugs. Under DSHEA, dietary supplements do not require FDA approval before they are marketed. The manufacturer is responsible for determining that the dietary supplements it manufactures or distributes are safe without claims that are false or misleading. DSHEA allows dietary supplements to bear statements of support that claim a benefit related to a classic nutrient deficiency disease, and allows the manufacturer to describe how ingredients affect the structure or function of the human body. The manufacturer may characterize the mechanism by which the ingredients act to maintain structure or function, and may specify that well-being may ensue from consumption of the supplements. The statement "calcium builds strong bones and teeth" is said to be a classic example of an allowable structure/function statement for a food. What constitutes an allowable statement for a supplement has not been established either by law or by regulation. To be legal under DSHEA, a nutritional support statement must not be a drug claim, and labels should not suggest that the product or ingredient is intended for prevention or treatment of disease.[26]

If the supplement bears the seal United States Pharmacopeia (USP), this indicates that the manufacturer has voluntarily submitted the product for validation of safety in manufacturing and that the product is pure and it's potency has been verified.

The decision to limit the FDA's regulation of supplements has resulted in a plethora of supplements and the market has exploded. Dietary supplements can be found in health food stores, supermarkets, and even corner convenience stores, leading to easy availability and subsequent high rates of use among adolescents.

In one adult study of military bodybuilders, weight lifters discussed the use of dietary supplements with physicians. They stated that they obtained most of their information on supplements and performance-enhancing substances from reading magazines.[27]

Creatine

Creatine is the most popular nutritional supplement, accounting for $400 million in sales annually. Despite recommendations against creatine use in adolescents younger than 18 years, its use is still common. In 2001, Metzl et al[28] questioned 1103 adolescents and found creatine use in 5.6%. Improved sports performance was cited as the main goal of use in 75% of those teens who used creatine.

Creatine is a nonessential amino acid that is produced in the liver, pancreas, and kidneys. Creatine can be found in meat, milk, and fish, among other foods. It assists in the formation of adenosine triphosphate. The total daily requirement of creatine is 2 g per day. Often, athletes use 2 to 3 times this amount when using creatine for improved sports performance.

Creatine is one of the most popular and widely researched natural supplements. Most studies have focused on the effects of creatine monohydrate on performance and health; however, many other forms of creatine exist and are commercially available in the sports nutrition/supplement market. Creatine has been shown to improve performance in brief, high-intensity exercises, including weight lifting, and to increase strength, fat free mass, and muscle morphology with heavy resistance training. Smaller benefits are found in endurance sports of longer duration. It is important to note that the effects of creatine diminish with longer hours spent training, and not all people have the same outcomes with creatine supplementation. Creatine supplementation increases creatine storage and promotes regeneration of adenosine triphosphate between high-intensity exercises. Technically, this will increase performance and longer training tolerance. Creatine-related adverse effects include weight gain, water retention, gastrointestinal cramping, fatigue, and diarrhea.[29]

Ephedrine/Stimulants

Stimulants such as ephedrine and caffeine are used by adolescent athletes for their ergogenic effects.[30] Stimulants are an attractive ergogenic option because they are widely available, easily accessible, and difficult to detect. Stimulants reduce the perception of fatigue and increase the time to exhaustion. They improve alertness as well as neurocognitive and aerobic performance. Ephedrine has been available in over-the-counter cough and cold remedies.

Ephedra was banned by the FDA in 2004 because of its numerous reported adverse effects, particularly strokes and psychosis. The drug has been implicated in the deaths of several athletes. Since its ban, ephedra has been replaced by other sympathomimetics with similar effects.

Caffeine is used in beverages, energy drinks, and over-the-counter pills. Caffeine for performance enhancement has been reported in 27% of adolescent athletes in the United States. Caffeine produces ergogenic effects at a dose as low as 250 mg (3.0-3.5 mg/kg). Caffeine may be effective for prolonged sports involving short bursts of activity, such as tennis and team sports.[31]

Other stimulants including methamphetamine may be used for performance enhancement. In the Monitoring the Future survey for 2010 and 2011, a representative sample of 8th- and 10th-grade students was surveyed regarding rates of use and motivations for using prescription stimulants, such as dextroamphetamine, for performance enhancement. Among 21,137 adolescent, past-year nonmedical use of Adderall was higher for male respondents who participated in lacrosse and wrestling. No particular sport among females was found to be associated with past-year nonmedical use of Adderall. The authors concluded that certain extracurricular activities, such as high-contact sports, may influence male participants to misuse prescription stimulants as performance enhancers either on or off the playing field.[32]

Beta-Blockers

Fear of performing, or stage fright, is a symptom suffered by many performers. It has been known for more than 30 years that among classical musicians, performance anxiety has affected the efforts of guitarist Andres Segovia, cellist Pablo Casals, and pianists Glenn Gould and Van Cliburn. In the past, the customary treatment for many was a "quick swig of alcohol," which now is not recommended. Today, the treatments include benzodiazepines (eg, diazepam), hypnotherapy, cognitive-behavioral therapy, meditation, and beta-blockers, widely known as the musician's underground drug.

In sports such as golf, archery, and pistol shooting, where a steady hand is critical, beta-blockers provide a performance-enhancing function that combats the normal physiologic tremor that is exacerbated in high-pressure situations.[33-35]

Side effects of beta-blockers include dizziness, fatigue, reactive airway disease, depression, and hypoglycemia.[36]

SUMMARY

Use of performance-enhancing drugs by adolescents is a complex health concern. Our societal drive to excel and to win has to be countered by the need to protect our children from dangerous and unhealthy practices. In order to alter the current use of performance-enhancing drugs by adolescents, we must come to grips with the importance we place on winning and appearance and with the health issues that may accompany these attempts to achieve perfection.[37]

Education of parents, coaches, physicians, and adolescents is paramount. There are existing concerns that medical students, residents, and other trainees receive minimal education in the field of sports medicine during both medical school and residency. An emerging issue for trainees is their education about the substances and supplements chosen by young athletes to improve athletic performance. This instruction should be added to the already existing focus of pediatric sports medicine on proper training and the management of common injuries.

Parents, coaches, physicians, and clinicians should carefully monitor the media and social networking sites for allegations of illicit substance use noted in multiple sports venues such as professional cycling, the Olympics, and Major League Baseball. These topics should be discussed, as they emerge in the media, with teens by parents, coaches, and their healthcare providers.

We know that conversations about the use of performance-enhancing substances range from the pragmatic to the philosophical, including discussions about whether such use is actual cheating or is a legitimate enhancement of human effort.

Beyond these philosophical arguments, the medical community is also concerned about the medical consequences associated with the use of illicit substances as well as supplements. Physicians and other clinicians need to offer alternatives to these practices, such as enhancing physical and psychological performance with adequate exercise, nutrition, sleep, and stress management. As advocates for children and teens, we also need to support sportsmanship, or excellence with integrity, rather than winning at all costs.[38]

RECOMMENDATIONS FOR PHYSICIANS

1. Open communication is mandatory with athletes, coaches and parents, since prevention begins in the community.
2. Provide up-to-date information regarding myths that adolescent athletes are exposed to on the Internet, in gyms, and in locker rooms.

3. Steer teens toward Web sites that provide information on supplements and other performance-enhancing supplements that is current and evidence based.
4. Speak to teachers, parents, and coaches about this information and be available to them for lectures, discussions, and forums on the use of performance-enhancing substances.

RESOURCES

http://www.drugfreesport.com
http://www.wada-ama.org
http://playhealthy.drugfree.org/
http://www.truesport.org
http://www.olympic.org/medical-commission?tab=medical-code

References

1. Goldman B, Klatz R. *Death in the Locker Room II: Drugs and Sports.* Chicago: Elite Sports Medicine Publications; 1992:23–24
2. Bamberger M, Yaeger D. Over the edge: special report. *Sports Illustrated.* 1997;86:64
3. Reider B. Now and Later. *Am J Sports Med.* 2008;36(9):1673–1674
4. Grivetti LE, Applegate EA. From Olympia to Atlanta: a cultural historical perspective on diet and athletic training. *J Nutr.* 1997;127(Suppl):860–868
5. Brown-Séquard CE. Note on the effects produced on man by subcutaneous injections of a liquid obtained from the testicles of animals. *Lancet.* 1889;2:105–107
6. Dotson JL, Brown RT. The history of the development of anabolic-androgenic steroids. *Pediatr Clin North Am.* 2007;54:761–769
7. American Academy of Pediatrics Committee on Sports Medicine and Fitness. Adolescents and anabolic steroids: a subject review. *Pediatrics.* 1997;99:904–908
8. Calfee R, Fadale P. Popular ergogenic drugs and supplements in young athletes. popular ergogenic drugs and supplements in young athletes. *Pediatrics.* 2006;117;e577–e589
9. Eaton DK, Kann L, Kinchen S, et al; Centers for Disease Control and Prevention. Youth risk behavior surveillance—United States, 2009. *MMWR Surveill Summ.* 2010;59(5):1–142
10. Johnston LD, O'Malley PM, Bachman G, Schulenberg JE. *Monitoring the Future National Results on Adolescent Drug Use: Overview of Key Findings, 2010.* Ann Arbor, MI: Institute for Social Research, The University of Michigan; 2011:77
11. Blashill AJ, Safren SA. Sexual orientation and anabolic androgenic steroids in US adolescent boys. *Pediatrics.* 2014;133(3):859–866
12. Dodge TL, Jaccard JJ. The effect of high school sports participation on the use of performance-enhancing substances in young adulthood. *J Adolesc Health.* 2006;39(3):367–373
13. Dandoy C, Gereige RS. Performance enhancing drugs. *Pediatr Rev.* 2012;33;265–272
14. Hartgens F, Kuipers H. Effects of androgenic-anabolic steroids in athletes. *Sports Med.* 2004;34:513–554
15. Fainaru-Wada M. Dreams, steroids, death: a ballplayer's downfall. *San Francisco Chronicle.* December 19, 2004:A1
16. Labrie F. DHEA, important source of sex steroids in men and even more in women. *Prog Brain Res.* 2010;182:97–148
17. Smurawa TM, Congeni JA. Testosterone precursors: use and abuse in pediatric athletes. *Pediatr Clin North Am.* 2007;54(4):787–796

18. Grimley Evans J, Malouf R, Huppert F, van Niekerk JK. Dehydroepiandrosterone (DHEA) supplementation for cognitive function in healthy elderly people. *Cochrane Database Syst Rev.* 2006;4:CD006221

19. Liu TC, Lin CH, Huang CY, Ivy JL, Kuo CH. Effect of acute DHEA administration on free testosterone in middle-aged and young men following high-intensity interval training. *Eur J Appl Physiol.* 2013;113(7):1783–1792

20. Fish L, Goldberg L, Spratt D. Supplements, steroid precursors, and adolescent health. *J Clin Endocrinol Metab.* 2005:90(9):1

21. Powers M. The safety and efficacy of anabolic steroid precursors: what is the scientific evidence? *J Athl Train.* 2002;37(3):300–305

22. Liu H, Bravata DM, Olkin I, et al. Systematic review: the effects of growth hormone on athletic performance. *Ann Intern Med.* 2008;148(10):747–758

23. Holt RI, Sönksen PH. Growth hormone, IGF-I and insulin and their abuse in sport. *Br J Pharmacol.* 2008;154(3):542–556

24. Hoffman JR, Kraemer WJ, Bhasin S, et al. Position stand on androgen and human growth hormone use. *J Strength Cond Res.* 2009;23(5 Suppl):S1–S59

25. Wu CH, Wang CC, Kennedy J. The prevalence of herb and dietary supplement use among children and adolescents in the United States: results from the 2007 National Health Interview Survey. *Complement Ther Med.* 2013;21(4):358–363

26. US Food and Drug Administration. Dietary Supplements. Available at: www.fda.gov/food/dietarysupplements. Accessed December 8, 2013

27. Kao TC, Deuster PA, Burnett D, Stephens M. Health behaviors associated with use of body building, weight loss, and performance enhancing supplements. *Ann Epidemiol.* 2012;22(5):331–339

28. Metzl JD, Small E, Levine SR, Gershel JC. Creatine use among young athletes. *Pediatrics.* 2001;108(2):421–425

29. Cooper R, Naclerio F, Allgrove J, Jimenez A. Creatine supplementation with specific view to exercise/sports performance: an update. *J Int Soc Sports Nutr.* 2012;9(1):9–33

30. Lattavo A, Kopperud A, Rogers PD. Creatine and other supplements. *Pediatr Clin North Am.* 2007;54(4):735–760

31. Ganio MS, Klau JF, Casa DJ, Armstrong LE, Maresh CM. Effect of caffeine on sport-specific endurance performance: a systematic review. *J Strength Cond Res.* 2009;23(1):315–324

32. Veliz P, Boyd C, McCabe SE. Adolescent athletic participation and nonmedical Adderall use: an exploratory analysis of a performance-enhancing drug. *J Stud Alcohol Drugs.* 2009;70(6):919–923

33. Lardon MT. Performance-enhancing drugs: where should the line be drawn and by whom? *Psychiatry (Edgmont).* 2008;5(7):58–61

34. Kruse P, Ladefoged J, Nielson U, et al. Beta-blockade used in precision sports: effect on pistol shooting performance. *J Appl Physiol.* 1986;61:417–420

35. Juhlin-Dannfelt A. Beta-adrenoceptor blockade and exercise: effects on endurance and physical training. *Acta Med Scand Suppl.* 1983;67:249–254

36. Barron AJ, Zaman N, Cole GD, et al. Systematic review of genuine versus spurious side-effects of beta-blockers in heart failure using placebo control: recommendations for patient information. *J Cardiol.* 2013;168(4):3572–3579

37. Yesalis CE, Bahrke MS. Doping among adolescent athletes. *Best Pract Res Clin Endocrinol Metab.* 2000;14(1):25–35

38. Greely H, Campbell P, Sahakian B, et al. Towards responsible use of cognitive-enhancing drugs by the healthy. *Scholarly Commons: Repository.* Available at: repository.upenn.edu/neuroethics_pubs/42. Accessed December 1, 2013

Adolesc Med 025 (2014) 126–156

Screening and Brief Intervention for Alcohol and Other Abuse

Sion Kim Harris, PhD, CPH[a*]; Jennifer Louis-Jacques, MD, MPH[b]; John R. Knight, MD[a]

[a]Center for Adolescent Substance Abuse Research, Boston Children's Hospital, Boston, Massachusetts;
[b]Craig Dalsimer Division of Adolescent Medicine, The Children's Hospital of Philadelphia, Philadelphia, Pennsylvania

INTRODUCTION

Substance abuse continues to be one of the leading public health problems in the United States.[1] More than 400,000 preventable deaths have been linked to substance use.[2] In addition, the treatment of associated medical and mental health problems places a major burden on the health care system.[2] In 2006, the total estimated societal costs of alcohol and drug use disorders reached more than $2 hundred billion.[3,4] Therefore, there is great need for a comprehensive public health approach to address substance abuse.

Most substance use begins during adolescence and young adulthood, with half of all lifetime cases of disorders developing by age 20.[5] Therefore, strategies for prevention, early identification, and interventions that target this age group are the logical ways to reduce costs and gain productive years of life. Interest in an integrated approach called Screening, Brief Intervention, and Referral to Treatment (SBIRT) has grown in recent years as a means to bridge the gap between universal prevention programs and specialty substance abuse treatment.[6,7] Facilitated by the development of rapid screening and assessment tools, physicians can quickly identify those patients who are using substances and assess the extent of their use, provide an immediate brief intervention (BI), and determine whether there is a need for follow-up or referral to treatment (RT).[8] Extensive research evidence supports the effectiveness of SBIRT for addressing hazardous alcohol use among adults seen in medical settings.[9-12] Based on the accumulated

*Corresponding author:
sion.harris@childrens.harvard.edu

evidence,[9] the US Preventive Services Task Force (USPSTF) recently renewed its recommendation that primary care physicians provide screening and brief counseling interventions to reduce alcohol misuse among nontreatment-seeking adults.[13] However, the USPSTF cited *insufficient evidence* ("I" grade) to recommend for or against screening and brief counseling for illicit drug use or medication misuse because of the relative paucity of studies in this area.[14]

Citing a similar lack of sufficient evidence, the USPSTF maintained an "I" grade for screening and brief counseling for adolescents in its updated recommendation statement.[13] However, recognition of and evidence for the potential utility of SBIRT for adolescents have been building in recent years. Initial research tended to concentrate on adolescent and young adult emergency department (ED) patients[15–18] and on college students.[19,20] Now, more research is focusing on the primary care setting because primary care offices offer ideal settings for implementing SBIRT with adolescents as part of a comprehensive public health strategy.[21,22] More than 80% of adolescents see a primary care physician yearly,[23] and many have established with their physicians trusting relationships that can be leveraged.[24]

Recognizing the important role that pediatricians can play in addressing adolescent substance use, the American Academy of Pediatrics (AAP) and the National Institute on Alcohol Abuse and Alcoholism (NIAAA) recommend that all pediatricians use SBIRT in their practices as part of routine care. Both the recent AAP policy statement on adolescent SBIRT[25] and the NIAAA guide on Alcohol Screening and Brief Intervention for Youth[26] offer physicians specific algorithm-based approaches for detecting and preventing adolescent alcohol and drug abuse in general medical settings. Physicians often note numerous barriers to screening in the office setting; the 2 most common are a lack of time and a lack of training to appropriately manage a positive screen.[27] These guides provide a structured method and brief practical tools that were derived from the accumulated evidence base and designed to be feasible for the busy physician. The objective of this report is to describe these new guidelines and present an updated review of the research available regarding adolescent substance abuse screening and BI in general medical settings. This review includes findings from a systematic electronic literature search conducted in December 2013 using PubMed and PsycINFO, as well as the reference lists of published studies and review articles.[18,21,22,28–31]

SCREENING

Adolescent self-report of substance use, within the context of a confidential assessment, is reliable[32,33] and compares favorably against bioassay results.[34–38] Therefore, physicians should begin asking adolescents about substance use and other sensitive questions as soon as the young person is old enough to be interviewed without the parent being present. No specific minimum age is given in either the AAP SBIRT or the Bright Futures child and adolescent health supervision guidelines[25,39] because the exact age will vary from patient to patient; it likely falls between 11 and 13 years for most adolescents. However, the NIAAA guide recommends screening children for alcohol use as young as age 9 years because 1 in 5 adolescents reports initiating drinking before the age of 13 years.[40] To begin the screening with younger patients (elementary and middle school-aged students), the NIAAA guide recommends starting with asking about friends' use as a nonthreatening way of opening the discussion about alcohol. Peer use is a strong risk factor for initiation of use, and a positive response presents an opportunity for anticipatory guidance to prevent initiation.[41,42]

After beginning with meeting the parent and adolescent together and reviewing the ground rules of confidentiality, the physician should ask the parent to leave the room in order to ask the adolescent personal questions.[43] In addition, before screening, the physician should emphasize that the details discussed will remain confidential unless he or she has acute safety concerns about the patient or others.[43] Screening for substance use should be considered during every clinical encounter throughout adolescence, even at sick visits, because adolescents who present for sick visits have been found to have higher rates of substance use problems than those who present for well-care visits.[44]

There are 3 main goals of screening within the SBIRT approach. The first is to determine whether a teen has used any alcohol or drugs, because *any* substance use, particularly among younger adolescents, is of concern. Substantial evidence indicates that earlier initiation of use increases the risk for addiction and associated physical and psychosocial health risks.[45-47] The second is to determine where the teens are located on the substance use spectrum (Table 1) and their level of risk (low, moderate, or high) for a substance use disorder, which then informs the physician's response. Third, screening provides a way for physicians to initiate a brief discussion with their teenage patients about substance use so that they can provide education and advice. As the AAP policy statement notes, screening is not sufficient to determine a diagnosis; this requires further assessment and history-taking.[25] Within the SBIRT algorithm, the screening step is intended to be a rapid, highly sensitive (ie, able to detect as many true-positive results as possible) decision support tool that informs next steps. For an initial screen, high sensitivity is preferred, even at the expense of lower specificity (ie, more false-positive results), to avoid missing anyone who may be at risk. False-positive results can be clarified with further assessment, whereas false-negative results represent a missed opportunity for early intervention and secondary prevention.

The ideal screening instrument for general medical settings must be brief and simple to score, developmentally appropriate for adolescents, assess all major substances of abuse, and accurately convey risk levels that will guide physician response. A structured screening tool with demonstrated reliability and validity among adolescents provides more accurate detection of adolescent substance abuse than tools developed for adults (eg, the CAGE) or a physician's own clinical impression, which often is wrong.[8,48,49] Table 2 lists the screening tools that cur-

Table 1
Substance use spectrum and goals for office intervention

Stage	Description	Office intervention goals
Abstinence	The time before an individual has ever used drugs or alcohol (more than a few sips)	Prevent or delay initiation of substance use through positive reinforcement and patient/parent education
Experimentation	The first 1-2 times that a substance is used and the adolescent wants to know how intoxication from using a drug(s) feels	Promote patient strengths; encourage abstinence and cessation through brief, clear medical advice and educational counseling
Limited use	Use together with ≥1 friends in relatively low-risk situations and without related problems; typically, use occurs at predictable times such as weekends	Promote patient strengths; further encourage cessation through brief, clear medical advice and educational counseling
Problematic use	Use in a high-risk situation, such as when driving or babysitting; use associated with a problem such as a fight, arrest, or school suspension; or use for emotional regulation such as to relieve stress or depression	As stated above, plus initiate office visits or referral for brief intervention to enhance motivation to make behavioral changes; provide close patient follow-up; consider breaking confidentiality
Abuse	Drug use associated with recurrent problems or that interferes with functioning	Continue as stated above, plus enhance motivation to make behavioral changes by exploring ambivalence and triggering preparation for action; monitor closely for progression to alcohol and other drug addiction; refer to comprehensive assessment and treatment; consider breaking confidentiality
Addiction (dependence)	Loss of control or compulsive drug use	As stated above, plus enhance motivation to accept referral to subspecialty treatment if necessary; consider breaking confidentiality; encourage parental involvement whenever possible

From American Academy of Pediatrics Committee on Substance Abuse. Substance use screening, brief intervention, and referral to treatment for pediatricians. *Pediatrics.* 2011;128(5):e1330–e1340.

rently hold the most promise for use in general medical settings. They all are brief, easy to administer and score, and delineate levels of risk for disorder. They can be administered alone or within the context of a more comprehensive psychosocial assessment, such as HEADSS (Home, Education, Activities, Drugs/Alcohol, Sex, Suicidality)[50] or SSHADESS (Strengths, School, Home, Activities, Drugs/Substance use, Emotions/Depression, Sexuality, Safety).[51] Also, these screens may be efficiently administered on paper or computer before the visit with the physician. A study of preferences for screening method among adolescent primary care patients found that they preferred, and reported being more likely to respond honestly on, a paper or computer questionnaire over a doctor or nurse interview.[52] Each of the tools listed in Table 2 is described in greater detail later.

Table 2
Adolescent substance problem screening tools

Tool (scoring; criteria for positive screen)	
Alcohol/drug screen	
CRAFFT[a] (each "yes" = 1 point on C,R,A,F,F,T items; ≥2 indicates high risk for substance use disorder)	*Introductory quick-screen for ANY use:* During the **past 12 months**, did you… 1. Drink any <u>alcohol</u> (more than a few sips)? (Do not count sips of alcohol taken during family or religious events.) 2. Smoke any <u>marijuana or hashish</u>? 3. Use <u>anything else</u> to <u>get high</u>? ("anything else" includes illegal, over-the-counter, and prescription drugs, and things that you sniff or "huff") *Question for ALL regardless of use:* 1. Have you ever ridden in a <u>C</u>AR driven by someone (including yourself) who was "high" or had been using alcohol or drugs? *Follow-up questions for those with ANY use:* 2. Do you ever use alcohol or drugs to <u>R</u>ELAX, feel better about yourself, or fit in? 3. Do you ever use alcohol or drugs while you are by yourself, or <u>A</u>LONE? 4. Do you ever <u>F</u>ORGET things you did while using alcohol or drugs? 5. Do your <u>F</u>AMILY or FRIENDS ever tell you that you should cut down on your drinking or drug use? 6. Have you ever gotten into <u>T</u>ROUBLE while you were using alcohol or drugs?
Alcohol screens	
AUDIT-C (≥5 for disorder)	1. How often do you have a drink containing alcohol? (0 = never; 1 = monthly or less; 2 = 2-4×/month; 3 = 2-3×/week; 4 = ≥4×/week) 2. How many standard drinks do you have on a typical day when you are drinking? (0 = 1 or 2; 1 = 3 or 4; 2 = 5 or 6; 3 = 7-9; 4 = 10 or more) 3. How often do you have 6 or more drinks on one occasion? (0 = never; 1 = less than monthly; 2 = monthly; 3 = weekly; 4 = daily or almost daily)
AUDIT[b] Among 14- to 18-year-olds: ≥2 for problem, ≥3 for disorder[c] Among 18- to 20-year-olds: ≥5 for males, ≥4 for females for disorder[d]	Items 1-3 above and the following: 4. How often during the last year did you find that you were unable to stop drinking once you had started? (Response scale for items 4-8: 0 = never; 1 = less than monthly; 2 = monthly; 3 = weekly; 4 = daily or almost daily) 5. How often during the last year did you fail to do what you were expected to do because of drinking? 6. How often during the last year did you need a drink in the morning after a heavy drinking session to get yourself going? 7. How often during the last year did you feel guilty or remorseful after drinking? 8. How often during the last year were you unable to remember what happened the night before because of drinking? 9. Have you or someone else been injured as a result of your drinking? (Response scale for items 9-10: 0 = no; 2 = yes, but not in the last year; 4 = yes, during the last year) 10. Has a relative or friend, or a doctor or other health care worker been concerned about your drinking or suggested you cut down?

NIAAA screening guide[e] (≤11-year-olds: any drinking is highest risk 12- to 15-year-olds: 1-5 days = moderate risk; 6+ days = highest risk 16-year-olds: 6-11 days = moderate risk; 12+ days = highest risk 17-year-olds: 6-23 days = moderate risk; 24+ days = highest risk 18-year-olds: 12-51 days = moderate risk; 52+ days = highest risk)

Elementary school age (9-11 years):
1. Do you have any friends who drank beer, wine, or any drink containing alcohol in the **past year**?
2. How about you—have you **ever** had more than a few sips of beer, wine, or any drink containing alcohol?

Middle school age (11-14 years):
1. Do you have any friends who drank beer, wine, or any drink containing alcohol in the **past year**?
2. How about you—in the **past year,** on **how many days** have you had more than a few sips of beer, wine, or any drink containing alcohol?

High school age (14-18 years):
1. In the **past year,** on **how many days** have you had more than a few sips of beer, wine, or any drink containing alcohol?
2. If your friends drink, **how many drinks** do they usually drink on an occasion?

Drug screen

Single-question screener for drug use[f] (≥1 time)

1. How many times in the past year have you used an illegal drug or used a prescription medication for nonmedical reasons (eg, for the experience or feeling it caused)?

Drug Abuse Screening Test-10,[g] modified for college students[h] (each "yes" = 1 point; 1-2 = low risk; 3-5 = moderate risk; 6-10 = high risk)

1. Have you used drugs other than those needed for medical reasons?
2. Have you used more than one drug at a time?
3. Are you always able to stop using drugs when you want to? (reverse score: no = 1, yes = 0)
4. Have you had "blackouts" or "flashbacks" as a result of drug use?
5. Have you ever felt bad or guilty about your drug use?
6. Have family members ever complained about your using drugs?
7. Have you ever stayed away from your family because of your drug use?
8. Have you engaged in illegal activities in order to obtain drugs?
9. Have you ever experienced withdrawal symptoms (felt sick) when you stopped taking drugs?
10. Have you had medical problems as a result of your drug use (eg, memory loss, hepatitis, convulsions, bleeding)?

[a]Knight JR, Shrier LA, Bravender TD, et al. A new brief screen for adolescent substance abuse. *Arch Pediatr Adolesc Med.* 1999;153(6):591–596. © 2013, John R. Knight, MD, Boston Children's Hospital. Used with permission.

[b]Babor TF, Higgins-Biddle JC, Saunders JB, Monteiro MG. *AUDIT: The alcohol use disorders identification test: guidelines for use in primary health care.* 2nd ed. Geneva, Switzerland: World Health Organization, Department of Mental Health and Substance Dependence; 2001

[c]Knight JR, Sherritt L, Harris SK, Gates EC, Chang G. Validity of brief alcohol screening tests among adolescents: a comparison of the AUDIT, POSIT, CAGE, and CRAFFT. *Alcohol Clin Exp Res.* 2003;27(1):67–73

[d]Kelly TM, Donovan JE, Chung T, et al. Brief screens for detecting alcohol use disorder among 18-20 year old young adults in emergency departments: comparing AUDIT-C, CRAFFT, RAPS4-QF, FAST, RUFT-Cut, and DSM-IV 2-Item Scale. *Addict Behav.* 2009;34(8):668–674

[e]National Institute on Alcohol Abuse and Alcoholism. *Alcohol screening and brief intervention for youth: practitioner's guide.* Washington, DC: National Institutes of Health, Department of Health and Human Services; 2011

[f]Smith PC, Schmidt SM, Allensworth-Davies D, Saitz R. A single-question screening test for drug use in primary care. *Arch Intern Med.* 2010;170(13):1155–1160

[g]Skinner H. The drug abuse screening test. *Addict Behav.* 1982;7:363–371

[h]McCabe SE, Boyd CJ, Cranford JA, Morales M, Slayden J. A modified version of the Drug Abuse Screening Test among undergraduate students. *J Subst Abuse Treat.* 2006;31(3):297–303

CRAFFT

The CRAFFT tool is a substance abuse screener specifically designed for use with adolescents to screen for both alcohol and drug use. It is brief enough to be practical for busy medical settings, is easy to remember using the CRAFFT mnemonic, and is simple to score (1 point for each "yes" answer).[53] It is the screening tool most thoroughly studied, with a recent review paper reporting 11 studies of its validity and 6 of its reliability among adolescents and young adults ages 12 to 26 years.[54] It has evidence of reliability and validity in multiple languages,[33,54,55] including Spanish,[56] Czech,[57] French,[58] and German,[59] as well as in diverse populations.[60-62] The CRAFFT is currently the most widely recommended tool for screening adolescents and is recommended in both the AAP policy statement and the NIAAA guide.

In the AAP SBIRT algorithm, the CRAFFT screen consists of 2 components: an initial set of 3 opening questions that ask about any past-12-month alcohol, cannabis, or other drug use and help to quickly determine how the screening and BI will proceed (Figure 1), and the 6 questions referred to by the mnemonic CRAFFT (Car, Relax, Alone, Forget, Family/friends, and Trouble; see Table 2). The opening questions were added by Knight et al[55] after the initial CRAFFT validation study in order to capture any substance *use* and to create efficiency in the screening process for adolescents who have never used. In a recent study of adolescent primary care patients, these initial past-12-month use questions, whether computer self-administered or physician-administered, were found to have moderate to strong criterion validity compared to a confidential Timeline Follow-Back calendar interview administered by a trained research assistant.[63] The responses to these opening questions dictate how the screening proceeds. Those who respond "no" to all 3 questions are additionally asked only the "C" (car) question about substance-related driving or riding risk. The screening continues with the remaining 5 questions (RAFFT) for adolescents who report any past-12-month use. All "yes" responses on the 6 CRAFFT items are then summed for a total score. Most CRAFFT validation studies have found a score of 2 or more to be the optimal cut point for identifying adolescents aged 18 years or younger with an alcohol or drug use disorder,[8,55,57,59-61] with sensitivities ranging from 0.68 to 1.00 and specificities from 0.33 to 0.97. Two studies by Kelly et al[64,65] examined the CRAFFT among 18- to 20-year-old ED patients and found the best cut point to be a score of 3 or more (sensitivity 0.82, specificity 0.67),[64] suggesting a slightly higher cut point for young adults compared to youth younger than 18 years. Studies to date have given no indication that there should be a different cut point by gender.

Unique to the CRAFFT is the "car" question. Motor vehicle-related injury is a leading cause of mortality and morbidity among adolescents and young adults worldwide.[66] Therefore, the car question should be asked regardless of past-year substance use because nonusing teenagers can be passengers in vehicles driven

Adolescent SBIRT Opening Questions

During the past 12 months, did you:
1. Drink any alcohol (more than a few sips)? **2.** Smoke any marijuana or hashish? **3.** Use anything else to get high?
("Anything else" includes illegal drugs, over the counter and prescription drugs, and things that you sniff or "huff.")

No to all

Yes to any

Praise and Encouragement
"You have made some very good decisions in your choice not to use drugs and alcohol. I hope you keep it up."
CRAFT "CAR" Question

If Yes to CAR

"Please don't ever ride with a driver who has had even a single drink, because people can feel that it's safe to drive even when it's not."
Offer a Contract for Life:
www.sadd.org/contract.htm

Administer CRAFFT
C = Have you ever ridden in a **CAR** driven by someone (including yourself) who was "high" or had been using alcohol or drugs?
R = Do you ever use alcohol or drugs to **RELAX**, feel better about yourself, or fit in?
A = Do you ever use alcohol or drugs while you are by yourself, or **ALONE**?
F = Do you ever **FORGET** things you did while using alcohol or drugs?
F = Do your family or **FRIENDS** ever tell you that you should cut down on your drinking or drug use?
T = Have you ever gotten into **TROUBLE** while you were using alcohol or drugs?

Brief Advice
"I recommend that you stop (drinking/smoking) and now is the best time. Alcohol/drugs kill brain cells and can make you do stupid things that you will regret. You are such a good (student/friend/athlete). I would hate to see anything interfere with your future."

CRAFFT = 0 or 1

CRAFFT ≥ 2

Brief Assessment
Tell me about your alcohol/substance use. Has it caused you any problems? Have you tried to quit? Why?

No Signs of Acute Danger or Addiction

Signs of Addiction

Signs of Acute Danger

Brief Negotiated Interview to stop or cut down.
Give brief advice and summary.
"As your physician, I recommend that you quit drinking entirely for the sake of your health and your brain, but we both know that decision is up to you. You said that all of your friends drink and you enjoy drinking at parties; on the other hand, you recently had a blackout and are not sure how you got home that night. What are your plans regarding alcohol use in the future?"
Give praise and encouragement of willing to quit. Plan follow-up.
"It sounds like you have already started thinking about how alcohol use is affecting your life and that it would be a really smart decision to cut down. Would you be willing to quit drinking entirely for one month and then check in again with me?"
If unwilling to quit, encourage to cut down. Plan follow-up.
"OK, it sounds like you're not willing to quit entirely, but you do want to cut down. Are you willing to limit yourself to one drink when you are at a party to make sure you don't have another blackout? I'd like you to come back in one month to see how that goes.

≤ 14 years, daily or near daily use of any substance, CRAFFT ≥ 5, alcohol related blackouts (memory lapses):
Refer to treatment.
Summarize
"I hear you saying that you depend on marijuana to help you concentrate and relax. You are frustrated because you are fighting with your parents all of the time and you were suspended from school. You tried quitting for a while, but that didn't last long. I am worried that you may be losing control over marijuana."
Refer
"I would like you to speak to someone to think more about the role marijuana is playing in your life, and the impact it could have on your future."
Invite parents
"Let's tell your parents that you have agreed to talk to someone about marijuana. They already know you use, and in my experience parents are usually relieved when their child agrees to speak to someone. I don't plan on saying much else, but is there anything you would like to be sure I keep confidential?"

Drug-related hospital visits; use of IV drugs; combining alcohol use with benzodiazepines, barbiturates or opiates; consuming potentially lethal volume of alcohol (14 or more drinks); driving after substance use.

Make an Immediate Intervention

Contract for safety:
"I am really worried about your drinking. Could you agree not to drink at all this weekend until you speak with your counselor/me again on Monday?"
Consider breaking confidentiality to ask parents to monitor and insure follow-through:
"I am going to tell your parents about our agreement so that they can support you."

Fig 1. AAP SBIRT algorithm. (From American Academy of Pediatrics Committee on Substance Abuse. Substance use screening, brief intervention, and referral to treatment for pediatricians. *Pediatrics.* 2011;128(5):e1330-e1340.)

by impaired drivers and thus be at risk. Because the car question can be positive for teens who do not use substances, this item tends to make CRAFFT's internal consistency reliability lower in comparison to other screening tools.[54,59] The recommended next step based on responses to the car and other screen items are described in the BI section.

Alcohol Use Disorders Identification Test

The Alcohol Use Disorders Identification Test (AUDIT) is another widely used brief screening tool that can be self- or interviewer-administered and has evidence for reliability and validity among adolescents.[8,59,67–69] Along with the CRAFFT, it is recommended by the NIAAA guide as a brief assessment tool for further clarifying an adolescent's need for referral and treatment after a rapid initial risk screen. Consisting of 10 items (see Table 2), it was developed by the World Health Organization[70,71] specifically to help identify problem drinking in primary care settings. However, because it solely targets alcohol, its utility is limited for situations where a comprehensive substance use screen is needed. Whereas studies of adults ages 18 years and older have generally used a sum score of 8 or more to indicate an alcohol use disorder (AUD), there is less agreement on a clear cut point across studies of adolescents.[69] Knight et al[8] found the optimal cut point to be 3 for detecting alcohol abuse or dependence (sensitivity = 0.88; specificity = 0.77) and 2 for identifying any drinking problem (sensitivity = 0.88, specificity = 0.81) among adolescent primary care patients aged 14 to 18 years. Among adolescents aged 13 to 19 years seen in the ED, Chung et al[67] found an optimal cut point of 4 for identifying a *Diagnostic and Statistical Manual of Mental Disorders* Fourth Edition (DSM-IV)–based AUD (sensitivity = 0.94; specificity = 0.80). However, they lowered the threshold for item 3 (frequency of ≥6 on 1 occasion) to 5 or more drinks.

Because the AUDIT's multiple response scales can be unwieldy for use in busy medical settings, researchers have examined various abbreviated versions, including the AUDIT-3 (item 3 only),[72] AUDIT-C (items 1-3),[73] and FAST (items 3, 5, 8, and 10),[74] as alternatives to the full AUDIT. AUDIT-C is the most widely tested of these short forms.[69,73,75–77] The 3 consumption items allow physicians to identify patients with dangerous drinking behaviors as well as active AUDs. In a meta-analysis of 14 adult studies directly comparing AUDIT-C with AUDIT in primary care settings, Kriston et al[77] found no significant differences in test characteristics (ie, sensitivity, specificity, positive and negative likelihood ratios) between the 2 in identifying unhealthy drinking (ie, risky drinking patterns or AUD). However, the full AUDIT tended to have higher specificity and positive likelihood ratios than AUDIT-C at similar levels of sensitivity, suggesting that the full AUDIT may be more accurate at assessing treatment need. AUDIT-C cut point scores with the best balance of sensitivity/specificity for detecting risky drinking or a current disorder in these studies tended to be 4 to 5 for men, and 3 to 4 for women.[69,77] Few studies to date have examined the performance of any

AUDIT short form among adolescents. McCambridge and Thomas[78] found that items 3, 4, 5, and 8 explained the most variance in total AUDIT scores among a Web-recruited sample of 16- to 24-year-olds, and existing AUDIT short forms such as the AUDIT-C were not superior to other possible combinations in predicting total AUDIT scores. Instead, they found that the combination of 3, 5, and 8 (1 item each on consumption, dependence, and problems) accounted for 82.3% of variance in full AUDIT scores (compared to 64.4% for AUDIT-C) and, at scores of 3 or more, had 87% sensitivity, 92% specificity, and correctly classified 89% of individuals with positive AUDIT screens (score ≥8). An optimal cut point of 3 or more was also found for AUDIT-C among 13- to 19-year-old ED patients,[79] whereas a study of 18- to 20-year-old ED patients found optimal cut points of 6 for males and 5 for females.[65]

NIAAA Screen

Recognizing the time pressures faced by busy physicians today, the NIAAA screen reflects the search for even briefer tools, such as a single consumption item,[80–82] to rapidly determine risk level and inform next steps (Figure 2). The NIAAA screen consists of 2 questions (a consumption item [use frequency] and a friends' use item) that differ slightly based on target age group (ie, elementary, middle, high school-age; see Table 2). The past-year frequency item (number of days of drinking) was selected over the past-30-day number of drinks per day and number of days of heavy episodic drinking (≥5 drinks on an occasion) because of better performance (highest area under the curve) in predicting any past-year AUD or AUD symptom in a large, nationally representative sample of adolescents aged 12 to 18 years.[80] However, the optimal cut points for the number of drinking days were found to vary by age and gender, resulting in the different thresholds for moderate and high risk across age-gender groups that are found in the NIAAA guide (see Table 2). The friends' use item serves both to facilitate opening a discussion about alcohol with younger adolescents as well as to identify youth at risk for any drinking and risky drinking, because peer drinking is one of the strongest predictors of adolescent drinking behavior.[83] Studies currently are underway to evaluate the psychometric properties of this screening tool.[84]

Drug Problem Screening

Among instruments assessing drug use problems, the Drug Abuse Screening Test is one of the oldest and most well studied.[85] Developed in 1982, the original Drug Abuse Screening Test[86] consists of 28 yes/no items that assess drug abuse and dependence symptoms as well as receipt of previous drug abuse treatment. A number of alternate versions have been developed and tested, including a modified 27-item version for adolescents (DAST-A),[87] on which a score of 7 or more was found to have the best test characteristics (positive predictive value of 82.3%, sensitivity 78.6%, and specificity 84.5%) for predicting a DSM-IV drug

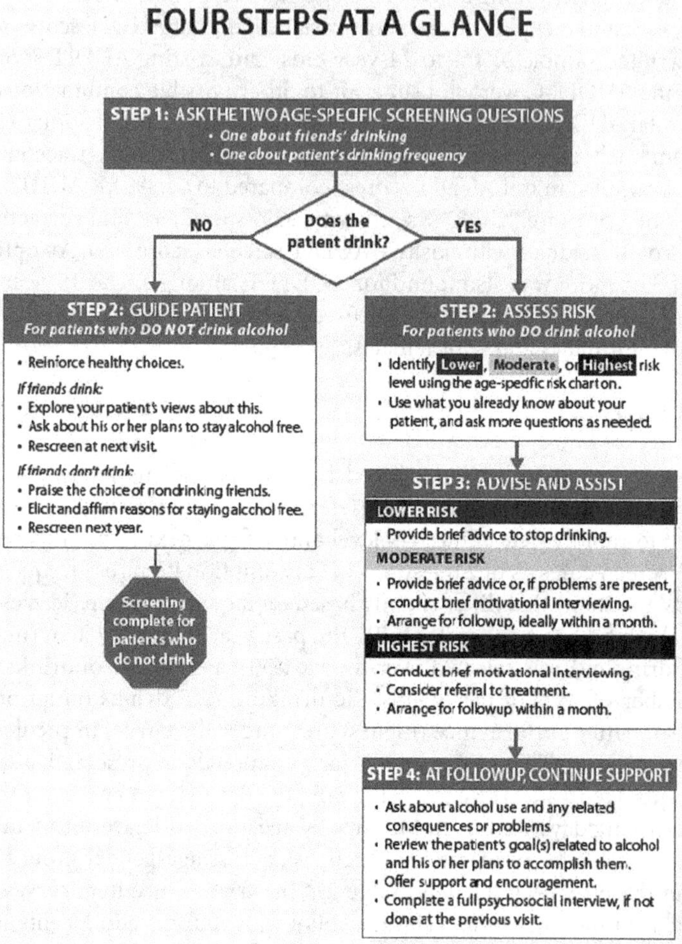

FOUR STEPS AT A GLANCE

STEP 1: ASK THE TWO AGE-SPECIFIC SCREENING QUESTIONS
- One about friends' drinking
- One about patient's drinking frequency

Does the patient drink?   NO   YES

STEP 2: GUIDE PATIENT
For patients who DO NOT drink alcohol

- Reinforce healthy choices.

If friends drink:
- Explore your patient's views about this.
- Ask about his or her plans to stay alcohol free.
- Rescreen at next visit.

If friends don't drink:
- Praise the choice of nondrinking friends.
- Elicit and affirm reasons for staying alcohol free.
- Rescreen next year.

Screening complete for patients who do not drink

STEP 2: ASSESS RISK
For patients who DO drink alcohol

- Identify Lower, Moderate, or Highest risk level using the age-specific risk chart on.
- Use what you already know about your patient, and ask more questions as needed.

STEP 3: ADVISE AND ASSIST

LOWER RISK
- Provide brief advice to stop drinking.

MODERATE RISK
- Provide brief advice or, if problems are present, conduct brief motivational interviewing.
- Arrange for followup, ideally within a month.

HIGHEST RISK
- Conduct brief motivational interviewing.
- Consider referral to treatment.
- Arrange for followup within a month.

STEP 4: AT FOLLOWUP, CONTINUE SUPPORT
- Ask about alcohol use and any related consequences or problems
- Review the patient's goal(s) related to alcohol and his or her plans to accomplish them.
- Offer support and encouragement.
- Complete a full psychosocial interview, if not done at the previous visit.

Fig 2. NIAAA screening guide. (From National Institute on Alcohol Abuse and Alcoholism. Alcohol Screening and Brief Intervention for Youth: Practitioner's Guide. Washington, DC: National Institutes of Health, Department of Health and Human Services; 2011.)

use disorder among adolescents aged 13 to 19 years admitted to a psychiatric facility.[87] We have been unable to find any other studies evaluating the DAST-A or its use in general medical settings. The DAST-10, a 10-item version of the original measure, is the most studied of the DAST short forms (see Table 2).[88–90] Because of its relative brevity and ease of scoring, it has recently been proposed by the National Institute on Drug Abuse (NIDA) for inclusion as one of the standard core data elements related to drug use in all electronic health record systems.[91,92] The NIDA consensus screening protocol involves asking an initial single past-year drug frequency item (see Table 2), first tested by Smith et al[93] in primary care. This is followed by, for those reporting drug use, the DAST-10 and a few additional questions on types of drugs used, frequency of use, any injection drug use, and substance use disorder treatment status.[91] Based on our literature review, the study by Smith et al is the only one to date that has tested both the single-item drug screen and the DAST-10 among primary care patients. This study found that any positive response to the single item had similar test characteristics to the DAST-10 (at its typical cut point ≥3), with both having 100% sensitivity for detecting a current drug use disorder. Specificity was slightly higher for the DAST-10 compared to the single item (77.1% vs. 73.5%), although confidence intervals (CIs) overlapped. However, this study included no participants younger than 21 years, and we have found no other published studies that tested these 2 tools among adolescents.

Future Directions for Screening

Widespread implementation of SBIRT is dependent on the availability of practical tools that can quickly and accurately triage patients into levels of risk and guide clinical decision-making and action. Work continues to identify the briefest possible tools for this purpose. As with attempts to shorten the AUDIT, Knight et al[94] examined whether the CRAFFT could be shortened. They found that a 5-item version without the Family/Friends item had acceptable properties, but shorter versions did not. Kelly et al[65] found that a 2-item screen assessing the DSM-IV alcohol abuse/dependence symptoms of "recurrent drinking in hazardous situations" and "drinking more than intended, or over a longer period than intended" had the best overall performance in identifying AUDs among 18- to 20-year-old ED patients compared to other brief screens, including the AUDIT-C and CRAFFT. Brown et al[95] found a 2-item conjoint screen for alcohol and drug problems ("In the past year, have you ever drunk or used drugs more than you meant to?" and "Have you felt you wanted or needed to cut down on your drinking or drug use in the last year?") showed promise for detecting disorders across most substances in family practice patients aged 18 years or older. However, these tools have not been tested with younger adolescents, and more studies are needed to evaluate the performance of such ultra-brief tools among adolescents, including single-question screens.

There has also been growing interest in the use of computer technology to increase efficiency and standardization of screening as well as to boost screening and documentation rates through integration with electronic health records.[49,92,96–99] Having an adolescent complete the screening on a computer device (eg, laptop, tablet) before seeing the physician may be helpful in providing some distance between the patient and physician about the disclosure of sensitive information and in leaving more time during the visit for the clinician to provide further assessment and counseling.[98] Studies of computerized screening of adolescents in medical settings generally show strong acceptability and feasibility among both patients and physicians.[49,98,100] Moreover, studies have found increased adolescent satisfaction with the office visit and more patient-physician discussion of substance use topics during the visit after a computerized system for screening adolescents and informing physicians of the results was implemented compared to before.[96,99,101] However, Chisolm et al[98] found that adolescent satisfaction with computerized screening and their perceptions about its usefulness and ease of use were highly correlated with their level of trust in the data remaining private and being used only for health care, as well as their comfort with having their data stored on computer. Consequently, attention should be paid to promoting adolescent trust in information confidentiality and security when implementing a computerized screening system in a medical office.

Initial evidence suggests that responses to computerized screening are reliable,[102,103] but evidence is mixed about the comparability of validity of computerized screening versus face-to-face interviewing. Some studies show similar performance,[63,104] whereas others have shown systematic differences (eg, computer assessment yielded lower use frequency for some substances and related problems than in-person interview).[103,105] Given increasing computerization in health care and its potential for improving efficiency and standardization, more studies are needed to elucidate the implications of computerized screening in adolescent SBIRT systems.

BRIEF INTERVENTIONS

Although the term *brief intervention* has been used to refer to shorter-duration substance abuse treatments as well as to opportunistic interventions provided to nontreatment-seeking individuals after screening, we will focus on the latter in this article and on those interventions that can practicably be used in general medical settings as part of an integrated SBIRT approach. Both the AAP policy statement and NIAAA guide lay out a screening outcome-dependent algorithm for BI that consists of either brief advice (ie, few minutes of assessment/feedback and structured advice) or brief motivational interventions (can be 15 minutes per session over multiple sessions) depending on where individuals fall on the substance use spectrum (see Table 1). These recommended counseling strategies, based on risk level, are described in brief.

Low Risk

For youth who are abstinent (no past-year use) and have never ridden with an impaired driver, both the AAP and NIAAA recommend giving positive reinforcement, such as praise and encouragement for healthy choices made (see sample "Praise and Encouragement" statement in Figure 1), and eliciting and affirming reasons for abstaining. However, within the primary care setting where patients are seen over time, physicians should emphasize confidentiality and leave an *open door* for patients to discuss and ask questions about substance use should the patients initiate use in the future. In addition, the NIAAA guide recommends, for abstinent youth who have friends who drink, exploring their attitudes about their friends' drinking and their plans for how to stay alcohol-free when friends drink.

To our knowledge, only one published study to date has examined the effects of brief physician advice, delivered during a single visit that included praise and encouragement for abstaining adolescents. In a large study of more than 2000 adolescent primary care patients in the United States and the Czech Republic, Harris et al[99] examined the effects of a less than 10-minute computer-facilitated screening and brief advice (cSBA) protocol delivered during a routine visit compared to a treatment-as-usual (TAU) control. The cSBA protocol consisted of adolescents completing a 5-minute computer program just before seeing their primary care physician (or nurse practitioner). This program included the CRAFFT screen, feedback about their CRAFFT score and risk level, and 10 interactive educational pages about the risks associated with substance use and about driving while intoxicated. Physicians in the cSBA condition were then given their patients' screening results and talking points for 2 to 3 minutes of brief advice, which included praise and encouragement for patients who had no use. Intervention effects on *initiation* (among baseline nonusers) and *cessation* (among baseline users) were examined separately. In confidential assessments conducted by research staff at 12-month follow-up, the study found that 44% fewer cSBA adolescents than TAU had *initiated* drinking since their baseline visit. This effect was not significant for cannabis use among US teens. On the other hand, in the Czech sample, the prevention effect was significant for cannabis but not for alcohol, with 53% fewer cSBA patients initiating cannabis use by 12 months compared to TAU. Although these effects cannot be attributed solely to physician praise and encouragement because there were other intervention components (computerized screening, feedback, and educational material), this study does suggest that, with the efficiencies that computer technology can provide for priming adolescents for the physician encounter, a few minutes of physician anticipatory guidance and positive reinforcement can be effective.

A few other studies have examined the effects of medical office BIs on *prevention* of adolescent substance use. The first study, conducted by De Micheli et al,[106] evaluated Brazilian adolescent outpatients (aged 13-19) who reported no substance use in the last month. They found that those randomly assigned to receive 2 to 3 minutes of physician brief advice about substance use effects and risks, and an information leaflet, had significantly less increase in substance use prevalence, frequency, and associated problems during the 6-month follow-up compared to youth in the no-intervention control group. A recent randomized controlled trial by Walton et al[107] of 714 cannabis-abstinent adolescents (aged 12-18) who presented to federally qualified health centers in the United States found that those who received a 40-minute computerized motivational intervention designed to promote self-efficacy and commitment to avoid substance use had a significantly lower cannabis initiation rate during the 12-month follow-up period and a lower frequency of cannabis use at 3 and 6 months compared to a control group receiving an information brochure along with standard care. In contrast, studies by Ozer et al[108] and Stevens et al[109] found no such preventive effects of brief medical office interventions on *initiation* rates of alcohol, tobacco, or drug use among adolescent primary care patients during 12 to 36 months of follow-up.

Driving/Riding Risk

All adolescents who have ever ridden with an intoxicated driver (regardless of their own substance use) or have driven after using substances should receive brief counseling about the associated risks and be asked to commit to avoiding such risks in the future. To promote avoidance self-efficacy, physicians are recommended to give teens and their parents the "Contract for Life," a harm-reduction document developed by the Students Against Destructive Decisions (available at www.sadd.org/contract.htm) that is intended to facilitate parent-teen communication on the topic and the development of a safety plan. By signing this document, teens commit to avoiding these risks, and parents commit to providing their child safe transportation home, if needed, without question. Physicians should explain that this document is intended to ensure safety, not to discourage conversation between parents and their children. Parents should be encouraged, should their child request such help, to praise their child for avoiding the riding/driving risk and to explore the event with their child at a later time when a calmer discussion is possible.

In the study by Harris et al,[99] physicians in the intervention phase were instructed to review the Contract for Life with all of their adolescent patients, in conjunction with giving such brief advice as "Please don't ever get in a car with someone who has been drinking or using drugs, and make arrangements ahead of time for safe transportation." Compared to the usual-care group, adolescents who received the intervention had a significantly lower rate at 3-month follow-up of any past-90-day driving after substance use/riding with an impaired driver, but the effect had dissipated by 12 months.[110] Two other studies conducted in primary care settings showed similar short-term effects of BI on adolescent substance-related driving/riding outcomes, with attenuation by 12 months, suggesting a need to identify ways to extend the effect over time.[37,111] Nearly all other adolescent/young adult BI studies that examined risky driving/riding outcomes were conducted in ED settings or trauma centers.[15,16,112–115] Most of the studies tested a brief motivational intervention among patients being treated for a substance-related injury/illness, thus taking advantage of a key teachable moment. However, the event precipitating the ED or trauma center visit in itself may be a strong change agent, as most of these studies found significant reductions in subsequent risky driving/riding frequency in both the intervention and control (eg, standard care plus information leaflet, screening feedback only, or brief advice) groups, with no difference between groups.[16,112–115]

Moderate Risk

Youth ages 12 years or older who have past-year substance use but score 0 or 1 on the CRAFFT are considered moderate risk in the AAP policy statement. For alcohol, however, the NIAAA recommends a gradation of risk based on age-dependent alcohol consumption thresholds (see Table 2). In either case, the practice recommendation is to give moderate-risk patients clear advice to avoid further substance use and to educate them about the health risks of substance use (example statement: "As your doctor, I recommend that you stop using. Alcohol can cause high blood pressure, heart problems, and liver problems, and both alcohol and drug use can harm brain development which continues into your mid-20s"). These statements can draw on knowledge of the patient's health concerns as motivating reasons for avoiding substance use. For example, a patient concerned about weight may find information about the caloric content of alcoholic beverages impactful or an athlete may find information on the effects of tobacco/marijuana on lung function motivational.

Several decades of research show support for brief patient-centered advice being a cost-effective, cost-saving intervention[116-120] among moderate-risk drinkers for reducing hazardous alcohol use and associated consequences such as ED visits, sick and hospital days, alcohol-related arrests, motor vehicle crashes, and mortality.[121-125] Some studies have found brief advice interventions as short as 5 minutes are as effective as longer interventions.[10,126-130] However, few of those studies were conducted with adolescents, particularly in primary care settings. Our review found only 5 controlled trials that reported the effects of BI in primary care samples of largely moderate-risk adolescents (any past-year use or CRAFFT score <2).[37,99,106,131,132] Two of the 4 tested interventions *primed* the adolescent before seeing the physician using screening and education by audio[131,133] or computer[99] program and *prompted* the physician with screening results and discussion points to guide a few minutes of brief counseling. Using computer-assisted priming, Harris et al[99] found a significant intervention effect on *cessation* of alcohol use at 3-month follow-up (no past-90-day use among baseline past-year drinkers) in the US sample and of cannabis use at 12-month follow-up (no past-12-month use among baseline past-year users). The alcohol cessation effect in the US sample had dissipated by 12 months. On the other hand, Boekeloo et al[131] found that patients randomized to receive an audio program promoting adolescent self-assessment and adolescent-physician communication about substance use reported higher rates of drinking and binge drinking at 12-month follow-up compared to a usual-care group. Paradoxically, intervention participants also reported increased rates of refusing to drink when offered drinks by friends. The authors hypothesized that the intervention may have increased willingness to disclose use at follow-up. The other 3 studies evaluated longer single-session interventions incorporating motivational interviewing (MI) strategies (described in the next section). De Micheli et al[106] found that, among adolescents with any past-month use, those randomized to receive a 20-minute motivational intervention had a significant decrease in scores on a drug-use problem measure by 6-month follow-up, whereas no such decline was seen in the usual-care group. The intervention group also showed a greater decline in past-month substance consumption compared to controls. Mason et al[132] pilot-tested a 20-minute motivational intervention that also addressed social network influences on behavior among moderate-risk (CRAFFT = 1) female adolescent patients of a primary care clinic. At 1-month follow-up, compared to usual-care controls the intervention group reported fewer alcohol-related problems, less substance use before sex, lower social stress, and fewer offers to use cannabis; however, substance use did not differ. Finally, Walton et al[37] examined the effects of their 40-minute computer- or therapist-delivered brief motivational intervention on past-year cannabis *users*. They found that adolescents randomized to computerized BI had decreased cannabis-related problems and other drug use at 3- or 6-month follow-up compared to standard-care controls, but both effects had dissipated by 12 months.

High Risk

Youth aged 12 years or older with CRAFFT scores of 2 or more and past-year use, and those aged 11 years or younger with *any* past-year use are considered high risk. Physicians should briefly conduct a further assessment that evaluates substance use history, usage patterns, any previous quit attempts, underlying reasons for use, problems experienced because of use, and presence of "red flags" that indicate acute risk of harm to themselves or others or addiction in order to determine need for RT services (see Figure 1). Example questions for alcohol include "What's the most number of drinks that you've had at any one time?" and "How often do you drink that much?"[26] The NIAAA guide provides new age- and gender-specific definitions for binge drinking (eg, 3 drinks for age ≤13) that account for differences in child/teen versus adult body composition and alcohol elimination.[134] Physicians also can use positive CRAFFT items as starting points for additional assessment, such as the "Trouble" or "Family/Friends" items to explore problems experienced or the "Forget" item to determine the types and amounts of substances used in those instances. The presence of any red flag warrants a consideration of breaking confidentiality to involve parents, both to protect patient safety and to begin the treatment referral process. Breaking confidentiality should proceed after a discussion with the patient about what can be disclosed versus what remains confidential, and how best to go about informing parents (see AAP policy statement for more detail).

This brief assessment can serve to identify factors that may promote a patient's ambivalence about substance use and enhance motivation for behavior change and help-seeking, which tends to be low among nontreatment-seeking individuals with hazardous or harmful substance use.[135] In a nationally representative sample of adolescents ages 12 to 17, only 3% of those with AUDs self-identified a need for alcohol treatment.[136] Consequently, BIs addressing substance use have predominantly been based on MI principles and strategies to enhance a person's intrinsic motivation for behavior change. MI is a patient-centered, semidirective counseling style characterized by collaboration, empathy, acceptance and affirmation, and evocation of a patient's own values and ideas (the "spirit" of MI).[137] Essential components of MI BIs are summarized by the acronym FRAMES (Feedback, Responsibility, Advice, Menu of options, Empathy, Self-efficacy) and are described in greater detail in a clinical guide for pediatricians by Gold and Kokotailo.[138] MI is seen as particularly useful with adolescents/young adults because it is compatible with their desire for autonomy and therefore may meet with less resistance.

There is a large body of research on MI-based BIs for moderate- to high-risk substance use encompassing both adults and adolescents, as described in several reviews and meta-analyses (eg, Jensen et al[30] and Smedslund et al[139]). A 2011 Cochrane meta-analysis of 59 studies concluded that, compared to no-treatment controls, MI-based interventions significantly reduced substance use and related problems, with effects strongest immediately postintervention (standardized mean difference [SMD] 0.79), weaker but still significant at 6- to 12-month follow-up (SMD 0.15-0.17), and nonsignificant at longer-term follow-up (≥ 12 months; SMD 0.06).[139] MI also tended to do better compared with an *assessment and feedback* control but not with other active conditions such as usual care. Similarly, the first meta-analysis of MI interventions for adolescent substance use, which included 21 studies published between 1998 to 2009, revealed a modest, but significant, effect of MI on adolescent alcohol, tobacco, and drug use outcomes posttreatment and at subsequent follow-up (mean effect size d = 0.173, 95% CI, 0.094-0.252).[30] Effects were strongest at short-term follow-up but retained significance over longer follow-up (mean d = 0.133, 95% CI, 0.023-0.244, for follow-up ≥ 6 months). Most interventions (13/21) involved a single MI session, but some ranged up to 9 sessions; effect size was not analyzed based on number of sessions. Acknowledging a potential bias toward positive findings in published studies,[140] the authors calculated that 105 null-finding studies would be required to reduce the observed omnibus effect size to zero.

The duration of MI sessions typically has ranged from 15 minutes to 1 hour, making them less practical for busy medical physicians to deliver along with screening in a single encounter. The brief negotiated interview (BNI) is a BI approach for addressing problematic substance use that combines MI and brief advice and, with screening, takes less than 10 minutes to conduct, making it more feasible for general medical settings. A BNI involves giving personalized feedback and advice based on screening and assessment, highlighting the problems that patients report experiencing because of their substance use, and using MI strategies to enhance motivation and planning for behavioral change.[141] Behavioral change goals are then negotiated and documented in a signed agreement. To date, BNIs have been primarily tested with youth in ED settings, where studies tend to show positive effects on substance-related problems and injury but mixed findings for substance use outcomes compared with standard care.[17,18,28,142,143]

REFERRAL TO TREATMENT

In our review, we found only 1 study each among adolescents[144] and adults,[145] both conducted with ED patients, that examined entry into substance abuse treatment following BI. In the study of adolescents, 127 Australian ED patients aged 12 to 19 years who presented for an alcohol/drug use-related cause were randomized to either standard care or a BI designed to identify and match patients to needed treatment services, enhance motivation to attend the treatment appointment, and ameliorate any barriers that might prevent attendance.[144] A phone call reminded patients of their appointment, and transportation and accompaniment to the appointment were offered. At 4-month follow-up, compared with controls, the BI group had higher rates of attending treatment (25% vs. 3% after accounting for loss to follow-up), and those who received treatment had greater reductions in overall consumption and hazardous substance use behaviors (eg, injection drug use) compared to those who did not. In the study of adults, ED patients who screened positive for problematic substance use were given a 5- to 10-minute BNI and a multisession MI-based brief treatment if the screening score was particularly high.[145] Compared with a propensity score-matched comparison group, patients who received BI or brief treatment (BT) had significantly higher rates of specialty treatment admission by 1-month follow-up among those with no prior substance use treatment. The effect was reduced among patients with prior substance use treatment. All effects were extinguished by 6 months. Given the paucity of studies in this area, it is difficult to determine what strategies may enhance the implementation and successful completion of the "RT" component of SBIRT. Interestingly, a study by Hassan et al[146] found that pediatricians tended to prefer to arrange follow-up care at their own offices for patients with problematic substance use rather than referring them to external counseling services or notifying parents.

BI MEDIATORS AND MODERATORS

Effect Mediators

Few studies to date have attempted to elucidate the mechanisms of effect for BIs for adolescent substance use (ie, the *active ingredients*). One qualitative study examined primary care physicians' views on the most promising components of brief alcohol interventions based on their clinical experience working with heavy-drinking college students.[147] There was consensus on 5 key components: providing a summary of the patient's drinking pattern, discussing drinking likes and dislikes, discussing life goals and effects of substance use, encouraging a risk-reduction agreement, and asking patients to track their drinking on diary cards. This last strategy, which promotes self-monitoring of substance use behavior, was found to have the largest effect on substance use across all behavioral change techniques examined in a meta-analysis of the effectiveness of specific BI components in alcohol BI trials.[148] However, the degree to which this finding applies to noncollege-aged adolescents is unclear because no studies in this age group were included in the meta-analysis.

Existing studies among adolescents all have focused on the active ingredients of brief MI. These studies have found that, similar to adult studies, physician fidelity to the *spirit* of MI and promotion of patient *change talk*, particularly statements about reasons and desire for, and ability, to change, are key to BI outcomes.[149-154] Other predictive components found in BI studies include the quality of the change plan[155] and the frequency of *complex* reflections made by the physician.[150] Finally, because of the robustness of substance use changes found in nonintervention control groups in many BI trials, it is suggested that simply assessing individuals for substance use and associated problems may in itself affect behavior by raising patients' awareness and initiating self-monitoring.[156-159]

Effect Moderators

Factors explored as potential moderators of BI effectiveness have included baseline substance use levels or problem severity, readiness to change, presence of co-occurring psychiatric concerns or other substance use disorders, and contextual risk factors such as peer substance use. A number of studies found that BI effectiveness was greater among patients who had heavier baseline use or had experienced more problems because of their use.[16,160-163] However, this finding may be attributed to a greater tendency for regression to the mean among those with use levels further away from the mean.[164] On the other hand, a recent review found little evidence of medical office BI effectiveness among patients with more severe levels of use such as dependence.[165] Most of the existing studies were conducted in general populations, where only small percentages of participants have abuse or dependence.

Baseline readiness to change was also found to moderate BI effectiveness in some studies, although the findings on whether BIs are more effective for those with greater readiness or less readiness are mixed.[154,166,167] The evidence is also mixed on whether BIs are as effective among patients who have problematic use of drugs other than alcohol or cannabis,[168-170] polysubstance use,[171,172] or comorbid psychiatric concerns.[173-177] Few of these studies involved adolescents, however[168,173,177]; thus, little can be said about how these factors may affect BI effectiveness among adolescents.

Finally, a study by Louis-Jacques et al[178] examined whether a primary care screening and physician brief advice intervention were as effective among teens who had a *risky* peer group (ie, friends who drink or approve of teen drinking) as among those who did not. They found a larger short-term BI effect on drinking *cessation* among teens *with* baseline peer risk than among those who did not. Their findings suggest that a primary care-based BI may be able to reduce teen drinking, even when there are social influences to the contrary. However, this is a single study, and much more work is needed to clarify for which types of adolescents, and under what circumstances, BIs in general medical settings may be more or less effective.

SUMMARY

Substance use is the most common health risk behavior among adolescents[40] and is one of the greatest threats to their current and future health. Universal screening of adolescents in general medical settings can be instrumental in identifying substance use early, before further problems develop and when BIs are more likely to be effective. Screening in and of itself may have some therapeutic effect.[157–159] Brief screening tools feasible for use by busy medical offices to quickly and reliably assess adolescent risk for a substance use disorder now are available. A recent study found that a physician-conducted CRAFFT screen interview required an average of 74 seconds to complete, whereas a computer self-administered version took an average of 49 seconds.[63] The CRAFFT and AUDIT tools currently have the most evidence for validity among adolescents, whereas the validity of other widely used tools such as DAST-10, NIDA-modified ASSIST (Alcohol, Smoking and Substance Involvement Screening Test), and ultra-brief screens (AUDIT-C, single-item screens) has yet to be established for adolescents. Studies are needed to identify effective strategies to promote universal adolescent screening and the use of valid screening tools in general medical settings. One statewide (Massachusetts) study found that although most (86%) primary care physicians seeing adolescents reported screening adolescents for substance use annually, only 1 in 3 reported using a validated tool (the CRAFFT). The remaining physicians reporting using informal screening procedures, their own questionnaire, or the CAGE.[179] Computerization of screening and integration into the electronic health record appear to be promising strategies to promote universal screening and standardized use of valid screening tools.[49,97,99,180]

Increasing adolescent screening rates necessitates supporting physicians' ability to respond effectively to the screen results. To that end, recent evidence-informed practice guides from the AAP and NIAAA provide a structured algorithm for specific recommended responses based on level of risk. Adolescents who are at low or moderate risk for a substance use disorder, who constitute most of those seen in general medical settings,[44] may be effectively counseled with a few minutes of brief advice, particularly after being primed with screening, feedback, and education before seeing their physician. High-risk patients (screen-positives) should receive a brief follow-up assessment to determine the appropriate level of care needed and a BI, using MI principles, to enhance motivation for behavioral change and help-seeking. Indications of acute danger or addiction may necessitate breaking confidentiality to protect patient safety and begin RT.

Our review shows a small but growing body of research on the effectiveness of *opportunistic* BIs following screening of adolescents in clinical settings. Studies to date have largely tested brief alcohol-focused MI-based interventions with adolescents in the ED or trauma care settings[17,18]; however, the number of studies conducted in primary health care settings is increasing.[37,99,106–108,131,181] The strongest BI effects found in these studies tend to be related to harm reduction, such as reduction of substance-related driving/riding, alcohol-related injuries, unplanned sex, and other negative consequences of use. Effects on substance *use* have been more modest and tend to be stronger at shorter (≤6 months) rather than longer follow-up (≥12 months). However, many of these studies compared BI to active control conditions, which often included elements of BI (eg, assessment, brief advice, informational handouts). Significant reductions in substance use and related harms were also seen in these control groups, likely making detection of a BI effect more difficult.[157,158] A few studies have shown initial support for a *prevention* effect of BI among abstinent adolescents. At the opposite end of the spectrum, little is known about the effects of BI for adolescents with dependence and needing RT because of a lack of studies. Other areas needing additional research are the effect of BI on adolescent drug use, particularly on use of drugs other than cannabis; the mediators and moderators of BI effects; ways to reinforce and sustain effects over time; and how best to increase SBI implementation in general medical settings and to effectively train physicians. The effect of efforts such as the Substance Abuse and Mental Health Services Administration-funded physician residency SBIRT training programs[182,183] remain to be determined.

There has been increasing investigation into the potential of interactive computer technologies to aid SBIRT delivery to adolescents and young adults.[184,185] A more detailed review of this area of research is beyond the scope of this article, but computer technology is proving to be an acceptable and effective tool in the delivery of BIs to young people, both as physician "extenders" in clinical settings and in the form of stand-alone self-guided programs. Computer technologies likely will play a critical role in promoting the expansion of SBIRT implementation for youth in general medical settings.

References

1. The National Center on Addiction and Substance Abuse (CASA). *Adolescent Substance Use: America's # 1 Public Health Problem.* New York; 2011
2. Horgan C, Skwara KC, Strickler G. *Substance Abuse: The Nation's Number One Health Problem.* Princeton, NJ: The Robert Wood Johnson Foundation; 2001
3. United States Department of Justice. *The Economic Impact of Illicit Drug Use on American Society.* Washington, DC: United States Department of Justice; 2011

4. Bouchery E, Harwood H, Sacks J, Simon C, Brewer R. Economic costs of excessive alcohol consumption in the U.S., 2006. *Am J Prev Med.* 2011;41(5):516–524

5. Kessler RC, Berglund P, Demler O, et al. Lifetime prevalence and age-of-onset distributions of DSM-IV disorders in the National Comorbidity Survey Replication. *Arch Gen Psychiatry.* 2005;62(6):593–602

6. Substance Abuse and Mental Health Services Administration. White Paper on Screening, Brief Intervention and Referral to Treatment (SBIRT) in Behavioral Healthcare. *SAMHSA.* 2011:1–30. Available at: www.samhsa.gov/prevention/sbirt/SBIRTwhitepaper.pdf. Accessed March 13, 2014

7. Babor TF, McRee BG, Kassebaum PA, et al. Screening, Brief Intervention and Referral to Treatment (SBIRT): toward a public health approach to the management of substance abuse. *Subst Abus.* 2007;28(3):7–30

8. Knight JR, Sherritt L, Harris SK, Gates EC, Chang G. Validity of brief alcohol screening tests among adolescents: a comparison of the AUDIT, POSIT, CAGE, and CRAFFT. *Alcohol Clin Exp Res.* 2003;27(1):67–73

9. Jonas D, Garbutt J, Amick H, et al. Behavioral counseling after screening for alcohol misuse in primary care: a systematic review and meta-analysis for the US Preventive Services Task Force. *Ann Intern Med.* 2012;157(9):645–654

10. Kaner EF, Beyer F, Dickinson HO, et al. Effectiveness of brief alcohol interventions in primary care populations. *Cochrane Database Syst Rev.* 2007;18(2):CD004148

11. Bertholet N, Daeppen JB, Wietlisbach V, Fleming M, Burnand B. Reduction of alcohol consumption by brief alcohol intervention in primary care: systematic review and meta-analysis. *Arch Intern Med.* 2005;165(9):986–995

12. O'Donnell A, Anderson P, Newbury-Birch D, et al. The impact of brief alcohol interventions in primary healthcare: a systematic review of reviews. *Alcohol Alcohol.* 2014;49(1):66–78

13. Moyer VA. Screening and behavioral counseling interventions in primary care to reduce alcohol misuse: U.S. Preventive Services Task Force recommendation statement. *Ann Intern Med.* 2013;159(3):210–218

14. Polen M, Whitlock E, Wisdom J, Nygren P, Bougatsos C. *Screening in Primary Care Settings for Illicit Drug Use: Staged Systematic Review for the U.S. Preventive Services Task Force. Evidence Synthesis No. 58, Part 1.* AHRQ Publication No. 08-05108-EF-S. Rockville, MD: Agency for Healthcare Research and Quality; 2008

15. Monti PM, Colby SM, Barnett NP, et al. Brief intervention for harm reduction with alcohol-positive older adolescents in a hospital emergency department. *J Consult Clin Psychol.* 1999;67(6):989–994

16. Spirito A, Monti PM, Barnett NP, et al. A randomized clinical trial of a brief motivational intervention for alcohol-positive adolescents treated in an emergency department. *J Pediatr.* 2004;145(3):396–402

17. Newton AS, Dong K, Mabood N, et al. Brief emergency department interventions for youth who use alcohol and other drugs: a systematic review. *Pediatr Emerg Care.* 2013;29(5):673–684

18. Yuma-Guerrero P, Lawson K, Velasquez M, et al. Screening, brief intervention, and referral for alcohol use in adolescents: a systematic review. *Pediatrics.* 2012;130(1):115–122

19. Carey K, Scott-Sheldon L, Carey M, DeMartini K. Individual-level interventions to reduce college student drinking: a meta-analytic review. *Addict Behav.* 2007;32(11):2469–2494

20. Fachini A, Aliane PP, Martinez EZ, Furtado EF. Efficacy of brief alcohol screening intervention for college students (BASICS): a meta-analysis of randomized controlled trials. *Subst Abuse Treat Prev Policy.* 2012;7:40

21. Mitchell S, Gryczynski J, O'Grady K, Schwartz R. Screening, brief intervention, and referral to treatment for adolescent drug and alcohol use: current status and future directions. *J Subst Abus Treat.* 2013;44(5):463–472

22. Agerwala S, McCance-Katz E. Integrating screening, brief intervention, and referral to treatment (SBIRT) into clinical practice settings: a brief review. *J Psychoactive Drugs.* 2012;44(4):307–317

23. Cherry DK, Hing E, Woodwell DA, Rechsteiner MS. *National Ambulatory Medical Care Survey.* Washington, DC: U.S. Department of Health and Human Services, Centers for Disease Control and Prevention, National Center for Health Statistics; 2008

24. Harris SK, Woods ER, Sherritt L, et al. A youth-provider connectedness measure for use in clinical intervention studies. *J Adolesc Health.* 2009;44(2 Suppl):S35–S36

25. American Academy of Pediatrics Committee on Substance Abuse. Substance use screening, brief intervention, and referral to treatment for pediatricians. *Pediatrics.* 2011;128(5):e1330–e1340

26. National Institute on Alcohol Abuse and Alcoholism. *Alcohol Screening and Brief Intervention for Youth: Practitioner's Guide.* Washington, DC: National Institutes of Health, Department of Health and Human Services; 2011

27. Van Hook S, Harris SK, Brooks T, et al. The "Six T's": barriers to screening teens for substance abuse in primary care. *J Adolesc Health.* 2007;40(5):456–461

28. Pilowsky D, Wu L. Screening instruments for substance use and brief interventions targeting adolescents in primary care: a literature review. *Addict Behav.* 2013;38(5):2146–2153

29. Boekeloo BO, Novik MG. Clinical approaches to improving alcohol education and counseling in adolescents and young adults. *Adolesc Med State Art Rev.* 2011;22(3):631–648, xiv

30. Jensen CD, Cushing CC, Aylward BS, et al. Effectiveness of motivational interviewing interventions for adolescent substance use behavior change: a meta-analytic review. *J Consult Clin Psychol.* 2011;79(4):433–540

31. Wachtel T, Staniford M. The effectiveness of brief interventions in a clinical setting in reducing alcohol misuse and binge drinking in adolescents: a critical review of the literature. *J Clin Nurs.* 2010;19(5-6):605–620

32. Knight JR, Goodman E, Pulerwitz T, DuRant RH. Reliability of the Problem Oriented Screening Instrument for Teenagers (POSIT) in adolescent medical practice. *J Adolesc Health.* 2001;29(2):125–130

33. Levy S, Sherritt L, Harris SK, et al. Test-retest reliability of adolescents' self-report of substance use. *Alcohol Clin Exp Res.* 2004;28(8):1236–1241

34. Schizer M, Sherritt L, Murphy D, Levy S. Self-report vs. bioassay for detecting substance use by adolescents. Paper presented at: Association for Medical Education and Research in Substance Abuse 36th Annual National Conference; November 1-3, 2012; Bethesda, MD

35. Zaldívar Basurto F, García Montes JM, Flores Cubos P, et al. Validity of the self-report on drug use by university students: correspondence between self-reported use and use detected in urine. *Psicothema.* 2009;21(2):213–219

36. Comasco E, Nordquist N, Leppert J, et al. Adolescent alcohol consumption: biomarkers PEth and FAEE in relation to interview and questionnaire data. *J Stud Alcohol Drugs.* 2009;70(5):797–804

37. Walton MA, Bohnert K, Resko S, et al. Computer and therapist based brief interventions among cannabis-using adolescents presenting to primary care: one year outcomes. *Drug Alcohol Depend.* 2013;132(3):646–653

38. Baer JS, Garrett SB, Beadnell B, Wells EA, Peterson PL. Brief motivational intervention with homeless adolescents: evaluating effects on substance use and service utilization. *Psychol Addict Behav.* 2007;21(4):582–586

39. Hagan JF, Shaw JS, Duncan P. *Bright Futures Guidelines for Health Supervision of Infants, Children, and Adolescents.* 3rd ed. Elk Grove Village, IL: American Academy of Pediatrics; 2008

40. Centers for Disease Control and Prevention. Youth Risk Behavior Surveillance—United States, 2011. *MMWR Surveill Summ.* 2012;61(SS-4):1–162

41. Duncan TE, Tildesley E, Duncan SC, Hops H. The consistency of family and peer influences on the development of substance use in adolescence. *Addiction.* 1995;90(12):1647–1660

42. Nash SG, McQueen A, Bray JH. Pathways to adolescent alcohol use: family environment, peer influence, and parental expectations. *J Adolesc Health.* 2005;37(1):19–28

43. Weddle M, Kokotailo P. Adolescent substance abuse: confidentiality and consent. *Pediatr Clin North Am.* 2002;49(2):301–315

44. Knight JR, Harris SK, Sherritt L, et al. Prevalence of positive substance abuse screen results among adolescent primary care patients. *Arch Pediatr Adolesc Med.* 2007;161(11):1035–1041

45. Hingson RW, Zha W. Age of drinking onset, alcohol use disorders, frequent heavy drinking, and unintentionally injuring oneself and others after drinking. *Pediatrics*. 2009;123(6):1477–1484
46. Hingson RW, Heeren T, Winter MR. Age at drinking onset and alcohol dependence: age at onset, duration, and severity. *Arch Pediatr Adolesc Med*. 2006;160(7):739–746
47. Winters KC, Lee CY. Likelihood of developing an alcohol and cannabis use disorder during youth: association with recent use and age. *Drug Alcohol Depend*. 2008;92(1-3):239–247
48. Wilson CR, Sherritt L, Gates E, Knight JR. Are clinical impressions of adolescent substance use accurate? *Pediatrics*. 2004;114(5):e536–e540
49. Stevens J, Kelleher KJ, Gardner W, et al. Trial of computerized screening for adolescent behavioral concerns. *Pediatrics*. 2008;121(6):1099–1105
50. Goldenring J, Rosen D. Getting into adolescent heads: an essential update. *Contemp Pediatr*. 2004;21:64
51. Ginsburg KR, Carlson EC. Resilience in action: an evidence-informed, theoretically driven approach to building strengths in an office-based setting. *Adolesc Med State Art Rev*. 2011;22(3):458–481, xi
52. Knight JR, Harris SK, Sherritt L, et al. Adolescents' preference for substance abuse screening in primary care practice. *Subst Abus*. 2007;28(4):107–117
53. Knight JR, Shrier LA, Bravender TD, et al. A new brief screen for adolescent substance abuse. *Arch Pediatr Adolesc Med*. 1999;153(6):591–596
54. Dhalla S, Zumbo BD, Poole G, Poolem G. A review of the psychometric properties of the CRAFFT instrument. *Curr Drug Abuse Rev*. 2011;4(1):57–64
55. Knight JR, Sherritt L, Shrier LA, Harris SK, Chang G. Validity of the CRAFFT substance abuse screening test among adolescent clinic patients. *Arch Pediatr Adolesc Med*. 2002;156(6):607–614
56. Pérez-Gómez A, Scoppetta-Díazgranados O. El Crafft/Carlos como instrumento para la identificación temprana de consumo de alcohol y otras SPA: una adaptación al Español. *Rev Colomb Psicol*. 2011;20(2):265–274
57. Csémy L, Knight JR, Starostova O, et al. Screening rizikového užívání návykových látek u dospívajících: zkušenosti s českou adaptací dotazníku CRAFFT (Screening for risk of substance use among adolescents: experience with the Czech adaptation of the CRAFFT questionnaire). *Vox Pediatr*. 2008;6:35–36
58. Bernard M, Bolognini M, Plancherel B, et al. French validity of two substance use screening tests among adolescents: a comparison of the CRAFFT and DEP-ADO. *J Subst Use*. 2005;10(6):385–395
59. Rumpf H-J, Wohlert T, Freyer-Adam J, Grothues J, Bischof G. Screening questionnaires for problem drinking in adolescents: performance of AUDIT, AUDIT-C, CRAFFT and POSIT. *Eur Addict Res*. 2013;19(3):121–127
60. Cook RL, Chung T, Kelly TM, Clark DB. Alcohol screening in young persons attending a sexually transmitted disease clinic: comparison of AUDIT, CRAFFT, and CAGE instruments. *J Gen Intern Med*. 2005;20(1):1–6
61. Cummins LH, Chan KK, Burns KM, et al. Validity of the CRAFFT in American-Indian and Alaska-Native adolescents: screening for drug and alcohol risk. *J Stud Alcohol*. 2003;64(5):727–732
62. Subramaniam M, Cheok C, Verma S, Wong J, Chong SA. Validity of a brief screening instrument-CRAFFT in a multiethnic Asian population. *Addict Behav*. 2010;35(12):1102–1104
63. Harris S, Knight J, Van Hook S, et al. Validity of computer vs. clinician screening of adolescents in primary care. Paper presented at: Association for Medical Education and Research in Substance Abuse 37th Annual National Conference; November 7-9, 2013; Bethesda, MD
64. Kelly TM, Donovan JE, Chung T, Cook RL, Delbridge TR. Alcohol use disorders among emergency department-treated older adolescents: a new brief screen (RUFT-Cut) using the AUDIT, CAGE, CRAFFT, and RAPS-QF. *Alcohol Clin Exp Res*. 2004;28(5):746–753
65. Kelly TM, Donovan JE, Chung T, et al. Brief screens for detecting alcohol use disorder among 18-20 year old young adults in emergency departments: comparing AUDIT-C, CRAFFT, RAPS4-QF, FAST, RUFT-Cut, and DSM-IV 2-Item Scale. *Addict Behav*. 2009;34(8):668–674

66. Peden M, Scurfield R, Sleet D, et al, eds. *World Report on Road Traffic Injury Prevention*. Geneva, Switzerland: World Health Organization; 2004
67. Chung T, Colby SM, Barnett NP, et al. Screening adolescents for problem drinking: performance of brief screens against DSM-IV alcohol diagnoses. *J Stud Alcohol*. 2000;61(4):579–587
68. Kelly TM, Donovan JE, Kinnane JM, Taylor DM. A comparison of alcohol screening instruments among under-aged drinkers treated in emergency departments. *Alcohol Alcohol*. 2002;37(5):444–450
69. Reinert DF, Allen JP. The Alcohol Use Disorders Identification Test: an update of research findings. *Alcohol Clin Exp Res*. 2007;31(2):185–199
70. Babor TF, Higgins-Biddle JC, Saunders JB, Monteiro MG. *AUDIT: The Alcohol Use Disorders Identification Test: Guidelines for Use in Primary Health Care*. 2nd ed. Geneva, Switzerland: World Health Organization, Department of Mental Health and Substance Dependence; 2001
71. Bohn MJ, Babor TF. The Alcohol Use Disorders Identification Test (AUDIT): validation of a screening instrument for use in medical settings. *J Stud Alcohol*. 1995;56(4):423–432
72. Gordon AJ, Maisto SA, McNeil M, et al. Three questions can detect hazardous drinkers. *J Fam Pract*. 2001;50(4):313–320
73. Bush K, Kivlahan DR, McDonell MB, Fihn SD, Bradley KA. The AUDIT alcohol consumption questions (AUDIT-C): an effective brief screening test for problem drinking. Ambulatory Care Quality Improvement Project (ACQUIP). Alcohol Use Disorders Identification Test. *Arch Intern Med*. 1998;158(16):1789–1795
74. Hodgson R, Alwyn T, John B, Thom B, Smith A. The FAST alcohol screening test. *Alcohol Alcohol*. 2002;37(1):61–66
75. Bradley KA, DeBenedetti AF, Volk RJ, et al. AUDIT-C as a brief screen for alcohol misuse in primary care. *Alcohol Clin Exp Res*. 2007;31(7):1208–1217
76. Dawson DA, Grant BF, Stinson FS, Zhou Y. Effectiveness of the derived Alcohol Use Disorders Identification Test (AUDIT-C) in screening for alcohol use disorders and risk drinking in the US general population. *Alcohol Clin Exp Res*. 2005;29(5):844–854
77. Kriston L, Hölzel L, Weiser A-K, Berner MM, Härter M. Meta-analysis: are 3 questions enough to detect unhealthy alcohol use? *Ann Intern Med*. 2008;149(12):879–888
78. McCambridge J, Thomas BA. Short forms of the AUDIT in a Web-based study of young drinkers. *Drug Alcohol Rev*. 2009;28(1):18–24
79. Chung T, Colby SM, Barnett NP, Monti PM. Alcohol use disorders identification test: factor structure in an adolescent emergency department sample. *Alcohol Clin Exp Res*. 2002;26(2):223–231
80. Chung T, Smith GT, Donovan JE, et al. Drinking frequency as a brief screen for adolescent alcohol problems. *Pediatrics*. 2012;129(2):205–212
81. Smith PC, Schmidt SM, Allensworth-Davies D, Saitz R. Primary care validation of a single-question alcohol screening test. *J Gen Intern Med*. 2009;24(7):783–788
82. Canagasaby A, Vinson DC. Screening for hazardous or harmful drinking using one or two quantity-frequency questions. *Alcohol Alcohol*. 2005;40(3):208–213
83. Brown S, Donovan J, McGue M, et al. Youth alcohol screening workgroup II: determining optimal secondary screening questions. *Alcohol Exp Res*. 2010;34(Supp S3):267A
84. Kelly S, O'Grady K, Gryczynski J, et al. Development and validation of a brief screening tool for adolescent tobacco, alcohol, and drug use. Paper presented at: Association for Medical Education and Research in Substance Abuse 37th Annual National Conference; November 7-9, 2013; Bethesda, MD
85. Yudko E, Lozhkina O, Fouts A. A comprehensive review of the psychometric properties of the Drug Abuse Screening Test. *J Subst Abus Treat*. 2007;32(2):189–198
86. Skinner H. The drug abuse screening test. *Addict Behav*. 1982;7:363–371
87. Martino S, Grilo CM, Fehon DC. Development of the drug abuse screening test for adolescents (DAST-A). *Addict Behav*. 2000;25(1):57–70
88. Bohn M, Babor T, Kranzler H. Validity of the Drug Abuse Screening Test (DAST-10) in inpatient substances abusers: problems of drug dependence. In: *Problems of Drug Dependence 1991: Pro-*

ceedings of the 53rd Annual Scientific Meeting of the Committee on Problems of Drug Dependence. Rockville, MD: Department of Health and Human Services; 1991;223

89. French MT, Roebuck MC, McGeary KA, Chitwood DD, McCoy CB. Using the drug abuse screening test (DAST-10) to analyze health services utilization and cost for substance users in a community-based setting. *Subst Use Misuse.* 2001;36(6-7):927–946

90. McCabe SE, Boyd CJ, Cranford JA, Morales M, Slayden J. A modified version of the Drug Abuse Screening Test among undergraduate students. *J Subst Abuse Treat.* 2006;31(3):297–303

91. Ghitza UE, Gore-Langton RE, Lindblad R, et al. Common data elements for substance use disorders in electronic health records: the NIDA Clinical Trials Network experience. *Addiction.* 2013;108(1):3–8

92. Tai B, Wu L-T, Clark H. Electronic health records: essential tools in integrating substance abuse treatment with primary care. *Subst Abuse Rehabil.* 2012;3:1–8

93. Smith PC, Schmidt SM, Allensworth-Davies D, Saitz R. A single-question screening test for drug use in primary care. *Arch Intern Med.* 2010;170(13):1155–1160

94. Knight JR, Sherritt L, Gates E, Harris SK. Should the CRAFFT substance abuse screening test be shortened? *J Clin Outcomes Manag.* 2004;11(1):19–25

95. Brown RL, Leonard T, Saunders LA, Papasouliotis O. A two-item conjoint screen for alcohol and other drug problems. *J Am Board Fam Pract.* 2001;14(2):95–106

96. Olson AL, Gaffney CA, Hedberg VA, Gladstone GR. Use of inexpensive technology to enhance adolescent health screening and counseling. *Arch Pediatr Adolesc Med.* 2009;163(2):172–177

97. Anand V, Carroll AE, Downs SM. Automated primary care screening in pediatric waiting rooms. *Pediatrics.* 2012;129(5):e1275–e1281

98. Chisolm D, Gardner W, Julian T, Kelleher K. Adolescent satisfaction with computer-assisted behavioral risk screening in primary care. *Child Adolesc Ment Health.* 2008;13(4):163–168

99. Harris SK, Csémy L, Sherritt L, et al. Computer-facilitated substance use screening and brief advice for teens in primary care: an international trial. *Pediatrics.* 2012;129(6):1072–1982

100. Kypri K, Langley JD, Saunders JB, Cashell-Smith ML, Herbison P. Randomized controlled trial of web-based alcohol screening and brief intervention in primary care. *Arch Intern Med.* 2008;168(5):530–536

101. Brown JD, Wissow LS. Discussion of sensitive health topics with youth during primary care visits: relationship to youth perceptions of care. *J Adolesc Health.* 2009;44(1):48–54

102. Thomas BA, McCambridge J. Comparative psychometric study of a range of hazardous drinking measures administered online in a youth population. *Drug Alcohol Depend.* 2008;96(1-2):121–127

103. Williams ML, Freeman RC, Bowen AM, et al. A comparison of the reliability of self-reported drug use and sexual behaviors using computer-assisted versus face-to-face interviewing. *AIDS Educ Prev.* 2000;12(3):199–213

104. McNeely J, Strauss S, Rotrosen J, Ramautar A, Gourevitch M. Validation of an audio computer assisted self-interview (ACASI) version of the Alcohol, Smoking, and Substance Involvement Screening Test (ASSIST) in primary care patients. Paper presented at: Association for Medical Education and Research in Substance Abuse 37th Annual National Conference; November 7-9, 2013; Bethesda, MD

105. Marshall G, Hays R, Nicholas R. Evaluating agreement between clinical assessment methods. *Int J Methods Psychiatr Res.* 1994;4:249–257

106. De Micheli D, Fisberg M, Formigoni ML. Study on the effectiveness of brief intervention for alcohol and other drug use directed to adolescents in a primary health care unit. *Rev Assoc Med Bras.* 2004;50(3):305–313

107. Walton MA, Resko S, Barry KL, et al. A randomized controlled trial testing the efficacy of a brief cannabis universal prevention program among adolescents in primary care. *Addiction.* 2013; doi: 10.1111/add.12469

108. Ozer EM, Adams SH, Orrell-Valente JK, et al. Does delivering preventive services in primary care reduce adolescent risky behavior? *J Adolesc Health.* 2011;49(5):476–482

109. Stevens MM, Olson AL, Gaffney CA, et al. A pediatric, practice-based, randomized trial of drinking and smoking prevention and bicycle helmet, gun, and seatbelt safety promotion. *Pediatrics.* 2002;109(3):490–497

110. Harris SK, Csemy L, Sherritt L, et al. Screening and brief physician's advice to reduce teens' risk of substance-related car crashes: an international trial. Paper presented at: Association for Medical Education and Research in Substance Abuse 35th Annual National Conference; November 3-5, 2011; Washington, DC

111. Knight JR, Sherritt L, Van Hook S, et al. Motivational interviewing for adolescent substance use: a pilot study. *J Adolesc Health*. 2005;37(2):167–169

112. Monti PM, Barnett NP, Colby SM, et al. Motivational interviewing versus feedback only in emergency care for young adult problem drinking. *Addiction*. 2007;102(8):1234–1243

113. Johnston BD, Rivara FP, Droesch RM, Dunn C, Copass MK. Behavior change counseling in the emergency department to reduce injury risk: a randomized, controlled trial. *Pediatrics*. 2002;110(2 Pt 1):267–274

114. Bernstein E, Edwards E, Dorfman D, et al. Screening and brief intervention to reduce marijuana use among youth and young adults in a pediatric emergency department. *Acad Emerg Med*. 2009;16(11):1174–1185

115. Bernstein J, Heeren T, Edward E, et al. A brief motivational interview in a pediatric emergency department, plus 10-day telephone follow-up, increases attempts to quit drinking among youth and young adults who screen positive for problematic drinking. *Acad Emerg Med*. 2010;17(8):890–902

116. Fleming MF, Mundt MP, French MT, et al. Brief physician advice for problem drinkers: long-term efficacy and benefit-cost analysis. *Alcohol Clin Exp Res*. 2002;26(1):36–43

117. Estee S, Wickizer T, He L, Shah MF, Mancuso D. Evaluation of the Washington state screening, brief intervention, and referral to treatment project: cost outcomes for Medicaid patients screened in hospital emergency departments. *Med Care*. 2010;48(1):18–24

118. Gentilello LM, Ebel BE, Wickizer TM, Salkever DS, Rivara FP. Alcohol interventions for trauma patients treated in emergency departments and hospitals: a cost benefit analysis. *Ann Surg*. 2005;241(4):541–550

119. Kraemer KL. The cost-effectiveness and cost-benefit of screening and brief intervention for unhealthy alcohol use in medical settings. *Subst Abus*. 2007;23(3):67–77

120. Tariq L, van den Berg M, Hoogenveen RT, van Baal PHM. Cost-effectiveness of an opportunistic screening programme and brief intervention for excessive alcohol use in primary care. *PLoS One*. 2009;4(5):e5696

121. Kristenson H, Ohlin H, Hulten-Nosslin MB, Trell E, Hood B. Identification and intervention of heavy drinking in middle-aged men: results and follow-up of 24-60 months of long-term study with randomized controls. *Alcohol Clin Exp Res*. 1983;7(2):203–209

122. Ockene JK, Reed GW, Reiff-Hekking S. Brief patient-centered clinician-delivered counseling for high-risk drinking: 4-year results. *Ann Behav Med*. 2009;37(3):335–342

123. Baer JS, Kivlahan DR, Blume AW, McKnight P, Marlatt GA. Brief intervention for heavy-drinking college students: 4-year follow-up and natural history. *Am J Public Health*. 2001;91(8):1310–1316

124. Blow FC, Barry KL, Walton MA, et al. The efficacy of two brief intervention strategies among injured, at-risk drinkers in the emergency department: impact of tailored messaging and brief advice. *J Stud Alcohol*. 2006;67(4):568–578

125. Bray JW, Cowell AJ, Hinde JM. A systematic review and meta-analysis of health care utilization outcomes in alcohol screening and brief intervention trials. *Med Care*. 2011;49(3):287–294

126. World Health Organization Brief Intervention Study Group. A cross-national trial of brief interventions with heavy drinkers. *Am J Public Health*. 1996;86:948–955

127. Kulesza M, Apperson M, Larimer ME, Copeland AL. Brief alcohol intervention for college drinkers: how brief is? *Addict Behav*. 2010;35(7):730–733

128. Kulesza M, McVay MA, Larimer ME, Copeland AL. A randomized clinical trial comparing the efficacy of two active conditions of a brief intervention for heavy college drinkers. *Addict Behav*. 2013;38(4):2094–2101

129. Soderstrom CA, DiClemente CC, Dischinger PC, et al. A controlled trial of brief intervention versus brief advice for at-risk drinking trauma center patients. *J Trauma*. 2007;62(5):1102

130. Yonkers KA, Forray A, Howell HB, et al. Motivational enhancement therapy coupled with cognitive behavioral therapy versus brief advice: a randomized trial for treatment of hazardous substance use in pregnancy and after delivery. *Gen Hosp Psychiatry.* 2012;34(5):439–449

131. Boekeloo BO, Jerry J, Lee-Ougo WI, et al. Randomized trial of brief office-based interventions to reduce adolescent alcohol use. *Arch Pediatr Adolesc Med.* 2004;158(7):635–642

132. Mason M, Pate P, Drapkin M, Sozinho K. Motivational interviewing integrated with social network counseling for female adolescents: a randomized pilot study in urban primary care. *J Subst Abuse Treat.* 2011;41(2):148–155

133. Boekeloo BO, Bobbin MP, Lee WI, et al. Effect of patient priming and primary care provider prompting on adolescent-provider communication about alcohol. *Arch Pediatr Adolesc Med.* 2003;157(5):433–439

134. Donovan JE. Estimated blood alcohol concentrations for child and adolescent drinking and their implications for screening instruments. *Pediatrics.* 2009;123(6):e975–e981

135. Substance Abuse and Mental Health Services Administration Office of Applied Studies. *The NSDUH Report: Young Adults' Need for and Receipt of Alcohol and Illicit Drug Use Treatment.* Rockville, MD: Substance Abuse and Mental Health Services Administration; 2009

136. Wu L-T, Ringwalt CL. Use of alcohol treatment and mental health services among adolescents with alcohol use disorders. *Psychiatr Serv.* 2006;57(1):84–92

137. Miller WR, Rollnick S. *Motivational Interviewing: Helping People Change.* 3rd ed. New York: The Guilford Press; 2012

138. Gold MA, Kokotailo PK. Motivational interviewing strategies to facilitate adolescent behavior change. *Adolescent Health Update.* 2007;20(1):1–8

139. Smedslund G, Berg RC, Hammerstrøm KT, et al. Motivational interviewing for substance abuse. *Cochrane Database Syst Rev.* 2011;(5):CD008063

140. Dickersin K. The existence of publication bias and risk factors for its occurrence. *JAMA.* 1990;263:1385–1389

141. D'Onofrio G, Fiellin DA, Pantalon MV, et al. A brief intervention reduces hazardous and harmful drinking in emergency department patients. *Ann Emerg Med.* 2012;60(2):181–192

142. Field CA, Baird J, Saitz R, Caetano R, Monti PM. The mixed evidence for brief intervention in emergency departments, trauma care centers, and inpatient hospital settings: what should we do? *Alcohol Clin Exp Res.* 2010;34(12):2004–2010

143. Cunningham RM, Chermack ST, Zimmerman MA, et al. Brief motivational interviewing intervention for peer violence and alcohol use in teens: one-year follow-up. *Pediatrics.* 2012;129(6):1083–1090

144. Tait RJ, Hulse GK, Robertson SI. Effectiveness of a brief-intervention and continuity of care in enhancing attendance for treatment by adolescent substance users. *Drug Alcohol Depend.* 2004;74(3):289–296

145. Krupski A, Sears JM, Joesch JM, et al. Impact of brief interventions and brief treatment on admissions to chemical dependency treatment. *Drug Alcohol Depend.* 2010;110(1-2):126–136

146. Hassan A, Harris SK, Sherritt L, et al. Primary care follow-up plans for adolescents with substance use problems. *Pediatrics.* 2009;124(1):144–150

147. Grossberg P, Halperin A, Mackenzie S, et al. Inside the physician's black bag: critical ingredients of brief alcohol interventions. *Subst Abus.* 2010;31(4):240–250

148. Michie S, Whittington C, Hamoudi Z, et al. Identification of behaviour change techniques to reduce excessive alcohol consumption. *Addiction.* 2012;107(8):1431–1440

149. Baer JS, Beadnell B, Garrett SB, et al. Adolescent change language within a brief motivational intervention and substance use outcomes. *Psychol Addict Behav.* 2008;22(4):570–575

150. McCambridge J, Day M, Thomas BA, Strang J. Fidelity to Motivational Interviewing and subsequent cannabis cessation among adolescents. *Addict Behav.* 2011;36(7):749–754

151. Campbell SD, Adamson SJ, Carter JD. Client language during motivational enhancement therapy and alcohol use outcome. *Behav Cogn Psychother.* 2010;38(4):399–415

152. Morgenstern J, Kuerbis A, Amrhein P, et al. Motivational interviewing: a pilot test of active ingredients and mechanisms of change. *Psychol Addict Behav.* 2012;26(4):859–869

153. Apodaca TR, Longabaugh R. Mechanisms of change in motivational interviewing: a review and preliminary evaluation of the evidence. *Addiction.* 2009;104(5):705–715
154. Barnett NP, Apodaca TR, Magill M, et al. Moderators and mediators of two brief interventions for alcohol in the emergency department. *Addiction.* 2010;105(3):452–465
155. Lee CS, Baird J, Longabaugh R, et al. Change plan as an active ingredient of brief motivational interventions for reducing negative consequences of drinking in hazardous drinking emergency-department patients. *J Stud Alcohol Drugs.* 2010;71(5):726–733
156. Walters ST, Vader AM, Harris TR, Jouriles EN. Reactivity to alcohol assessment measures: an experimental test. *Addiction.* 2009;104(8):1305–1310
157. Jenkins RJ, McAlaney J, McCambridge J. Change over time in alcohol consumption in control groups in brief intervention studies: systematic review and meta-regression study. *Drug Alcohol Depend.* 2009;100(1-2):107–114
158. Bernstein JA, Bernstein E, Heeren TC. Mechanisms of change in control group drinking in clinical trials of brief alcohol intervention: implications for bias toward the null. *Drug Alcohol Rev.* 2010;29(5):498–507
159. McCambridge J, Kypri K. Can simply answering research questions change behaviour? Systematic review and meta analyses of brief alcohol intervention trials. *PLoS One.* 2011;6(10):e23748
160. McCambridge J, Strang J. The efficacy of single-session motivational interviewing in reducing drug consumption and perceptions of drug-related risk and harm among young people: results from a multi-site cluster randomized trial. *Addiction.* 2004;99(1):39–52
161. Palfai TP, Zisserson R, Saitz R. Using personalized feedback to reduce alcohol use among hazardous drinking college students: the moderating effect of alcohol-related negative consequences. *Addict Behav.* 2011;36(5):539–542
162. Blow FC, Ilgen MA, Walton MA, et al. Severity of baseline alcohol use as a moderator of brief interventions in the emergency department. *Alcohol Alcohol.* 2009;44(5):486–490
163. Field CA, Caetano R. The effectiveness of brief intervention among injured patients with alcohol dependence: who benefits from brief interventions? *Drug Alcohol Depend.* 2010;111(1-2):13–20
164. Finney JW. Regression to the mean in substance use disorder treatment research. *Addiction.* 2008;103(1):42–52
165. Saitz R. Alcohol screening and brief intervention in primary care: absence of evidence for efficacy in people with dependence or very heavy drinking. *Drug Alcohol Rev.* 2011;29(6):631–640
166. Walker DD, Stephens R, Roffman R, et al. Randomized controlled trial of motivational enhancement therapy with nontreatment-seeking adolescent cannabis users: a further test of the teen marijuana check-up. *Psychol Addict Behav.* 2011;25(3):474–484
167. Korcha RA, Cherpitel CJ, Moskalewicz J, et al. Readiness to change, drinking, and negative consequences among Polish SBIRT patients. *Addict Behav.* 2012;37(3):287–292
168. Srisurapanont M, Sombatmai S, Boripuntakul T. Brief intervention for students with methamphetamine use disorders: a randomized controlled trial. *Am J Addict.* 2007;16(2):111–116
169. Zahradnik A, Otto C, Crackau B, et al. Randomized controlled trial of a brief intervention for problematic prescription drug use in non-treatment-seeking patients. *Addiction.* 2009;104(1):109–117
170. Bernstein J, Bernstein E, Tassiopoulos K, et al. Brief motivational intervention at a clinic visit reduces cocaine and heroin use. *Drug Alcohol Depend.* 2005;77(1):49–59
171. Magill M, Barnett NP, Apodaca TR, Rohsenow DJ, Monti PM. The role of marijuana use in brief motivational intervention with young adult drinkers treated in an emergency department. *J Stud Alcohol Drugs.* 2009;70(3):409–413
172. Klimas J, Field C-A, Cullen W, et al. Psychosocial interventions to reduce alcohol consumption in concurrent problem alcohol and illicit drug users. *Cochrane Database Syst Rev.* 2013;2(1):3
173. Stein LAR, Clair M, Lebeau R, et al. Motivational interviewing to reduce substance-related consequences: effects for incarcerated adolescents with depressed mood. *Drug Alcohol Depend.* 2011;118(2-3):475–478
174. Satre DD, Delucchi K, Lichtmacher J, Sterling SA, Weisner C. Motivational interviewing to reduce hazardous drinking and drug use among depression patients. *J Subst Abuse Treat.* 2013;44(3):323–329

175. Penberthy JK, Hook JN, Hettema J, Farrell-Carnahan L, Ingersoll K. Depressive symptoms moderate treatment response to brief intervention for prevention of alcohol exposed pregnancy. *J Subst Abuse Treat.* 2013;45(4):335–342

176. Martino S, Carroll KM, Nich C, Rounsaville BJ. A randomized controlled pilot study of motivational interviewing for patients with psychotic and drug use disorders. *Addiction.* 2006;101(10):1479–1492

177. Hides L, Carroll S, Scott R, et al. Quik Fix: a randomized controlled trial of an enhanced brief motivational interviewing intervention for alcohol/cannabis and psychological distress in young people. *Psychother Psychosom.* 2013;82(2):122–124

178. Louis-Jacques J, Knight JR, Sherritt L, Van Hook S, Harris SK. Do risky friends change the efficacy of a primary care brief intervention for adolescent alcohol use? *J Adolesc Health.* 2013; S1054-139X(13)00510-7. doi: 10.1016/j.jadohealth.2013.09.012

179. Harris SK, Herr-Zaya K, Weinstein Z, et al. Results of a statewide survey of adolescent substance use screening rates and practices in primary care. *Subst Abus.* 2012;33(4):321–326

180. Ozer EM, Adams SH, Lustig JL, et al. Increasing the screening and counseling of adolescents for risky health behaviors: a primary care intervention. *Pediatrics.* 2005;115(4):960–968

181. D'Amico EJ, Miles JN, Stern SA, Meredith LS. Brief motivational interviewing for teens at risk of substance use consequences: a randomized pilot study in a primary care clinic. *J Subst Abuse Treat.* 2008;35(1):53–61

182. Pringle JL, Kowalchuk A, Meyers JA, Seale JP. Equipping residents to address alcohol and drug abuse: the National SBIRT Residency Training Project. *J Grad Med Educ.* 2012;4(1):58–63

183. Ryan SA, Martel S, Pantalon M, et al. Screening, brief intervention, and referral to treatment (SBIRT) for alcohol and other drug use among adolescents: evaluation of a pediatric residency curriculum. *Subst Abus.* 2012;33(3):251–260

184. Marsch LA, Bickel WK, Grabinski M. Application of interactive, computer technology to adolescent substance abuse prevention and treatment. *Adolesc Med State Art Rev.* 2007;18(2):342–356, xii

185. White A, Kavanagh D, Stallman H, et al. Online alcohol interventions: a systematic review. *J Med Internet Res.* 2010;12(5):e62

Adolesc Med 025 (2014) 157–171

Treatment of Adolescent Substance Use Disorders

Consuelo C. Cagande, MD[a],[*]; Basant K. Pradhan, MD[b]; Andres J. Pumariega, MD[c]

[a]*Associate Professor of Psychiatry,* [b]*Assistant Professor of Psychiatry,* [c]*Professor and Chair, Psychiatry, Department of Psychiatry, Cooper University Hospital and Cooper Medical School of Rowan University, Camden, New Jersey*

INTRODUCTION AND OVERVIEW

Treating substance use is challenging, even more so in adolescents. Risk for substance use (legal and illicit) peaks between the ages of 18 and 22 years, except for cocaine. However, those who begin using substances before the age of 15 years are at the greatest risk for developing long-lasting patterns of abuse and dependence.[1]

The most recent findings from the Monitoring the Future Survey raises significant concerns about future increases in the most serious addictions.[2] The survey indicates that alcohol and cigarette use among adolescents has decreased, but use of illicit drugs, which declined in the late 1990s and early 2000s, has been increasing in recent years. After marijuana, there has been an increasing trend in use of prescription and over-the-counter medications, which account for most of the top drugs abused by 12th graders in the past year. Alarmingly, use of bath salts and resulting presentations to the emergency department have increased, and bath salts were included in the 2012 survey for the first time.

Given these findings, a comprehensive evaluation of biologic, psychological, and social factors should be considered when choosing an appropriate and effective treatment plan for adolescents. Different levels of care for treatment and prevention in this population will be discussed here.

---

*Corresponding author:
cagande-consuelo@cooperhealth.edu

Biologic Factors

Adult models of addiction have been primarily used to study biologic risk factors for the adolescent population. However, a focus on developmental processes and co-occurring psychiatric conditions in the adolescent population is vital and requires further research.

Significant evidence in monozygotic twins and adopted siblings raised apart has revealed the strong heritability of alcohol use and abuse.[1] Studies also have revealed a 3- to 4-fold increase of alcohol and substance abuse disorders in those with a positive family history of addiction and a greater prevalence of use of gateway drugs in those with a paternal history of substance abuse disorder. A family history of psychiatric illness with or without substance use in the family also predisposes the adolescent to a co-occurring psychiatric disorder. Early onset of psychiatric disorders such as anxiety and depression predisposes adolescents to maladaptive coping through self-medication with gateway drugs of nicotine, alcohol, and marijuana.[2]

There is now strong evidence that the adolescent brain is highly vulnerable not only from its environment but also because of its developmental process. Adolescence is a transitional period of development when many changes are experienced concomitantly, including physical maturation, drive for independence, increased salience of social and peer interactions, and brain development. This developmental period is also characterized by a marked increase in risky behaviors, including experimentation with drugs and alcohol, criminal activity, and unprotected sex. Understanding the neurobiologic basis of these risky behaviors is key to identifying which teens may be at greatest risk for poor outcomes.[3,4] This can lead to more effective treatment at this age.

Prominent developmental transformations are seen in the prefrontal cortex and limbic brain regions of adolescents across a variety of species. These alterations include an apparent shift in the balance between mesocortical and mesolimbic dopamine systems. Developmental changes in these stressor-sensitive regions, which are critical for attributing incentive salience to drugs and other stimuli, likely contribute to the unique characteristics of adolescent substance abuse.[4]

Although results of studies on the dopamine D2 receptor gene as a biologic marker for alcoholism were not significant, other receptors may show some genetic evidence. The 5-HT-1B receptor, which is implicated in various psychiatric illnesses, has an 861C allele that is specifically associated with substance abuse.[1] Genetic factors are also influenced by the environment. Thus, treatment of adolescent substance use, as in adults, must consider neurodevelopmental and genetic factors in addition to other domains (discussed later). A history of genetic predisposition should help the physician formulate and initiate an early intervention and prevention treatment plan.

Another significant biologic factor in substance abuse risk in adolescents is the development of cue-based cravings for various substances. These are learned associations between the state of well-being and heightened arousal associated with given substances and environmental cues ("people, places, and things") involved in their use. Kilgus et al[5,6] demonstrated how cravings are found frequently among adolescent users and are associated with relapse and negative outcomes.

Psychological and Behavioral Factors

Cognitively, adolescents are less likely to be aware of the negative consequences of using drugs. They have fewer negative perceptions of risks and attitudes about substances. They believe these substances are part of their normal recreational culture, and they are highly influenced by their peers. Their decision-making capacity and emotional intelligence are far from mature and predispose them to impulsive and poor decisions.[1]

Poor self-image, low self-confidence or self-esteem, and low assertiveness are some personality and psychological traits that make adolescents more vulnerable.[1] Poor impulse control is a core behavioral feature of substance use disorders (SUDs).[7] Aggressiveness, poor interpersonal skills, and precocious sexuality are other characteristics to be considered. Early onset of any psychopathology compounded by stressful life events, early novelty seeking, and early disruptive behavioral patterns are additional risk factors.[1] Early age at onset of drug use has been shown to be associated with a longer duration of untreated illness and poorer clinical and functional outcomes.[8] Therefore, it should be considered when developing and implementing early prevention and intervention programs as well as comprehensive treatment plans.

An age group that deserves special consideration is the transitional group of 18 to 22 year-olds who are still using substances. This age group tends to have an earlier onset of substance use, which has a major effect on their brain development and coping capacity. Persistent use by youth in this age group may place them at greater risk for substance dependence and addiction as adults. This is an age cohort that often is neglected or forgotten unless the legal system is involved.

Social Factors

Social factors are powerful predictors of youth substance use. In addition, peer influence is a major factor in adolescent behavior. Family values, parenting styles (ie, inconsistent disciplinary management between caregivers), parental substance use, permissive or tolerant attitudes about substance use by parents, and quality of the parent-child relationship all are implicated in adolescent substance use.

Patterns of drug use may vary by gender as well as by drug type. Boys tend to report more use than girls, particularly as they get older. They also report more use of many different drugs.[1] Boys may have more opportunities to initiate drug use than girls; however, when the opportunity to use was controlled, boys and girls were equally likely to use.[9]

History of trauma (eg, loss of a loved one; physical, sexual, or emotional abuse) is strongly associated with substance use. Neglect, low socioeconomic strata, domestic violence, and children who stay home alone after school while parents work predispose these children to substance use. Social factors should be considered when formulating a comprehensive treatment plan.[1] Parents are integral to the management of SUDs in adolescents. Knowing the family history of substance use provides an understanding of the youth's struggles with substance use. Family dysfunction and conflict can be additional risk factors leading to a reduced resiliency factor in preventing adolescent substance abuse. Family therapy with strength building and support is crucial.[10]

PHILOSOPHY OF TREATMENT

Pediatricians are positioned to have an ongoing relationship with both the adolescent and the family, and they are able to detect changes over time. However, pediatricians usually do not have sufficient time for assessing the presence of substance use or identifying the at-risk adolescent user and family. Adolescents who go to the pediatrician for routine visits do not necessarily present with signs and symptoms of substance use. They more commonly present in the emergency room. Basic data obtained should include physical findings (eg, weight loss, needle tracks, nasal irritation), changes in personal habits (eg, altered sleep pattern, new friends or interests, change in dress), changes in academic performance, and behavioral and psychological symptoms (eg, affective dysregulation, risk taking, stealing).[1]

Treatment of adolescent substance use should take into account age, sex, ethnicity, cultural background, and readiness for change. A treatment team of health care professionals, family, and community members should be assembled to provide an effective therapeutic system. Parents and community supports are integral parts of every treatment plan and modality. Greater adolescent self-disclosure and parental warmth are associated with lower adolescent substance use. These findings underscore the need to facilitate parents' access to and involvement in treatment of adolescents. The parent-adolescent relationship and the mental health of parents are essential aspects to consider for interventions.[11]

Unfortunately, effective treatment typically is not initiated until after years of substance use. Increasing evidence suggests that intervention during the early stages of an SUD may help reduce the severity and persistence of the initial or primary disorder and prevent secondary disorders. Additional research on appropriate treatments for early-stage cases, the long-term effects of early intervention, and appropriate service design for those in the early stages of a mental illness is needed. This means not only strengthening and reengineering existing systems but also, crucially, constructing new streams of care for young people transitioning to adulthood.[8]

The most promising models being promoted for timely identification and treatment are the medical home and integrated behavioral care models, which are central parts of the Affordable Care Act. The medical home model makes the primary care pediatric practice the hub of all health and mental health care for youth. It provides early access to services and care management designed to prevent more advanced morbidities and costs. The integrated behavioral care model within the medical home provides the primary care pediatrician with screening and assessment tools, psychiatric consultation, and access to treatment resources (co-located or by referral) for early identification and timely behavioral health care within the pediatric office. The option for referral to specialized behavioral health services remains but is closely coordinated with the medical home. With implementation of mental health parity under the Affordable Care Act, such services should be better funded, thus reducing financial barriers.[12,13]

In order to implement timely treatment, comprehensive screening and assessment are imperative. The Screening, Brief Intervention, and Referral to Treatment (SBIRT) model promoted by the Substance Abuse and Mental Health Administration fits well into the integrated behavioral health model. Screening tools are available, and the CRAFFT questionnaire, the Substance Abuse Subtle Screening Inventory (SASSI), and the CAGE-AID can be administered routinely during adolescent well visits or indicated visits.[2,14] After brief screening and diagnostic assessment when indicated, the initial intervention typically focuses on education, motivation for change, and consideration of treatment options.[15] Drug testing is commonly used but is not routinely recommended for adolescents. The therapeutic alliance is a priority in adolescents, and forcing urine drug testing may disrupt the relationship. A toxicology screen as part of a routine assessment is not endorsed by the American Academy of Pediatrics (AAP). This includes home- or school-based drug testing. Furthermore, the AAP advocates against involuntary testing in adolescents who have decisional capacity, even if parental consent is given, unless there are strong medical or legal reasons to do so. Drug screening can be important as part of ongoing assessment and treatment.[1]

All adolescents should be screened concurrently for psychiatric disorders, such as depression, anxiety, and even psychosis. Self-medicating with drugs is common among substance users. In addition, there is significant risk of kindling or aggravating an underlying psychopathology by substance use. Examples include the aggravating and disinhibiting effects of alcohol and benzodiazepines on mood disorders (increasing risk for suicidality) and the more recently discovered kindling effects of cannabis on early-onset psychosis.[16,17] If the underlying co-occurring psychiatric disorder is not treated, then accomplishing either decreased use or recovery will be more difficult. Any assessment should include ongoing suicide risk assessment. Adolescents are impulsive, and those with substance use and depression (double jeopardy) are at higher risk for impaired judgment, suicide, and causing harm to others through accidents and violence. Questions should be asked about plans, attempts, or interrupted behaviors with intent to either commit suicide or harm others. Access to guns or other weapons should be questioned, and parents should be advised to remove the adolescent's access to firearms.[10] Prescreening for comorbid psychiatric disorders can be accomplished in the pediatric office by using a broad-based screening scale such as the Pediatric Symptom Checklist, which is part of Bright Futures.[18]

TREATMENT MODALITIES

Treatment interventions and programs should take into account developmental issues that are influenced by cultural values, such as the importance of the peer group; degree of autonomy from parents and the community; family boundaries and hierarchies; limit testing and risk taking; immediate time orientation; failure to anticipate consequences; and culturally normative cognitive skills. Family- and community-based interventions designed for youths of particular cultural backgrounds are available.[1]

Psychological and Social Interventions

The primary goal of any treatment model is patient-physician therapeutic alliance. Motivational enhancement techniques help form therapeutic alliances and patient-generated goals. Individual and peer-enhanced motivational interviewing can be effective with adolescents. It can be readily initiated in the pediatric office and built on by substance abuse counseling.[1]

Cognitive behavioral therapy (CBT) is one of the best evidence-based treatment approaches to treatment of adolescent SUD. Adolescents learn how to identify triggers in certain stress-provoking situations and how to use positive coping skills that will deter them from succumbing to cue-based cravings for substances that can lead to relapse. Anticipatory guidance can be used as a technique for relapse prevention. There is much evidence supporting CBT for psychiatric disorders that co-occur with SUDs.[1]

Family therapy, combined CBT and family therapy, and group interventions improve treatment outcome. Family, especially parents if available, is vital to the management of adolescent SUD. History of family substance use should be elicited. Parents who are actively using should be referred to an adult treatment program. Family therapy is crucial, and family support and strength building are well within the realm of primary care practice.[1]

Family-based therapies, such as multifamily group therapy, improve treatment outcomes and lead to better patient prognosis. Family members are encouraged to be assertive and self-sufficient. Multidimensional family therapy (MDFT) is based on the theory that multiple ecologic factors and abnormal development maintain drug use and other problem behaviors. MDFT focuses on 4 areas of adolescent life: (1) the individual (developing a sense of self, self-efficacy); (2) parents and family; (3) transactional patterns; and (4) family interactions (relationships) with extrafamilial systems.[1] Brief strategic family therapy addresses adolescent-parent conflicts that can be generational or cultural in nature and focuses on developing an empathic bridge between youth and parents within the context of consistent structure.[19]

Peer groups play a vital role in promoting abstinence as well as abuse. In an unsupervised setting, adolescents are vulnerable to negative peer influences. While undergoing treatment, patients should be involved with new peer groups that are trying to achieve the same goal of abstinence and can support each other in remaining sober. The adolescent should be encouraged to participate in school activities that can provide more positive peer interactions and healthier lifestyles.[10] Adolescent-specific help groups may not be available in most communities but can be valuable treatment resources. Modified 12-step programs (Alcohol Anonymous [AA], Narcotics Anonymous [NA]) and relapse prevention groups for adolescents are available. Twelve-step groups for youths improve outcome primarily by increasing motivational factors as opposed to improving coping or self-efficacy.[1] Adolescents usually will develop positive coping skills in a group setting. These skills include relaxation therapy, recreation and various leisure skills, social skills, relationship enhancement, and other coping strategies with extensive opportunities for practice.[1]

A traditional technique or skill that is gaining more attention is mindfulness meditation. Mindfulness is defined as *a mental state achieved by focusing one's awareness on the present moment while calmly acknowledging and accepting one's feelings, thoughts, and bodily sensations, used as a therapeutic technique.* It is based on the concept of mindfulness in Buddhist meditation. This technique can be used both to target enhanced self-awareness of distress or cravings and to master anxiety associated with their cravings without the use of substances. It is a skill that can be taught to persons of all ages and can be integrated into cognitive-behavioral interventions.[20]

Evidence supports the use of behavioral therapy, such as contingency management, in overcoming 2 major challenges that permeate SUD: poor retention rates because of compromised motivation and reliance on subjective measures to assess treatment outcomes. Rewards are provided for objective evidence of sobriety, changes in behavior associated with drug use, improved family functioning, school attendance, socialization, and treatment plan adherence.[1]

Multisystemic therapy addresses the multiple risk factors for SUD in a highly individualized and strategic fashion. Some factors are individual youth characteristics, family functioning, caregiver functioning, peer relations, school performance, indigenous family supports, and neighborhood characteristics. Assessment and treatment are in manual form (written systematic protocols) and focus on 9 treatment principles with performance-based outcome criteria. These principles are as follows: (1) behavior makes sense in its context; (2) strengths as levers for change; (3) increasing responsible behavior; (4) present focused, well defined, and action oriented; (5) target sequences of behaviors; (6) developmentally appropriate; (7) continuous effort; (8) evaluation and accountability; and (9) generalization.[21,22]

Programs and Levels of Care

A range of programs and levels of care are used to treat adolescent substance abuse. They include detoxification (DT), inpatient hospitalization, residential treatment centers (RTCs), outpatient programs (OPs), and self-help. Matching adolescents to an appropriate level of care is based on considerations of severity of symptoms and behaviors, level of function, degree of comorbidity, available services and support resources, financial status, legal mandates, as well as factors such as age, gender, and ethnicity/cultural background.[1]

The goal of DT is to terminate substance use and medically treat the withdrawal symptoms in a safe and supervised setting. Adolescents who have less complicated withdrawal symptoms can be detoxified in the outpatient setting by an experienced DT specialist. Most DT programs are conducted on an outpatient basis. DT is the first step in a more comprehensive treatment plan. It also involves counseling, support, and group work.[1]

Hospitalization in a psychiatric unit provides a structured therapeutic environment. It includes services by psychiatric care practitioners, addiction counselors, and therapists. The initial step is a comprehensive assessment that may include psychiatric evaluation as well as assessment of the family by the treatment team. The focus is not solely on the substance use but also on co-occurring psychiatric disorders. Inpatient programs for adolescents are strict, with detailed daily activity schedules and intensive therapeutic interventions. Lengths of stay have been reduced and typically do not exceed 2 weeks before the adolescent steps down to a lower level of care.[1]

RTCs originally were more confrontational and had more stringent codes of behavior. Now they are more supportive, are more empathically confrontational, and have greater treatment flexibility. The adolescent who is more antisocial and behaviorally disruptive would be the best match for an RTC.[1] RTCs allow the adolescent with an SUD to be removed from factors that influence substance use, such as peers and the environment. This drug-free setting teaches the adolescent drug-free ways of coping using the different psychotherapy or psychological and behavioral models mentioned earlier, including family-based therapy. Other goals are to build self-esteem, develop social skills, and educate and train the individual for work. Life skills training is essential in RTCs because the adolescent's development is often arrested as a result of substance use. Attention to multifactorial dimensions (eg, biologic, psychological, social, cultural, spiritual) will help individualize the adolescent's treatment plan. Treatment in the RTC typically is voluntary and usually lasts for several weeks to months. Most people who enter such programs leave before completing their course of treatment because of financial pressures or intense cravings.[1]

OPs constitute the level of care that includes most substance use treatment programs. Adolescents who have just finished an inpatient program or RTC most likely will be stepped down to an OP, although most youths receive treatment solely at this level of care. Modalities include behavioral or programmatic structure, counseling, and family therapy. OPs start as partial hospitalization programs, where the adolescent spends most of the day at the program (including schooling) and spends the night at home, often as an alternative to inpatient hospitalization. The adolescent and parents or family must be motivated and cooperative with the treatment program. Youths should be willing to submit to random drug testing. Other therapeutic modalities, such as behavior therapy, skills development, hypnosis, biofeedback, and crisis programs (eg, telephone hotlines, walk-in centers, referral services, and emergency interventions), are available.[1]

Other OPs include intensive outpatient program models, after school programs, and evening treatment. The latter allows parents to be involved but with less interference with daily life. School-based programs hold considerable promise for early treatment intervention in SUDs. Programs should be flexible by offering convenient times and places, and choice of formats (group or individual sessions) in order to minimize barriers to treatment success.[1]

Two effective tools that have evidence supporting their use in determining the level of care needed for adolescent substance abuse treatment are the American Society of Addiction Medicine (ASAM) Adolescent Criteria and the Child and Adolescent Level of Care Intensity Instrument (CASII) by the American Academy of Child and Adolescent Psychiatry. The CASII is based on the ASAM criteria. It has the advantages of ease of use, orientation to service intensity independent of location, and ability to accommodate dual treatment (mental health and addiction), which are essential for adolescent substance abuse treatment.[23]

Pharmacology and Co-occurring Disorders

There are few studies on the use of medications in adolescents for treatment of primary SUDs. In adolescents, pharmacotherapy for an alcohol use disorder (AUD) may target alcohol withdrawal symptoms, alcohol consumption reinforcement properties, craving, or comorbid mental disorders. Although uncommon among adolescents, severe alcohol withdrawal may require closely monitored application of benzodiazepines. Disulfiram alters alcohol metabolism and increases abstinence in adolescents with AUD; however, sufficient motivation to maintain abstinence is needed for this approach to be successful. Medications to reduce alcohol craving, including naltrexone and acamprosate, may assist some adolescents in maintaining abstinence.[24] In a randomized, double-blind, placebo-controlled crossover study comparing naltrexone (50 mg/day) and placebo in 22 adolescent problem alcohol drinkers aged 15 to 19 years, naltrexone reduced drinking and alcohol cravings. It also altered subjective responses to alcohol in a sample of adolescent problem drinkers, but given the small sample, a larger clinical trial with long-term follow-up is suggested.[25]

A systematic review of 23 randomized control trials included opioid-dependent participants with a mean age older than 16 years who received opioid DT using buprenorphine, methadone, clonidine, or lofexidine. The study comprised a total of 2112 participants. The review found buprenorphine and methadone were the most effective DT treatments. Although the analysis suggests buprenorphine is the most effective method of DT, there is some uncertainty about whether it is more effective than methadone; therefore, this therapy requires further research.[26] A retrospective quality improvement study of men aged 18 to 55 years found that buprenorphine with naloxone (Suboxone) treatment decreased premature termination of opioid DT completion compared with clonidine, which has been the traditional supportive treatment of opioid withdrawal.[27]

More than 70% of adolescents with SUD are diagnosed with 1 or more comorbid psychiatric disorders.[28] Adolescents may have similar patterns as adults in terms of self-medicating with substances for their psychiatric symptoms. However, a meta-analysis concluded that there is little evidence supporting this theory.[29] On the other hand, there is empirical support for the rebound effects (ie, symptom exacerbations) of substance use on symptom severity in youth with comorbid psychiatric illness.[30]

Anxiety, depression, and impulsive and disruptive disorders are common comorbid diagnoses with SUDs. Early identification of the symptoms of these disorders can be helpful in preventing relapse or worsening use. Abstinence from substance use for at least 1 month can help determine whether the SUD or psychiatric diagnosis is primary. However, it is best not to delay treatment for psychiatric diagnoses such as depression, psychosis, or bipolar disorder (BPD) with psychotropic medications in adolescents, especially if safety or lethality is a concern. It is imperative that there be collaboration between a child and adolescent psychiatrist or therapist and a family physician or pediatrician when a psychiatric consultation is not readily available.[10,31]

Selective serotonin reuptake inhibitors (SSRIs) are the first choice of medications for treatment of major depressive episodes (MDE), anxiety, and trauma-related disorders. They have safer side effects and drug-to-drug interaction profiles. The downside of SSRIs is that they may take up to 4 to 6 weeks to be effective. It is important to monitor and, if possible, collaborate with a child and adolescent psychiatrist when starting SSRIs. Careful monitoring is imperative, especially if suicidality or suicidal behavior is reported. It also is important to screen for possible symptoms of underlying BPD, which could kindle mania or hypomania.[10,31]

Caution should be exercised in prescribing other classes of antidepressants for youth with SUD. Specifically, the combination of tricyclic antidepressant (TCA) and alcohol or marijuana can cause more interactions than others. Effects include mental status changes consistent with delirium and tachycardia possibly as a result of metabolism of both cannabis and TCAs by similar hepatic mitochondrial enzymes. Cannabis and TCAs are both cholinergic and adrenergic, which could be responsible for the elevated heart rate.[32] It is vital to educate and inform the adolescent and parents about the potential risks of combining prescription medications with drugs of abuse.

Dicola et al[33] studied the treatment rates among adolescents with co-occurring MDE. They concluded that there were exceptionally low rates of SUD treatment in their high-risk sample. They found less than half (48%) of adolescents received any form of MDE treatment in the past year, and only 10% received any form of SUD treatment. Only 16% of adolescents who received MDE treatment also received SUD treatment. Compared to having no insurance, having public insurance was associated with an increased likelihood of receiving MDE treatment alone but was not associated with an increased likelihood of receiving both MDE and SUD treatment. Adolescents with private insurance who were part of a high-risk population did not have significantly higher rates of MDE or SUD treatment. Involvement in the criminal justice system was the major factor affecting the likelihood that an adolescent would receive both MDE and SUD treatment as opposed to either no treatment or treatment for MDE alone.[33]

Treatment of disruptive and impulsive behaviors depends on the psychiatric diagnosis. Adolescents with SUD have a high rate of comorbid diagnosis of attention-deficit/hyperactivity disorder (ADHD). ADHD is known to be a strong risk factor for SUD in adolescence. Research has shown that stimulant treatment does not increase the risk of SUD in adolescents or adults with ADHD; rather, stimulant treatments may have a protective or risk reduction effect. However, 2 in 10 youths with ADHD misuse their medication. There is evidence that slow uptake of medication in the brain allows for effective treatment without patients experiencing the euphoric qualities of immediate-release agents that lead to abuse or diversion. As a result, extended-release products and different formulations, such as lisdexamfetamine dimesylate (LDX), are less likely to be misused and diverted and may have lower abuse potential.[34] A single-center, randomized, double-blind, placebo-controlled 6-period crossover study evaluated the abuse potential of single oral doses of 50, 100 (equivalent to 40 mg d-amphetamine), and 150 mg LDX, 40 mg d-amphetamine, and 200 mg diethyl-propion in 36 individuals with a history of stimulant abuse. They concluded that at an equivalent amount of amphetamine base taken orally, LDX 100 mg had attenuated responses on measures of abuse liability compared with immediate-release d-amphetamine 40 mg.

After oral administration, LDX must be enzymatically converted to its active moiety, d-amphetamine, and the naturally occurring essential amino acid, l-lysine. Because of these properties, LDX cannot be mechanically manipulated to extract d-amphetamine. The attenuation of maximum liking effects and the delay of time to peak effects on the measures of abuse liability, combined with the inability to easily extract d-amphetamine, suggest that LDX has a reduced risk for drug tampering and may have the potential for a decreased risk of oral abuse compared to d-amphetamine.[35]

An alternative nonstimulant medication for treatment of ADHD is atomoxetine. The antidepressant bupropion is another nonstimulant medication for adolescents with SUD and comorbid depressive episode or ADHD. It has also been shown to reduce cravings and is indicated for smoking cessation. A naturalistic study suggests that bupropion is well tolerated and may be an effective medication for treatment of substance-abusing adolescents with comorbid mood disorders and ADHD.[36] Humphrey et al[37] performed a meta-analysis of stimulant medication and substance use outcomes. They concluded that treatment of ADHD with stimulant medication neither protects nor increases the risk of later SUD. This finding suggests there are multiple biopsychosocial predisposing factors that need attention throughout adolescent development.

Mood stabilizers can treat severe mood dysregulation or diagnosed BPD. When treating dually diagnosed disorders such as BPD and SUD, physicians should consider a simultaneous approach. Given the limited but important data on the effects of medication treatment reducing SUD in BPD, both psychosocial and medication strategies should be considered simultaneously in these comorbid adolescents. There is evidence that pharmacologic interventions are effective for youth with SUD and BPD. Two studies, including one randomized controlled study, have reported that mood stabilizers, specifically lithium and valproic acid, significantly reduced substance use in bipolar youth.[38] A controlled, 6-week study of treatment with lithium in youth with affective dysregulation and substance dependence reported a clinically significant decrease in the number of positive urine tests as well as a significant increase in overall global functioning.[39] In a 5-week open trial of valproic acid in adolescent outpatients with marijuana abuse/dependence and "explosive mood disorder," Donovan and Nunes[40] reported significant improvement in marijuana use and affective symptoms. The use of atypical neuroleptics as mood-stabilizing agents in comorbid SUD-BPD remains understudied but compelling, and further work in this area is needed.

The potential for interactions between prescribed medications and alcohol or illicit substances necessitates patient education and monitoring. Although there is a paucity of empirical information on the applicability of these pharmacotherapy approaches in adolescents, cautious application of these medications in select cases in the context of systematic psychosocial interventions is warranted to promote abstinence and address associated problems. However, the risk of not treating adolescent psychiatric disorders will impede SUD treatment initiation, precipitate early dropout or relapse, or interfere with achievement of abstinence.[10,28] The well-documented adverse outcomes associated with prolonged duration of untreated illness in psychosis underscore the need for far greater identification and intervention in emerging psychiatric disorders associated with adolescent SUD.[8]

CONCLUSION

The preadolescent and adolescent years are potentially the most vulnerable periods of development. Prevention and identification of early substance use and associated psychiatric disorders as well as early and timely treatment are crucial. Understanding the biopsychosocial factors of development and treatment can guide the physician and improve outcomes and prevent relapse.

There are many effective psychosocial treatments, particularly models of multidimensional family therapy and motivational enhancement therapy. Unfortunately, medications do not necessarily treat the substance use directly but can address underlying psychiatric disorders. An integrated collaborative plan of care involving primary care physicians, child and adolescent psychiatrists or addiction psychiatrists, and other addiction and mental professionals is essential for treatment of this population.

References

1. Pumariega AJ, Kilgus MD, Rodriguez L. Adolescence. In: Ruiz, P. (ed). *Lewinsohn's Textbook on Addictions.* Philadelphia, PA: Lippincott, Williams, & Williams; 2005:1021–1037
2. Johnston LD, O'Malley JL, Bachman JG, Schulenberg JE. *Monitoring the Future: National Survey Results on Drug Use, 1975 – 2011. Volume I: Secondary School Students.* Ann Arbor, MI: Institute for Social Research, The University of Michigan; 2012
3. Casey BJ, Jones RM. Neurobiology of adolescent brain and behavior. *J Am Acad Child Adolesc Psychiatry.* 2010;49(12):1189–1201
4. Spear LP. The adolescent brain and age-related behavioral manifestations. *Neurosci Biobehav Rev.* 2000;24(4):417–463
5. Kilgus MD, Pumariega AJ, Seidel RW. Experimental manipulation of cocaine craving in adolescents by videotaped environmental cues. *Addictive Disord Treat.* 2009;8(2):80–87
6. Kilgus MD, Pumariega AJ, Rea W. Physiological and cognitive changes that accompany cocaine craving in adolescents. *Addictive Disord Treat.* 2009;8(3):128–137
7. Moeller FG, Dougherty DM, Barratt ES, et al. The impact of impulsivity on cocaine use and retention in treatment. *J Subst Abuse Treat.* 2001;21(4):193–198
8. McGorry PD, Purcell R, Goldstone S, Amminger GP. Age of onset and timing of treatment for mental and substance use disorders: implications for preventive intervention strategies and models of care. *Curr Opin Psychiatry.* 2011;24(4):301–306

9. Van Etten ML, Neumark YD, Anthony JC. Male-female differences in the earliest stages of drug involvement. *Addiction.* 1999; 94:1413–1419
10. Griswold KS, Aronoff H, Kernan JB, Kahn LS. Adolescent substance use and abuse: recognition and management. *Am Fam Physician.* 2008;77(3):331–336
11. BertrandK, Richer I, Brunelle N, Beaudoin I, Lemieux A, Ménard JM. Substance abuse treatment for adolescents: how are family factors related to substance use change? *J Psychoactive Drugs.* 2013;45(1):28–38
12. Sia C, Tonniges T, Osterhus E, Taba S. History of the medical home concept. *Pediatrics.* 2004;113;1473–1478
13. Campo J, Shafer S, Strohm J, et al. Pediatric behavioral health in primary care: a collaborative approach. *J Am Psychiat Nurses Assoc.* 2005;11:276–282
14. Mitchell SG, Gryczynski J, Gonzales A, et al. Screening, brief intervention, and referral to treatment (SBIRT) for substance use in a school-based program: services and outcomes. *Am J Addict.* 2012;21(Suppl 1):S5–S13
15. Clark DB, Gordon AJ, Ettaro LR, Owens JM, Moss HB. Screening and brief intervention for underage drinkers. *Mayo Clinic Proc.* 2010;85(4):380–391
16. Longo LP, Johnson B. Addiction: part I. Benzodiazepines—side effects, abuse risk and alternatives. *Am Fam Physician.* 2000;61(7):2121–2128
17. Arseneault L, Cannon M, Witton J, Murray R. Causal association between cannabis and psychosis: examination of the evidence. *Br J Psychiatry.* 2004;184:110–117
18. Jellinek M, Murphy J, Little M, et al. Use of the Pediatric Symptom Checklist to screen for psychosocial problems in primary care: a national feasibility study. *Arch Pediatr Adolesc Med.* 1999;153: 254–260
19. Santisteban DA, Coatsworth JD, Perez-Vidal A, et al. Efficacy of brief strategic family therapy in modifying Hispanic adolescent behavior problems and substance use. *J Fam Psychol.* 2003;17:121–133
20. Pradhan BK. *Yoga and Mental Health: De-Mystification, Standardization and Application.* Lanham, MD: Rowman Littlefield Publishers; 2014
21. Henggeler SW, Pickrel SG. Brondino MJ. Multisystemic treatment of substance-abusing and -dependent delinquents: outcomes, treatment, fidelity, and transportability. *Mental Health Serv Res.* 1999;1:171–184
23. Pumariega A, Winters N, Chenven M, et al. Child and Adolescent Level of Care Utilization System (CALOCUS), later titled Child and Adolescent Service Intensity Instrument (CASII). Washington, DC: American Academy of Child and Adolescent Psychiatry; 2007
24. Clark DB. Pharmacotherapy for adolescent alcohol use disorder. *CNS Drugs.* 2012;26(7):559–569
25. Miranda R, Ray L, Blanchard A, et al. Effects of naltrexone on adolescent alcohol cue reactivity and sensitivity: an initial randomized trial. *Addict Biol.* 2013 Mar 13.1-142013;[Epub ahead of print]
26. Meader N. A comparison of methadone, buprenorphine and alpha(2) adrenergic agonists for opioid detoxification: a mixed treatment comparison meta-analysis. *Drug Alcohol Depend.* 2010;108(1–2):110–114
27. Steele A, Cunningham F. A comparison of suboxone and clonidine treatment outcomes in opiate detoxification. *Arch Psychiatr Nurs.* 2012;26(4):316–323
28. Kaminer Y, Bukstein OG. *Adolescent Substance Abuse: Psychiatric Comorbidity and High Risk Behaviors.* New York: Routledge/Taylor & Francis; 2008
29. Degenhardt L, Hall W, Lynskey M. Exploring the association between cannabis use and depression. *Addiction.* 2003;98:1493–1504
30. Tomlinson KL, Tate SR, Anderson KG, McCarthy D, Brown SA. An examination of self-medication and rebound effects: psychiatric symptomatology before and after alcohol or drug relapse. *Addic Behav.* 2005;31:461–574
31. Riggs PD, Davies RD. A clinical approach to integrating treatment for adolescent depression and substance abuse. *J Am Acad Child Adolesc Psychiatry.* 2002;41:1253–1255

32. Wilens TE, Monuteauz MC, Snyder LE, et al. The clinical dilemma of using medications in substance-abusing adolescents and adults with ADHD: what does the literature tell us? *J Child Adolesc Psychopharm.* 2005;15:787–798

33. Dicola LA, Gaydos LM, Druss BG, Cummings JR. Health insurance and treatment of adolescents with co-occurring major depression and substance use disorders. *J Am Acad Child Adolesc Psychiatry.* 2013;52(9):953–960

34. Faraone SV, Upadhyaya HP. The effect of stimulant treatment for ADHD on later substance abuse and the potential for medication misuse, abuse and diversion. *J Clin Psychiatry.* 2007;68(11):e228

35. Jasinski DR, Krishnan S. Abuse liability and safety of oral lisdexamfetamine dimesylate in individuals with a history of stimulant abuse. *J Psychopharm.* 2009;23(4):419–427

36. Solhkhah R, Wilens TE, Daly J, et al. Bupropion SR for the treatment of substance-abusing outpatient adolescents with attention-deficit/hyperactivity disorder and mood disorders. *J Child Adolesc Psychopharm.* 2005;15(5):777–786

37. Humphreys KL, Eng T, Lee SS. Stimulant medication and substance use outcomes: a meta-analysis. *JAMA Psychiatry.* 2013;70(7):740–749

38. Joshi G, Wilens T. Comorbidity in pediatric bipolar disorder. *Child Adolesc Psychiatr Clin N Am.* 2009;18(2):291–319

39. Geller B, Cooper TB, Sun K, Zimerman B, Frazier J, Williams M, Heath J. Double-blind and placebo-controlled study of lithium for adolescent bipolar disorders with secondary substance dependency. *J Am Acad Child Adolesc Psychiatry.* 1998;37(2):171–178

40. Donovan S. Nunes E. Treatment of co-morbid affective and substance use disorders: therapeutic potential of anticonvulsants. *Am J Addict.* 1998;7(3):210–220

Adolesc Med 025 (2014) 172–183

Substance Abuse Among Culturally Diverse Youth

Basant K. Pradhan, MD[a*]; Consuelo C. Cagande, MD[b];
Andres J. Pumariega, MD[c]

[a]Assistant Professor of Psychiatry, [b]Associate Professor of Psychiatry,
[c]Professor and Chair, Department of Psychiatry, Cooper University Hospital
and Cooper Medical School of Rowan University, Camden, New Jersey

INTRODUCTION

Adolescence, a developmental period of physical and psychological changes, marks the commencement of greater independence, increased experimentation, and risk taking among youth between the ages of 12 and 18 years.[1] Experimentation with illicit substances (eg, marijuana, nonmedical use of prescription medications, hallucinogens) and licit substances (eg, alcohol, tobacco, prescription drugs) has its onset primarily during the adolescent years, with noticeable peaks at young adult ages.[2] Substance use causes a number of adverse physical (ie, death from injury and increased participation in risky behaviors), mental (ie, depression, personality disorders, and developmental lags), and social (ie, poor academic performances, withdrawal, delinquency, and disengagement from family and peers) health effects among adolescents.[3] Furthermore, research has revealed that adolescent substance use problems increase the risk of developing substance use disorders (SUDs) later in life.[4]

Traditionally the United States has been the land of immigrants, and in the last few decades it has faced a rapidly changing demographic and cultural landscape. Culturally diverse children and youth are a growing sector of the population. By the year 2019, most children and youth aged 17 years and younger will be non-white, and all ethnic and racial groups in this population will comprise a plurality.[5] As a consequence, cultural factors relating to mental illness and substance abuse-related emotional disturbances deserve closer attention. For obvious reasons, including stigma itself (which often is culturally based), the process of

---

*Corresponding author:
pradhan-basant@cooperhealth.edu

evaluating and treating substance abuse becomes even more daunting in culturally diverse youth and requires added expertise and unique approaches.

PREVALENCE OF SUBSTANCE USE DISORDERS AMONG CULTURALLY DIVERSE YOUTH

Current information about adolescent substance use disorders (SUDs in the
United States is largely derived from the annual Monitoring the Future (MTF)
survey,[6] the Youth Risk Behavior Survey (YRBS),[7] Healthy People 2020 Objective SA-13.1 Reports,[8] regional school studies, studies on various treatment programs for SUD, and national household surveys. Despite prevention efforts by
health professionals, recent estimates from national surveys suggest that adolescent substance use and abuse continue to be persistent and commonly widespread public health issues.[6]

In the YRBS, more than 15,000 US high school students from 43 states and 21
large urban school districts are surveyed nationally.[7] This report primarily examines rates of substance use in white, black, and Latino youth. It demonstrates
that Latino and black youth use substances at significantly higher rates. For
example, the percentage of lifetime alcohol use was highest in Latinos (73.2%),
followed by whites and blacks, whereas binge drinking was equal in Latinos and
whites (24%), followed by blacks (12.4%). Current cannabis use is highest among
blacks (25.4%) and Latinos (24.4%) and lower in whites (21.7%). Lifetime use of
cocaine is significantly higher in Latinos (10.2%) compared to whites (6.7%) and
blacks (2.6%). This predominance of substance use among Latinos is also seen
with a number of other substances: lifetime inhalant use (Latinos 14.4% vs.
whites 10.7% and blacks 9.2%); lifetime use of ecstasy (Latinos 10.6% vs. whites
7.7% and blacks 6.0%); and lifetime use of methamphetamine (Latinos 4.6% vs.
whites 3.7% and blacks 2.6%). The exception is the abuse of prescription medications, for which lifetime use is highest in whites (22.9%) compared to Latinos
(19.4%) and blacks (14.7%).

The MTF Survey, which has surveyed more than 45,000 8th-graders and high
school students annually from 1992 through 2012, reports the use of alcohol,
cigarette, and illicit drugs. It has shown that black students have lower reported
lifetime annual prevalence rates for virtually all drugs compared to whites and
Latinos, whereas the latter have the highest lifetime and annual prevalence rates
for cocaine and crack, confirming what has been reported in the MTF surveys.

The Healthy People 2020 Objective SA-13.1 is one of the leading health indica-
tors for substance abuse. It tracks annually the proportion of adolescents aged 12
to 17 years who reported using alcohol or illicit drugs in the past 30 days.[8] This
2011 report demonstrates that diversities do exist in the past-month use of alcohol or illicit drugs by adolescents with respect to age, race and ethnicity, and
country of birth. Among age groups, the youngest adolescents (12-13 years) had

the lowest rate of alcohol or illicit drug use (5.1%) in 2011. Rates for the other age groups generally increase with age: 16.0% of adolescents aged 14 to 15 years reported using alcohol or illicit drugs during the past 30 days, and 31.8% of adolescents aged 16 to 17 years reported using alcohol or illicit drugs during the past 30 days. Adolescents born outside the United States reported a lower rate of alcohol or illicit drug use (13.7%) than adolescents born in the United States (18.3%). Among racial and ethnic groups within the United States, Asian adolescents aged 12 to 17 years reported the lowest rates of alcohol or illicit drug use (10.3%). Rates for adolescents in other racial and ethnic groups were 17.2% for blacks, 17.9% for Latino adolescents, 18.4% for white, non-Latino adolescents, 20.2% for American Indian or Alaska Native adolescents, and 25.1% for adolescents who identify with 2 or more races. All disparities described are statistically significant at the 0.05 level of significance.[8]

IMMIGRATION AND DRUG ABUSE

In the context of elaborating on an explanatory model of SUD in youth, Miller[9] notes that when unusually stress-sensitive children encounter the normative helplessness and struggle for autonomy that attends adolescence, they may engage in maladaptive coping behaviors such as drug abuse. These problems always occur within a social, economic, and cultural context as well, beginning with the immediate ecology of the family and household living environment and later becoming generalized to the larger surroundings, including the school and peer groups. Added to this, immigration and acculturation stress can create a vicious circle of further maladaptation to ongoing stress and may contribute to SUD in these already vulnerable youth. Further, trauma experiences associated with the history or daily experiences of adolescents of particular racial and ethnic groups are often associated with higher risk for adolescent substance abuse.[10]

Pumariega and Rothe[11] outlined how the stresses related to immigration and acculturation may be associated with SUD in youth in the United States, particularly second-generation youth. Migration stress can be divided into premigration stress (including exposure to violence, persecution, and torture in the country of origin); migration stress (including the disruption and separation of families, traumatic journeys, detention in refugee camps, and various forms of victimization during the journey); and postmigration and acculturation stress (resulting from the process of adaptation to the host culture, low levels of education and job skills, living in high-risk neighborhoods, and overcrowded, poor-quality inner-city schools). In addition, immigrant children and their families often face the stressors of prejudice and discrimination against immigrants, especially if they are racially different from the majority culture.[12] For some children and youth, this situation may lead to poor academic functioning, low self-esteem, depression, and suicidality.[11] Some minority youth may adopt a position of defiance against the dominant culture by joining gangs,[13] which increases their vulnerability to peer influence to use substances. As a result of these stressors, second-generation children of immigrants are generally at increased risk for mental health problems, including anxiety, depression, and substance abuse.[11,14] The linkage between depressive symptomatology, substance abuse, and suicide among immigrant youth, particularly Latinos, has been documented in a number of studies.[15-18] Most of these studies suggest that suicides in these youth tend to occur as an outcome of underlying depressive illness, often interacting with alcohol and drug abuse and precipitated by stressful life events.

The role of acculturation stress in SUD has been well studied in adult populations and, to some extent, in immigrant youth. Researchers have reported links between acculturation stress and drug abuse in Latino adolescents, with additional risk factors for substance abuse being depression, and the absence of family protective factors.[19-21] They also note that the higher rates of substance abuse and suicidality are correlated with higher levels of assimilation by immigrant youth, as evidenced by their adoption of more *Americanized* patterns of activities and relationships, such as greater media exposure, lower levels of family activity, and higher levels of independent peer activities. When assimilating Latino youth attempt to *fit in* with mainstream American peer culture, they may lose a sense of their original identity and heritage. In addition, the phenomenon of acculturative family distancing (ie, when an acculturating youth adapts more rapidly than the immigrant parents to the host culture, thus resulting in intergenerational conflict) has been associated with an increased risk of substance abuse in second-generation youth.[19] However, Pumariega et al[20,21] found that although culturally determined factors are associated with higher risk for adolescent substance abuse, psychological distress and depressive symptomatology along with demographic factors contribute greatest risk. Swanson et al[18] found a correlation between depressive symptoms and substance use reported by adolescents along the United States-Mexico border, and Sanchez-Barker[22] explains that substance abuse can be a sign of depression among Latino youth.

MENTAL HEALTH DISPARITIES AND SUD IN DIVERSE YOUTH

The studies cited earlier not only support the findings of higher levels of mental health problems in second-generation immigrants but also clarify the processes through which these generational disparities arise. For example, substance abuse was found to be higher among Mexican-origin youth living on the US side of the border than among Mexican youth, with second-generation status, depression, male gender, cultural factors (lack of family cohesion, unsupervised time with friends, no religious ties, media exposure), and school problems being predictors of higher risk.[19] It also has been shown that the development of particular psychopathology seems to follow a multigenerational pattern. For example, Latino children suffer from higher levels of anxiety than European-origin or black children, with significantly higher anxiety symptoms in second-generation versus first-generation Latino youth.[23] Similarly, Pina and Silverman[24] found a differential expression of anxiety symptoms in Latino youth. In a study of Japanese, Chinese, and Korean immigrant youth, age, acculturation, and cultural adjustment difficulties significantly predicted mental health symptoms.[25]

Disparities in Provision and Utilization of Mental Health Services

In addition to acculturation stress and other differential stressors, disparities in service use may contribute to the increasing risk for psychopathology found among diverse youth, including SUD. For example, Pumariega et al[26] and Juszczak et al[27] found that Latino youth used half as many counseling services as whites and blacks and that first-generation Latino immigrants used even fewer services. A number of studies have similarly shown lower levels of utilization of mental health services by Russian, Bosnian, and southeast Asian immigrants.[28–30] Yeh et al[31] found that Latinos and Asian youth showed higher levels of unmet mental health needs than white youth, but parents endorsed fewer barriers to care because cultural factors influenced parental perceptions of barriers. A result of such disparities may be a high risk of referral of black and Latino youth to juvenile authorities for behavioral difficulties, with similar high rates for southeast Asian immigrant youth.[32]

Rates of prescribing psychotropic medication are lower for black, Latino, and Asian youth than for white youth.[33,34] Various studies also have found significant disparities in the delivery of psychotherapy services among immigrant groups. Alegria et al[35] outlined various factors contributing to ethnic-racial disparities in adolescent SUD treatment, including health service policies, operation of the health care and school-based services systems, provider-level factors (eg, stereotyping, bias, lack of cultural sensitivity), and community, family, and individual factors (eg, stigma, greater threshold for tolerance of symptoms).

Psychopharmacogenomic Factors

Psychopharmacogenomic research specifically addressing diversity in SUD is in its infancy. However, it is important to be aware of the various recent biologic and genetic factors that may serve the goal of addressing health disparities.[36,37] The relative proportion of functional genetic variants for any given gene may vary by ancestry. In theory, this can lead to different patterns of medication metabolism, activity, and risk for side effects.

Ethnopsychopharmacology has focused on the study of pharmacogenomic risk alleles, which vary in frequency across different ethnic and racial populations, thus raising questions about the importance of these factors when prescribing medications. These factors include the distribution of rapid, slow, and super-slow activity of cytochrome P450 (CYP) isoenzymes (especially CYP2D6 and CYP2D19) across different racial and ethnic populations and polymorphisms of the serotonin 2A and dopamine D3 receptors related to antipsychotic and antidepressant treatment response. These differences have been associated with reports of blacks (and Caribbean Latinos with African heritage) experiencing a lower clinical response to serotonin reuptake inhibitors and more frequent extrapyramidal side effects with antipsychotics. Asians have a larger percentage of slow metabolizers of isoenzymes and often experience western medicines as being too strong, with many side effects. One relevant finding is the slower metabolism of alcohol and benzodiazepines by Asians and American Indians because they have a metabolizing version of aldehyde enzymes that places them at higher risk for intoxication.[37]

Despite extensive pharmacogenomic research, few genetic variants with definitive clinical utility have been identified. One meta-analytic review of ethnic differences in tolerability of psychotropic drugs did not find significant differences.[38] However, to date there has been significant underrecruitment of diverse populations into randomized controlled studies, thus limiting the validity and generalizability of such results.

APPROACHES TO SUD AMONG DIVERSE YOUTH

Medications do not necessarily treat the substance use directly, except for initial detoxification. The primary role of psychotropic medications in SUD is treatment of comorbid psychiatric illness, and the ethnopharmacologic factors discussed earlier should be considered. Considering the huge role of psychotherapy and psychosocial interventions in managing the SUD, we will focus on the psychotherapy aspects only.

Culturally Competent Standards and Practice Guidelines

In the last 15 years, an increasing number of culturally competent guidelines and documents have addressed health and behavioral health services. They include the Surgeon General's supplement on mental health, race, and ethnicity,[39] cultural competence standards from the Center for Mental Health Services,[40] the Institute of Medicine report titled *Unequal Treatment*,[41] and many state cultural competence standards.

The most recent set of clinically oriented practice guidelines is the *Practice Parameter for Cultural Competence in Child and Adolescent Psychiatric Practice* from the American Academy of Child and Adolescent Psychiatry.[42] This document makes 13 recommendations for culturally informed and appropriate behavioral health practice based on a comprehensive review of the literature:

1. Evaluate and address barriers (eg, economic, geographic, bureaucratic, insurance, cultural beliefs, stigma) that may prevent culturally diverse children and their families from obtaining mental health services.
2. Evaluate children and families in the language they are proficient in.
3. Recognize the effect of dual language competence on the child's adaptation and functioning.

4. Physicians should be aware of their own cultural biases to prevent stereo-typing or cognitive shortcuts that may interfere with objective clinical judgment.

5. Physicians should be aware of cultural differences in developmental pro-gression, idiomatic expressions of distress, and symptomatic presentation for different disorders and consider them when reaching a formulation and diagnosis.

6. Evaluate the history of immigration-related trauma and community trauma (eg, violence, abuse, domestic violence) experienced by the child and family, and incorporate approaches to address them in treatment.

7. Evaluate the level of acculturation and presence of acculturation stress and intergenerational acculturation family conflict in diverse children and families, and address these in treatment.

8. Make special efforts to include family members and key members of tradi-tional extended families (eg, grandparents, other elders) in assessment, treatment planning, and treatment.

9. Evaluate and incorporate cultural values, beliefs, and attitudes in their treatment interventions that can enhance the child's and family's partici-pation in and effectiveness of treatment.

10. Physicians should treat culturally diverse children and their families in familiar settings within their communities whenever possible.

11. Support parents to develop appropriate behavioral management skills consonant with their cultural values and beliefs.

12. Preferentially use psychological and pharmacologic interventions with evidence for the ethnic/racial population to which the child and family belong.

13. Address ethnopharmacologic factors (eg, pharmacogenomic, dietary, use of herbal cures) that may influence the child's response to medications or experience of side effects.

Role of Collaboration with the Traditional or Indigenous Healers

Diverse cultural groups' explanatory models for mental health and illness can vary, invoking spiritual, supernatural, sociologic, and interpersonal explanatory models. Such explanatory models often lead families to seek help for their chil-dren's problems from a spiritual healer, church elder, community leader, or rela-tive, rather than from health professionals. Reasons for such preferences include greater acceptability of the healer's explanatory model of illness, greater family support, less stigma for seeking services, and perceived greater rapidity of effec-tiveness. This preference is seen particularly among first-generation immigrants and refugees, including Latinos, Asian-origin, American Indian, and some European-origin groups.[34]

Physicians should consider consulting and collaborating with traditional healers (eg, curanderos, santeros, shamans) and including rituals and ceremonies in psychotherapy with children from more traditional backgrounds. Collaboration with indigenous traditional healers can ameliorate cultural loyalty conflicts within families and children and improve access to care in populations unfamiliar with or even mistrusting of the medical/psychiatric model. This is typically feasible when traditional healing methods complement or enhance (and do not directly conflict with) the effectiveness of Western psychotherapeutic and pharmacologic interventions. Traditional healers are often reticent to identify themselves as collaborating with Western-trained physicians. However, mutual respect and education in exchanging information and perspectives can foster collaboration.[34]

Culturally Informed Intervention Models

The crucial role of various culturally informed psychotherapies in the treatment of diverse populations with their added complexities cannot be overemphasized. Recent studies report that the mental health services in the United States are culturally mismatched with the treatment preferences of ethnic minority clients.[43] This calls for the strong need to develop culturally competent practices that consider language, culture, and contextual issues consistent with the cultural values and beliefs of their clients and to incorporate culturally adapted evidence-based practices (CA-EBPs) in mental health services.

A number of culturally informed evidence-based interventions have been developed to address the special mental health needs of immigrant populations. Promising studies had demonstrated the efficacy of brief motivational enhancement therapies with minority youth, including 1 study in a primary care setting.[44,45] Multisystemic therapy, which is a community-based approach for substance abuse that combines individual cognitive-behavioral therapy, family behavioral therapy, and community resource development and integration, has shown significant effectiveness in various ethnic groups (blacks, Asian Pacific Islanders, and Latinos).[46] School-based substance use prevention approaches have the potential to reach ethnic minority youth who otherwise might not be able to access clinic-based treatment. For example, Botvin et al[47] achieved 1-year decreases in polysubstance use and 2-year decreases in binge drinking among black and Latino inner-city youth by using a culturally adapted cognitive-behavioral, school-based program. A prospective, randomized controlled trial of a culturally adapted prevention curriculum among Alaskan youth showed 6-month decreases in use of inhalants and medications.[48]

Brief strategic family therapy (BSFT), a family-based intervention that focuses on acculturating family distancing (the distancing that occurs between immigrant parents and children that is a result of immigration, cultural differences, and differing rates of acculturation) has demonstrated significant improvements in addressing youth substance abuse and conduct disturbance, and it has been adopted as a National Institute for Drug Abuse (NIDA)-endorsed evidence-based practice.[49] It is a short-term, problem-focused therapeutic treatment intervention designed for children and adolescents aged 6 to 17 years and their families. BSFT uses reduction or elimination of illegal drug use to address problem behaviors. Family involvement is a key part of the therapy, which includes establishing a healthy relationship with both the client and the family. The therapist works with the family to identify times in the family's life when youth has the most acting-out behaviors. After these patterns are identified, the therapist assists the family in changing these patterns and encourages more positive family time. Specific strategies are used to assist the family with making the changes necessary, such as *reframing* (finding and stating something positive about a negative statement); *changing alliances* (avoiding the situation where 2 in the family gang up on another); *building conflict resolution skills* (learning better ways to solve problems); and *empowering parents* (parents learning to take some control of their children's lives). A major focus of BSFT is also bridging youth and family cultural and generational differences, thus addressing conflicts arising from acculturative family distancing.

Role of Traditional Interventions

American Indian communities have long used traditional healing methods for the treatment of adolescents with SUD. Programs such as Project Venture (National Indian Youth Leadership Project) and American Indian Life Skills are recognized evidence-based interventions for American Indian youth that have benefit for adolescent SUD and comorbidities.[50,51] Investigators have started to discuss treatments for Asian Americans that fit with cultural conceptions of mental health. For example, the concept of mindfulness has roots in Buddhism and Asian traditions, and it has been gaining momentum in western psychology as a viable treatment of depression, anxiety, trauma, and other mental health problems. Mindfulness and acceptance techniques (eg, mindfulness-based cognitive therapy, mindfulness-based stress reduction) have been included in the categorization of the "third wave" of cognitive-behavioral therapies.[52] There has also been recent interest in exploring mindfulness as an intervention strategy of cultural fit for Asian Americans. Villareal Armas[53] discussed mindfulness interventions as an appropriate intervention for trauma in Thai survivors of modern-day slavery. However, few existing studies have empirically investigated the efficacy of mindfulness-based treatments with Asian American populations.

Pradhan[54] developed an integrative and strength-based model of psychotherapy called yoga-mindfulness based cognitive therapy (Y-MBCT) which integrates the concepts and techniques from the Eastern mindfulness philosophy with elements from the Western cognitive behavioral therapies (CBT) and motivational interviewing (MI) principles. Its efficacy currently is being tested in various psychiatric disorders, including SUD in youth. These are combined to target specific symptoms reported by youth in order to reduce stress, craving, impulsivity, anxiety, depression, and psychosomatic symptoms as well as to enhance coping, resiliency factors, and quality of life.

CONCLUSION

Given the rapid growth of our diverse population, the science behind understanding risk factors and treatment approaches for adolescent SUD needs to have a much greater cultural focus. This includes examining factors that lead to disparities and addressing differential treatment outcomes for different ethnic and racial populations. Because early age of onset of SUD has been associated with a longer duration of untreated illness and poorer clinical and functional outcomes, it is critical to begin this work as soon as possible in order to prevent an even greater rise in adolescent SUD in the future.[55] A greater emphasis on the prevention, early identification, and treatment of child and adolescent mental and emotional disturbances in diverse populations will be central to these efforts. The approaches of modifying existing evidence-based treatments, bridging mental health services with other more culturally sanctioned services, and providing interventions that match cultural factors will be crucial in further advancing the treatment options available for treatment of SUDs. There is much room for innovation and expansion within these areas in order to increase our knowledge about, and availability of, culturally congruent services.

References

1. Burrow-Sanchez JJ. Understanding adolescent substance abuse: prevalence, risk factors, and clinical implications. *J Couns Dev.* 2006;84:283–290
2. Greydanus DE, Patel DR. The adolescent and substance abuse: current concepts. *Curr Probl Pediatr Adolesc Health Care.* 2005;35:78–98
3. Hawkins JD, Catalano RF, Miller JY. Risk and protective factors for alcohol and other drug problems in adolescence and early adulthood: implications for substance abuse prevention. *Psychol Bull.* 1992;112:64–105
4. Chen C-Y, Storr CL, Anthony JC. Early-onset drug use and risk for drug dependence problems. *Addict Behav.* 2009;34:319–322
5. US Bureau of the Census. International migration is projected to become primary driver of U.S. population growth for first time in nearly two centuries. May 15, 2013. Available at: www.census.gov/newsroom/releases/archives/population/cb13-89.html. Accessed December 8, 2013
6. Johnston LD, O'Malley PM, Bachman JG., Schulenberg J. *The Monitoring the Future: National Survey Results 1975-2012, Volume 1.* Rockville, MD: National Institute on Drug Abuse; 2013
7. Eaton D, Kann L, Kinchen S, et al. Youth Risk Behavior Surveillance—United States, 2011 Centers for Disease Control and Prevention. *MMWR Morb Mortal Wkly Rev.* 2012;61(4):1–166
8. US Department of Health and Human Services. Healthy People 2020. Available at: healthypeople.gov/2020/default.aspx. Accessed March 19, 2014
9. Miller BC, McCoy JK, Olson TD, Wallace CM. (1986). Parental discipline and control attempts in relation to adolescent sexual attitudes and behavior. *J Marriage Fam.* 1986;48:503–512
10. Fletcher AC, Jefferies BC. Parental mediators of association between perceived authoritative parenting and early adolescent substance abuse. *J Early Adolesc.* 1999;19:465–487
11. Pumariega AJ, Rothe EM. Leaving no children or families outside: the challenges of immigration. *Am J Orthopsychiatry.* 2010;80:506–516
12. Rothe EM, Lewis J, Castillo-Matos H, et al. Post traumatic stress disorder in Cuban children and adolescents after release from a refugee camp. *Psychiatr Serv.* 2002;53:970–976
13. Vigil D. *Barrio Gangs: Street Life and Identity in Southern California.* Austin: University of Texas Press; 1988

14. Hovey J, King C. Acculturative stress, depression, and suicidal ideation among immigrant and second-generation Latino adolescents. *J Am Acad Child Adolesc Psychiatry.* 1996;35:1183–1192

15. Deykin EY, Levy JC, Wells V. Adolescent depression, alcohol and drug abuse. *Am J Public Health.* 1987;77:178–182

16. Harlow LL, Newcomb MD, Bentler PM. Depression, self-derogation, substance abuse, and suicide ideation: lack of purpose in life as meditational factor. *J Clin Psychol.* 1986;42:5–21

17. Heberman HM, Garfinkel BD. Completed suicide in youth. *Can J Psychiatry.* 1988;33:494–504

18. Swanson JW, Linskey AO, Quintero-Salinas R, et al. Depressive symptoms, drug use, and suicidal ideation among youth in the Rio Grand Valley: a bi-national school survey. *J Am Acad Child Adolesc Psychiatry.* 1992;31:669–678

19. Szapocznik J, Kurtines W. *Breakthroughs in Family Therapy with Drug Abusing And Problem Youth.* New York: Springer; 1989

20. Pumariega A, Swanson J, Holzer C, Linskey A, Quintero-Salinas R. Cultural context and substance abuse in Hispanic adolescents. *J Child Fam Stud.* 1992;1:75–92

21. Pumariega AJ, Millsaps U, Rodriguez L, Moser M, Pumariega JB. Substance abuse in immigrant Latino youth in Appalachia: preliminary findings. *Addict Disord Treat.* 2007;6(4):157–165

22. Sanchez-Barker TN. Coping with depression: adapted for use with incarcerated Hispanic youth. *Diss Abstr Int B Sci Eng.* 2003;64:2403

23. Glover S, Pumariega A, Holzer C, Rodriguez M. Anxiety symptomatology in Mexican-American adolescents. *J Child Fam Stud.* 1999;8:47–57

24. Pina A, Silverman W. Clinical phenomenology, somatic symptoms, and distress in Hispanic/Latino and European American youths with anxiety disorders. *J Clin Child Adolesc Psychol.* 2004;33:227–236

25. Yeh C. Age, acculturation, cultural adjustment, and mental health symptoms of Chinese, Korean, and Japanese immigrant youths. *Cult Div Ethnic Minority Psychol.* 2003;9:34–48

26. Pumariega A, Glover S, Holzer C, Nguyen N. Utilization of mental health services in a tri-ethnic sample of adolescents. *Community Ment Health J.* 1998;34:145–156

27. Juszczak L, Melinkovich P, Kaplan D. Use of health and mental health services by adolescents across multiple delivery sites. *J Adolesc Health.* 2003;32(6 Suppl):108–118

28. Chow J, Jaffee K, Choi D. Use of public mental health services by Russian refugees. *Psychiatr Serv.* 1999;50:936–940

29. Hsu E, Davies C, Hansen D. Understanding mental health needs of Southeast Asian refugees: historical, cultural, and contextual challenges. *Clin Psychol Rev.* 2004;24:193–213

30. Weine S, Razzano L, Brkic N, et al. Profiling the trauma related symptoms of Bosnian refugees who have not sought mental health services. *J Nerv Ment Dis.* 2000;188:416–421

31. Yeh M, McCabe K, Hough R, Dupuis D, Hazen A. Racial/ethnic differences in parental endorsement of barriers to mental health services for youth. *Mental Health Serv Res.* 2003;5:65–77

32. Vander Stoep A, Evens C, Taub J. Risk of juvenile justice systems referral among children in a public mental health system. *J Mental Health Admin.* 1997;24:428–442

33. Leslie L, Weckerly J, Landsverk J, Hough R, Hurlburt M, Wood P. Racial/ethnic differences in the use of psychotropic medication in high-risk children and adolescents. *J Am Acad Child Adolesc Psychiatry.* 2003;42:1433–1442

34. Martinez C, McClure H, Eddy J. Language brokering contexts and behavioral and emotional adjustment among Latino parents and adolescents. *J Early Adolesc.* 2009;29:71–98

35. Alegria M, Carson N, Goncalves M, Keefe K. Disparities in treatment for substance use disorders and co-occurring disorders for ethnic/racial minority youth. *J Am Acad Child Adolesc Psychiatry.* 2011;50(1):22–31

36. Shields A, Fortun M, Hammonds E, et al. The use of race variables in genetic studies of complex traits and the goal of reducing health disparities: a transdisciplinary perspective. *Am Psychol.* 2005;60:77–103

37. Malik M, Lawson W, Lake J, Joshi S. Culturally adapted pharmacotherapy and the integrated formulation. *Child Adolesc Psychiatr Clin N Am.* 2010;19:791–814

38. Ormerod S, McDowell SE, Coleman JJ, Ferner RE. Ethnic differences in the risks of adverse reactions to drugs used in the treatment of psychoses and depression: a systematic review and meta-analysis. *Drug Saf.* 2008;31:597–607

39. US Office of the Surgeon General. *Mental Health: Culture, Race, and Ethnicity. A Supplement to: Mental Health: A Report of the Surgeon General.* Rockville, MD: US Department of Health and Human Services, Substance Abuse and Mental Health Services Administration, Center for Mental Health Services, National Institutes of Health, National Institute of Mental Health; 2001

40. *Cultural Competence Standards for Managed Care Mental Health for Four Racial/Ethnic Underserved/Underrepresented Populations.* Rockville, MD: Center for Mental Health Services, Substance Abuse and Mental Health Administration, US Department of Health and Human Services; 1999

41. Institute of Medicine. *Unequal Treatment: Confronting Racial and Ethnic Disparities in Health Care.* Washington, DC: National Academies Press; 2002

42. Pumariega AJ, Rothe E, Mian A, et al; Committee on Quality Issues. Practice parameter for cultural competence in child and adolescent psychiatric practice. *J Am Acad Child Adolesc Psychiatry.* 2013;52(10):1101–1115

43. Chu J P, Sue S. Asian American mental health: what we know and what we don't know. Online Readings in Psychology and Culture, Unit 3. 2011. Available at: scholarworks.gvsu.edu/orpc/vol3/iss1/4. Accessed December 7, 2013

44. Gil AG, Wagner EF, Tubman JG. Culturally sensitive substance abuse intervention for Hispanic and African American adolescents: empirical examples from the Alcohol Treatment Targeting Adolescents in Need (ATTAIN) Project. *Addiction.* 2004;99(s2):140–150

45. D'Amico E, Miles J, Stern S, Meredith L. Brief motivational interviewing for teens at risk of substance use consequences: a randomized pilot study in a primary care clinic. *J Subst Abuse Treat.* 2008;35:53–61

46. Henggeler SW, Clingempeel WG, Brondino MJ, Pickrel SG. Four-year follow-up of multisystemic therapy with substance-abusing and substance-dependent juvenile offenders. *J Am Acad Child Adolesc Psychiatry.* 2002;41(7):868–874

47. Botvin GJ, Griffin KW, Diaz T, Ifill-Williams M. Preventing binge drinking during early adolescence: one-and two-year follow-up of a school-based preventive intervention. *Psychol Addict Behav.* 2001;15(4):360–365

48. Johnson KW, Shamblen SR, Ogilvie KA, Collins D, Saylor B. Preventing youths' use of inhalants and other harmful legal products in frontier Alaskan communities: a randomized trial. *Prev Sci.* 2009;10(4):298–312

49. Santisteban D, Coatsworth J, Perez-Vidal A, et al. Brief structural/strategic family therapy with African American and Hispanic high-risk youth. *J Community Psychol.* 1997;25:453–471

50. Carter S, Straits KJE, Hall M. Project venture: evaluation of an experiential, culturally-based approach to substance abuse prevention with American Indian youth. *J Exp Educ.* 2007;29(3):397–400

51. LaFromboise TD, Bigfoot DS. Cultural and cognitive considerations in the prevention of American Indian adolescent suicide. *J Adolesc.* 1988;11:139–153

52. Brown LA, Gaudiano BA, Miller IW. Investigating the similarities and differences between practitioners of second- and third-wave cognitive-behavioral therapies. *Behav Modif.* 2011;35:187–200

53. Villareal Armas G. Cultural competence in the trauma treatment of Thai survivors of modern-day slavery: the relevance of Buddhist mindfulness practices and healing rituals to transform shame and guilt of forced prostitution. In: Kalayjian A, Eugene D, eds. *Mass Trauma and Emotional Healing Around the World: Rituals and Practices for Resilience and Meaning-Making, Volume 2: Human-Made Disasters.* Santa Barbara, CA: Praeger; 2010:269–285

54. Pradhan BK. *Yoga and Mental Health: De-mystification, Standardization and Application.* Lanaham, MD: Rowman Littlefield Publishers. In press

55. McGorry PD, Purcell R, Goldstone S, Amminger GP. Age of onset and timing of treatment for mental and substance use disorders: implications for preventive intervention strategies and models of care. *Curr Opin Psychiatry.* 2011;24:301–306

Adolesc Med 025 (2014) 184–214

Evolving Array of Substances Used by Adolescents

Janet F. Williams, MD[a]*; Leslie H. Lundahl, Phd[b]; Rachel S-D Fortune, MD[c]

[a]Professor of Pediatrics, Distinguished Teaching Professor, Department of Pediatrics, Associate Dean for Faculty and Diversity, School of Medicine Office of the Dean, University of Texas Health Science Center, San Antonio, Texas; [b]Assistant Professor, Department of Psychiatry and Behavioral Neurosciences, Wayne State University School of Medicine, Detroit, Michigan; [c]Instructor, Adolescent Medicine, Yale University School of Medicine, Department of Pediatrics, New Haven, Connecticut

INTRODUCTION

As a recognizable pattern of adolescent and young adult drug use emerged more than 2 decades ago among attendees of all-night dance parties, called *raves* or *trances*, the National Institute on Drug Abuse (NIDA) began designating the most common stimulants, depressants, and hallucinogens used in those settings as *club drugs*. This label and genre became increasingly mainstream as underground rave music and culture moved from the margins of alternative society into popular teen and young adult culture. The typical rave held at a club or bar, empty warehouse, or rural space consisted of a large tightly packed crowd of perspiring dancers engaged in a feverish marathon of sensory stimuli, including loud, pulsating techno-rock music, flashing laser lights, and waving glow-in-the-dark light sticks. In this setting, stimulant club drugs helped participants stay awake all night while inducing intense feelings of elation and well-being, with heightened sensory perceptions and hallucinatory effects. Sedative club drugs helped rave attendees *come down* in the morning. In this and other settings, club drugs are among the predatory drugs used to facilitate sexual assault (date rape). The club drug category most often has consisted of 6 of the drugs discussed in this article: Rohypnol, gamma-hydroxybutyrate (GHB), methamphetamine, 3,4-methylenedioxymethamphetamine (MDMA, or Ecstasy), ketamine, and lysergic acid diethylamide (LSD). Cocaine also can be included but is not discussed here.

*Corresponding author:
jawilliams@uthscsa.edu

The drugs discussed in this article share the distinction of comprising the evolving array of substances most popular for abuse by adolescents and young adults. Each of the categories (club drugs, dissociative anesthetics, hallucinogens, and inhalants) contains diverse substances that differ in pharmacology, effects, and routes of use, yet they share the single distinctive characteristic for which each category is named. More recent emerging substances of abuse include synthetic cathinones, synthetic cannabinoids, *Salvia divinorum* (salvia), and dextromethorphan (DXM). Confusion can arise from the fact that many drug categories overlap, and several of these substances belong to more than 1 category. The designer drug Ecstasy is a club drug as well as a hallucinogen and stimulant. Ketamine is both a dissociative and a club drug. Inhalant use falls into over-the-counter (OTC) substance abuse, another broad category that includes DXM abuse. Natural plant-based or herbal medicinal substances of abuse, including salvia, marijuana, psilocybin mushrooms, and peyote cactus, have psychoactive or hallucinogenic effects. As designer drug laboratories strive to improve nature and people seek *better living through chemistry*, abusable chemicals, including synthesized cannabinoids and cathinones, will continue to emerge.

EPIDEMIOLOGY

The Monitoring the Future (MTF) survey and other studies have shown that current adolescent and young adult annual and lifetime use prevalence rates for all substances are lower than those in the peak use years of the 1990s.[1-4] Illicit drug use rates are lower among students than those of age-matched peers not in school.[3,5] Among 12th-graders, college students, and young adults aged 19 to 30 years, males are more likely than females to use any type of illicit drug.[1-3] Use of any of the drugs discussed in this article, similar to any substance use, crosses every demographic boundary and occurs in rural as well as urban settings and among all ethnic groups in the United States. The prevalence of any substance use is consistently lower for black 12th-graders than for white or Hispanic 12th-graders.[1] Any inexpensive and highly accessible substance of abuse, such as inhalants or alcohol, has greater use prevalence among geographically isolated and socioeconomically disadvantaged populations, such as more often occurs on American Indian reservations and among Alaska Native youth.[1,5-7] MTF trend data for *annual* or past-year use by US adolescents are listed in Table 1.[4]

Since initial inclusion in the 2002 MTF survey, GHB, Rohypnol, and ketamine annual use rates have trended considerably lower for both young adults and 12th-graders so that rates declined by nearly half. According to the Drug Abuse Warning Network (DAWN) reports, 58% of emergency department visits in 2001 involving GHB were for 18- to 25-year-old patients.[8] In 2011, GHB use detection patterns suggested the user cohort has aged.[9] In 2012, 19- to 30-year-olds reported a lifetime phencyclidine (PCP) use prevalence of 1.2%, down from the 8.4% peak in 1986.[3] MDMA use rose rapidly beginning in 1997, peaked between 2000 and 2002, then declined sharply, resulting in large age group

Table 1
Monitoring the Future: prevalence of annual substance use

Twelfth-grader trends in use plus 2013 grades 10 and 8

Drug Used	Peak Year Since 1991*	Annual	12th-Graders → 2011 Annual	2012 Annual	2013 Annual	10th-Graders 2013 Annual	8th-Graders 2013 Annual
Rohypnol	2002	1.6	1.3	1.5	0.9	0.6	0.4
Gamma-Hydroxybutyrate (GHB)	2004	2	1.4	1.4	1	—	—
Phencyclidine (PCP)	1996	2.6	1.3	0.9	0.7	—	—
Ketamine	2002	2.6	1.7	1.5	1.4	—	—
Lysergic acid diethylamide (LSD)	1996	8.8	2.7	2.4	2.2	1.7	1
3,4-Methylenedioxymethamphetamine (MDMA)	2001	9.2	5.3	3.8	4	3.6	1.1
Methamphetamine	1999	4.7	1.4	1.1	0.9	1	1
Bath salts	2012†	1.3	—	1.3	0.9	0.9	1
Synthetic marijuana	2011†	11.4	11.4	11.3	7.9	7.4	4
Inhalants	1995	8	3.2	2.9	2.5	3.5	5.2
Inhalants: nitrites	1996	1.6	0.9‡	—	—	—	—
Salvia	2011	5.9	5.9	4.4	3.4	2.3	1.2
Dextromethorphan (DXM)	2006	6.9	5.3	5.6	5.0	4.3	2.9

Annual = Percent who "used in past year."

*Or a later Monitoring the Future survey inclusion date.

†First year asked.

‡2009—not asked/tabulated.

Adapted from *American teens more cautious about using synthetic drugs*. Ann Arbor, MI: University of Michigan News Service. Available at: monitoringthefuture.org//pressreleases/13drugpr_complete.pdf. Accessed March 19, 2014.

differences in reported *lifetime* or ever use of this drug.[3] MDMA use rates are so low among MTF respondents older than 30 years that this age group is no longer asked about this drug. Methamphetamine annual use was reported by 1% of 12th-graders and by 0.2% of 18- to 30-year-olds, with distinct age cohort differences in lifetime use rates similar to MDMA findings.[1,3]

Questions introduced in the 2012 MTF survey indicated relatively limited use of synthetic cathinones or *bath salts* among 8th-, 10th-, and 12th-graders, use by 1.3% of 19- to 20-year olds, and use by less than 0.5% of those aged 27 to 30 years.[3] The 2012 annual use of synthetic marijuana was 8.8% among 10th-graders and 11.3% among 12th-graders, ranking second to marijuana use. The 2012 rate of 4.4% for 8th-graders ranked it third behind marijuana and inhalant use. The largest annual use rate of 7.0% was reported by 19- to 20-year-olds.[2] The 2013 MTF results show US adolescents became increasingly cautious about synthetic drug use.[4] Perceived risk of LSD use has dropped, although use rates have remained low for a decade.

Inhalants do not attract as much attention from media or health professionals compared with other drugs, despite being a more prevalent problem, so inhalant use remains largely underrecognized. Both MTF and National Survey on Drug Use and Health (NSDUH) studies have demonstrated how inhalant use differs from other drug use. Most notably, use decreases with increasing age, which is a consistent pattern opposite that of nearly all other abused substances. Much of the decline in use with age has already occurred by 10th grade, and by about age 20 years, active inhalant use is almost nil.[1-3] NSDUH data in 2012 showed that 62.5% of the 594,000 new volatile substance abusers aged 12 to 49 years were younger than 18 years.[2] Inhalant use is slightly higher among females than males in grades 8 and 10, but boys show higher rates by grade 12 and thereafter.[3]

Since MTF began to track salvia use in 2009, declining use rates suggest that the popularity of this drug may have peaked around 2011. Slightly more than 1% of 19- to 30-year-old young adults reported annual salvia use in 2012.[3] The use prevalence of DXM, a cough suppressant found in many OTC cough and cold preparations, has changed little since it was first added to the MTF survey in 2006.[4]

An increasingly important influence on drug use epidemiology has been the burgeoning connectivity of the Internet. The Internet has become an extensive and readily accessible source of scientific facts and research-based antidrug messaging as well as nonrefereed opinion and misinformation about the gamut of substance use topics. Internet and other media usage has become a norm of daily life and thus a major influence on adolescent and young adult behavior, including a broad range of drug use behaviors.[10] Particularly for adolescents and young adults, sites touting safe drug abuse and offering specific how-to tips and instructions plus access to online sale of drugs and precursors may be difficult to resist.[10-12]

DETECTION

Because every patient population includes substance users, it is incumbent on all physicians and other healthcare professionals to stay abreast of the ever-evolving drug use scene in their locale. Users infrequently present to the medical home with obvious drug use symptoms, so health care professionals must have the knowledge and skills to screen for substance use, recognize telltale signs and symptoms of use or addiction, and pursue effective management steps. The Internet is another resource where health care personnel can find current drug use information, follow trends, identify reliable resources, and learn about sites accessed by patients.

Screening as a routine part of all health maintenance visits and relevant acute care patient visits can be accomplished efficiently and effectively using a confidential and nonconfrontational approach and a structured psychosocial interview format combined with validated substance use screening tools. For adolescent patient care, the HEADSS mnemonic, or the strengths-based SSHADESS, helps the physician or nonphysician clinician broach the topic of drug use among other potential risk areas.[13,14] Routine use of screening, brief intervention, and referral to treatment (SBIRT) tools and skills can quickly determine the extent of patient drug use and guide physician response accordingly, including reinforcing healthy decision-making and patient strengths and applying brief intervention and enhancing motivation for behavioral change and treatment acceptance.[15]

Specific questions that may relate to the likelihood of substance use include asking about drug availability, perception of harm from use, academic and employment functioning, depression and mental health, and drug use by peers or family. Patients who engage in risk-taking behaviors, such as early or risky sexual activity or early use of any drug, including nicotine or alcohol, are more likely to have ongoing substance use. General behavioral changes, including apathy, malaise, poor appetite and weight loss, or change in peer group or activities, may indicate substance use. Whenever social ills such as crime, unemployment, child neglect/abuse, or domestic violence affect a patient's life, there is greater likelihood that substance use is a contributing or complicating factor, so screening is essential. Consider multiple drug use whenever *any* substance use is suspected or detected, particularly the drugs discussed in this article.

Health care professionals should become familiar with the drug testing methods used by local hospitals and reference laboratories in order to know which drugs are included in their routine laboratory screening panels, as well as the limitations of this technology.[16] Urine drug testing does not usually detect GHB, ketamine, LSD, synthetic cannabinoids, inhalants, or salvia, and can easily miss Rohypnol and even MDMA, depending on the dosage used and the type of assay. Hair analysis is fraught with problems and is not recommended. Specific gas chromatography and mass spectrometry (GC/MS) testing of blood, urine, or body tissue samples can detect Rohypnol, GHB, LSD, inhalants and more, including synthetic cannabinoid metabolites, but this testing is most often reserved for special forensic purposes.[16]

MANAGEMENT

Most patients using the drugs discussed in this article come to medical attention through an acute or emergency care setting because they have experienced acute adverse drug effects or related injury. All acute care must start with the *ABC*'s of life support to assess, stabilize, and monitor the patient's general hydration and cardiorespiratory status as well as address any specific acute injury or toxicity. Monitoring vital signs is crucial to confirming stability or complications, such as hypertension or hyperthermia. Despite the cause, all intoxicated patients respond best in a calm and supportive environment. Clinical toxicology consultation with local experts and a regional Poison Control Center can help identify any specifically indicated or contraindicated medications and other treatment.

No medications reverse acute intoxication by any of the drugs discussed in this article, with one exception: short-acting benzodiazepine antagonist use can help counteract Rohypnol intoxication. Rapid rehydration, core cooling, and fluid and electrolyte manipulation are essential to combat the heat injury and rhabdomyolysis associated with MDMA, methamphetamine, or PCP use. A benzodiazepine, such as diazepam, helps with agitation, panic, seizure control, and intubation of patients showing stimulant drug effects, but neuromuscular blocking agents can exacerbate these effects. Pressor medications and bronchodilators are relatively contraindicated. Adding a ß-blocking agent can seriously complicate hypertension caused by the central nervous system (CNS) stimulant drugs of abuse, such as amphetamine analogs and synthetic cathinones.

Adolescents and club drug users more often use multiple drugs together, intentionally or unintentionally, so they may present with nonspecific symptoms or with mixed or potentiated symptomatology (eg, when a depressant drug or inhalant is used with alcohol).[17] Laboratory testing helps monitor oxygenation, assess general health, diagnose pregnancy, and other concurrent conditions as well as detect abuse of multiple substances. Extensive testing for organ system damage is appropriate for those patients with specific indications or a history of regular and long-term drug use. Once stability is ensured, the patient needs a comprehensive medical evaluation in order to transition to the indicated inpatient or outpatient care, which includes psychosocial and mental health support to meet the management plan goals.

Few programs are designed specifically for treating adolescents or those individuals abusing the substances addressed in this article, so the range of treatment methods used for other addictive disorders has been tried with these drugs.[18-20] Neuroleptics and other pharmacotherapies are indicated in the treatment of comorbid conditions. Treatment challenges are posed by the diversity of abused substances and polydrug use as well as the diversity of user populations. Although the principles of effective substance abuse treatment in general apply to the treatment of these patients, any treatment regimen must address the gamut of potential contributory and comorbid factors, including physical, physiologic, pharmacologic, developmental, socioemotional, mental health, neurocognitive, cultural, academic, and demographic factors. In addition, the pessimistic attitudes that the public, health care professionals, and even the patient and family may have about recovery must be overcome.[19,20]

ROHYPNOL (FLUNITRAZEPAM)

Selected Street Names: Circles, Forget Pill, Forget-Me-Pill, La Rocha, Lunch Money Drug, Mexican Valium, Pingus, R2, Reynolds, Roach, Roach 2, Roaches, Roachies, Robutal, Rochas Dos, Roche, Roofies, Rophies, Rope, Ropies, Roples, Row-Shay, Ruffies, Wolfies

Flunitrazepam (Rohypnol), a benzodiazepine that is 10 times more potent than diazepam, has similar anxiolytic, muscle relaxant, sedative-hypnotic, amnestic, and anticonvulsant effects.[21-24] Flunitrazepam, although not approved for use in the United States, is used in Europe, Asia, and Latin America for treating insomnia and as a sedative, anticonvulsant, or presurgical anesthetic. Currently a schedule IV drug, Rohypnol is under national Drug Enforcement Administration (DEA) consideration to become a schedule I drug, the designation given to drugs with high abuse potential and no accepted therapeutic use in the United States. Because of its specific ability to produce anterograde amnesia, flunitrazepam is one of the date rape drugs used to intoxicate unsuspecting victims. In response, the drug manufacturer, Roche, reformulated Rohypnol tablets to contain a dye that turns blue upon contacting a liquid. The popularity of flunitrazepam among cocaine and heroin users comes from its ability to potentiate heroin's depressant effects as well as to mitigate the *crash* after cocaine use.

Rohypnol is sold as individually wrapped tablets (and sometimes capsules) in doses ranging from 0.5 to 1.0 mg, and as a 2.0 mg/mL injectable solution. Rohypnol pills readily dissolve in carbonated beverages. They remain odorless and tasteless, so they are most often ingested, but they can be pulverized and insufflated. Drug effects begin within 30 minutes, peak at 2 hours, and last about 8 hours. A dose as small as 1 mg can impair the user for 8 to 12 hours. The half-life of Rohypnol ranges between 9 and 25 hours with renal excretion of metabolites.

Clinical Consequences: Acute Effects and Presentations

At low doses, Rohypnol, a CNS depressant, produces effects similar to those of alcohol, namely, reduced anxiety, disinhibition, muscle relaxation, drowsiness, slurred speech, ataxia, and slowing of psychomotor function. Higher doses can result in bradycardia, respiratory depression, confusion, hallucinations, lack of muscle control, loss of consciousness, and amnesia. Paradoxical effects, including aggressive, violent, or erratic behavior, have been reported. Other adverse effects associated with Rohypnol include hypotension, visual disturbances, dizziness, gastrointestinal disturbances, and urinary retention.

Chronic Effects and Presentations

Similar to other benzodiazepines, chronic Rohypnol use leads to tolerance and dependence. Withdrawal symptoms range from vague restlessness and anxiety to more bothersome headache, myalgia, photosensitivity, numbness and tingling of extremities, and increased seizure potential that can manifest as frank tremors, hallucinations, and convulsions. Seizures from Rohypnol withdrawal may occur more than a week after use has stopped.

Additional Management Considerations

- When an alert patient presents within 1 hour of a known Rohypnol ingestion, reduce absorption by inducing emesis, then administer oral activated charcoal and a cathartic.
- For an unconscious patient, consider airway protection and gastric lavage.
- Standard urine drug tests detect benzodiazepines, but Rohypnol is used in such small dosages and is distributed so rapidly that routine screens often fail to detect it. After a dose as low as 1 mg, Rohypnol (and its active metabolite 7-amino-flunitrazepam) can be detected by gas chromatography/mass spectroscopy (GC/MS) of blood or urine for up to 72 hours postingestion.
- The antidote for confirmed benzodiazepine toxicity is the short-acting benzodiazepine antagonist flumazenil. Start with 0.2 mg intravenously (IV). If no response is seen in 1 minute, give 0.3 to 0.5 mg IV. Because the effects of flumazenil are short lived compared to those of Rohypnol sedation, it can be readministered as long as the cumulative dose is less than 3 mg. Midazolam can be used to reverse benzodiazepine effects in severe cases.
- Flumazenil use can precipitate withdrawal in benzodiazepine-dependent patients. It may induce seizures in patients receiving benzodiazepines for epilepsy or those who overdosed on a tricyclic antidepressant.
- Combined use of Rohypnol and other depressant drugs, including alcohol, potentiates sedative and toxic effects and can be lethal.
- Treatment for Rohypnol dependence follows standard benzodiazepine detoxification protocol, which is usually a 3- to 5-day inpatient program with intensive medical monitoring and management of withdrawal symptoms.
- Benzodiazepine withdrawal can be life threatening. Treat similar to alcohol withdrawal, using replacement with a long-acting benzodiazepine (eg, diazepam) followed by a gradual dose taper.

GAMMA-HYDROXYBUTYRATE (GHB)

Selected Street Names: Cherry Meth, Easy Lay, Fantasy, G, Georgia Home Boy, Goop, Grievous Bodily Harm, G-Riffick, Growth Hormone Booster, Liquid E, Liquid Ecstasy, Liquid X, Organic Quaalude, Salty Water, Scoop, Soap

GHB Precursors and Selected Names

- **Gamma-Butyrolactone (GBL):** Brand names: Blue Nitro, Blue Nitro Vitality, Gamma G, GH Revitalizer, RenewTrient, Remforce, Revivarant, Revivarant G
- **1,4-Butanediol (BD):** Brand names: Enliven, GHRE, NRG3, Revitalize Plus, Serenity, Somatopro, Thunder Nectar, Weight Belt Cleaner
  - **Street names:** Cherry fX Bombs, Lemon fX Drops, Orange fX Rush

GHB is a synthetically produced CNS depressant that is also endogenously present in the brain as an active metabolite of the inhibitory neurotransmitter gamma-aminobutyric acid (GABA).[21-24] GHB acts on the dopamine system, mediating sleep cycles, temperature regulation, memory, emotional control, cerebral blood flow, and glucose metabolism. Originally available OTC in health food stores during the 1980s, GHB was used by bodybuilders as a dietary supplement for its alleged growth hormone-releasing role in fat reduction and muscle growth stimulation. In 1990, after reports of adverse events, GHB was removed from the US market and in 2000 was listed as a schedule I drug. GHB was approved by the US Food and Drug Administration in 2002 for highly restricted use as the schedule III drug Xyrem, an oral solution used for treating narcolepsy-associated cataplexy and for opioid or alcohol withdrawal. As a club drug, GHB is used for its purported safety while causing euphoria, disinhibition, sedation, and enhanced sex drive. It is commonly taken to help the user come down from an Ecstasy high and often is combined with alcohol, which compounds the toxicity. With anesthetic properties similar to flunitrazepam, GHB is 1 of the most commonly used date rape drugs. When GHB is slipped in a drink, it is referred to as being *scooped*.

On the illicit market, GHB is sold in vials as a salty or soapy-tasting clear liquid, or as a white powder, tablet, or capsule that is tasteless when mixed in beverages. GBL (an industrial solvent and floor stripper) and BD (a dietary supplement), legally available precursor substances that are enzymatically converted to GHB in the body, also are abused. BD can be purchased from health food stores and Web sites or ordered from bodybuilding magazines or gyms. GHB can be produced in a clandestine or home laboratory by reacting GBL with either sodium or potassium hydroxide. Chemical kits, reagents, and recipes are readily available on the Internet.

Clinical Consequences: Acute Effects and Presentations

GHB produces dose-dependent depressant effects similar to those of the barbiturates and methaqualone; however, drug purity and strength vary considerably, and drug effects are highly inconsistent among individual users. Drug effects begin about 10 to 20 minutes after ingestion and last 2 to 6 hours and possibly up to 10 hours. The half-life is 27 minutes, and it is eliminated relatively quickly as carbon dioxide. A dose of 10 mg/kg typically causes euphoria, amnesia, and hypotonia. Drowsiness, dizziness, headache, bradycardia, nausea, and somnolence result from 20 to 30 mg/kg dosages. At 30 to 40 mg/kg, hallucinations, sleep paralysis, or myoclonic jerking movements can occur. Other reported effects include delusions, depression, vertigo, ataxia, vomiting, excess salivation, transient metabolic acidosis, hypotension, hypothermia, memory impairment, agitation, loss of airway reflexes, respiratory depression, apnea, coma, and death. The user may lose peripheral vision and have nystagmus, mydriasis, or miosis. When in deep coma, pupillary light reflexes may be lost. GHB overdose overwhelms the body's ability to eliminate the drug, causing greater and longer-lasting effects, namely, sudden onset of coma and possible respiratory arrest. The classic symptom triad of GHB toxicity is coma, bradycardia, and myoclonus. As a patient starts to recover, an *emergence phenomenon* of myoclonic jerking, transient confusion, and combativeness followed by rapid recovery to normal over 2 to 3 hours may occur. A drug-specific feature of GHB is the spontaneous remission of coma to a normal or hyperalert state of arousal. Treatment predominantly consists of monitored supportive care with aspiration precautions.

Chronic Effects and Presentations

Persons who regularly use GHB commonly present with mild-to-moderate symptoms, including insomnia, anxiety, irritability, mood swings, aggression, behavioral changes, and hallucinations. Both tolerance to GHB effects and dependence can develop rapidly. Cessation of chronic GHB use leads to withdrawal symptoms nearly indistinguishable from those of alcohol dependence, except for the rapid onset of symptoms within 1 to 6 hours of last GHB use. Withdrawal presents as nausea, vomiting, diaphoresis, restlessness, insomnia, irritability, anxiety, tremor and delirium. Severe withdrawal is characterized by visual and auditory hallucinations, paranoia, and psychotic thoughts. Signs of life-threatening withdrawal include hypertension, tachycardia, and seizures. The mean duration of GHB withdrawal ranges from 9 to 14 days.

Additional Management Considerations

- Suspect GHB intoxication when a patient has the following symptoms:
  - Unexplained or sudden coma with no evidence of head trauma, elevated intracranial pressure, or other known cause
  - Apparent alcohol intoxication with unusually dramatic symptomatology
  - The *classic triad* of coma, bradycardia, and myoclonus
  - Spontaneous and complete resolution of unexplained coma
- Suspect GHB withdrawal in the following cases:
  - Serious bodybuilder or weight trainer presents with agitation or delirium

- Patient presents with psychotic features in the absence of a past history of a psychiatric disorder
- Urine drug screens do not detect GHB use. GC/MS of urine collected within 12 hours of GHB ingestion or blood collected within 4 to 5 hours can detect GHB and metabolites.
- Severe toxicity warrants intensive care. Consider succinylcholine paralysis and intubation. Use postintubation sedation for patients who become agitated as they emerge from sedation.
- Administer atropine for persistent symptomatic bradycardia.
- GHB withdrawal and detoxification require close medical supervision, usually through a 1- to 2-week hospitalization.
- For mild withdrawal symptoms, try a closely monitored outpatient regimen using 20 to 40 mg of diazepam orally, tapered daily over 1 week. However, symptoms may escalate to delirium with psychosis within a few hours, even after beginning the benzodiazepine regimen.
- For severe GHB withdrawal symptoms, sedation with high-dose benzodiazepines, usually diazepam or parenteral lorazepam, and barbiturates may be indicated. Use benzodiazepines to stop withdrawal seizures.
- Life-threatening GHB withdrawal symptoms can arise even after the first 2 weeks of detoxification.
- Inpatient intensive care detoxification is indicated for patients using more than 30 g of GHB per day because they are at risk for hyperthermia and possible rhabdomyolysis. Another indication is treatment of GHB-dependent patients prescribed benzodiazepines for more than 72 hours because drug metabolism slows.
- Outpatient aftercare is necessary.

PHENCYCLIDINE AND KETAMINE

Selected Street Names for Phencyclidine: Angel, Angel Dust, Boat or Love Boat, Dummy Dust, Embalming Fluid, Hog, Ozone, Peace, Rocket Fuel, Superweed, Tac, Tic, Zombie

Selected Street Names for Ketamine: Bump, Cat Valium, Green, Honey Oil, Jet, Jet K, K, Ketalar, Ketaject, Kit Kat, New Ecstasy, Psychedelic Heroin, Purple, Special K, Special la Coke, Super Acid, Super C, Super K, Vitamin K

Phencyclidine (PCP) is a schedule II (high abuse potential) dissociative anesthetic that was developed and used in veterinary medicine as an IV surgical anesthetic. It was never approved for human use because of its high frequency of severe intraoperative and postanesthesia agitation, hallucinations, and prolonged psychotic reactions that last hours to days.[21,22,25,26] In the 1960s, the popularity of abusing PCP in a pill form was limited by the slow onset of effects, which were unpredictable and often violent in nature. Over the next decade, a more versatile powdered form of PCP led to greater use through snorting or by smoking with tobacco, marijuana, or herbs. Snorted or smoked PCP rapidly disrupts the brain's N-methyl-D-aspartate (NMDA) receptor complexes where the excitatory neurotransmitter glutamate binds and plays a key role in pain perception, emotion, learning, and memory. PCP also causes important dopamine and serotonin system effects and induces potent anticholinergic activity.

Ketamine is the dissociative anesthetic developed in 1963 to replace PCP. It is a schedule III drug still used for human and veterinary anesthesia. Although ketamine very closely resembles PCP's structure and actions, its shorter action and lower potency make it more attractive for abuse than PCP. Users consider ketamine to have minimal overdose risk because its desired effects occur at a dose about half of its anesthetic dose and many times lower than the lethal dose. Ketamine in liquid form can be abused by intramuscular or IV injection but is more often ingested. The white powder form is either snorted or smoked with tobacco or marijuana. Because this odorless and slightly bitter-tasting drug can be ingested unknowingly in a beverage and cause amnesia, it is also considered a date rape drug.

Clinical Consequences: Acute Effects and Presentations

Dissociative anesthetics distort perceptions of sight and sound. They produce feelings of being detached or disconnected from the environment and physical self, but not true hallucinations. The onset, duration, and effects of these drugs are somewhat unpredictable, whether comparing use by different individuals or different use episodes by 1 person, an experience some users find especially attractive. Effects are typically felt within 2 to 15 minutes, depending on the route of use, and are sustained for several hours but have been reported to last days. One episode of PCP use may cause a sense of detachment from reality, including distorted space, time, and body image. Another episode may cause intense terror and panic with a feeling of almost complete sensory detachment. During the next episode, the user may feel invulnerable with superhuman strength. Users have become completely disoriented, violent, or suicidal.

The threshold effects of ketamine use are cognitive and emotional changes that stem from behavioral disinhibition. They manifest as belligerence, aggressiveness, impulsivity, unpredictability, psychomotor agitation, as well as impaired judgment and social functioning. Using a low dose of 5 mg or less of PCP generally causes confusion, inability to concentrate, dysarthria, illogical speech, nystagmus (horizontal, vertical, or rotary), variable or miotic pupils and a blank stare, tachypnea, tachycardia, hypertension, ataxia, nausea and vomiting, flushing, sweating and drooling, impaired motor function, and decreased pain awareness. The user may experience unintentional injuries yet remain unaware of them until the drug effects subside. Muscle rigidity and spasms cause grimacing, bruxism, ataxia, and bizarre uncoordinated or repetitive movements. Taking a PCP dose up to about 20 mg exacerbates vital sign elevations and causes the classic wide-awake stupor, a fixed stare or disconjugate and roving gaze, midposition reactive pupils, as well as muscle twitching, myoclonus, and seizures. Significant myoclonus, spasticity, and rigid posturing can lead to fractures, rhabdomyolysis, and renal compromise. High-dose intoxication causes critical elevations of pulse, blood pressure, and temperature, as well as a deep coma that can last up to several days depending on the dosage used. Severe and potentially fatal hyperthermia has occurred acutely or after a delay. Severe toxicity causes diaphoresis, disconjugate gaze with dilated pupils, absent deep pain response, periodic respirations, and apnea. Dose-dependent neuronal hyperexcitability ranges from hyperreflexia, opisthotonus, and focal or generalized seizures to status epilepticus. Short-term psychological effects include depression, delirium, and amnesia.

The lower potency of ketamine usually causes the desired feeling of being relaxed and floating or being separated from the body. Tingling sensations may precede the *trip* to *K-land*, which may include hallucinations, visual distortions, altered time perception, and a sense of heightened ability to discern causal connections. Flash-backs have been reported. A ketamine user will appear catatonic with rigid postur-ing and flat facies, have an open mouth, mydriasis, and a fixed sightless stare. High doses cause social withdrawal, autistic behavior, and impaired cognitive function-ing with bizarre thought patterns and responses. Users in a *K-hole* exhibit true cata-tonia or marked motor impairment, which they perceive as a near-death experience with terrifying sensations of loss of time and identity. Ketamine use while taking any of a broad range of medications or illicit drugs increases seizure risk.

Chronic Effects and Presentations

Chronic use of dissociative drugs leads to tolerance and addiction with recog-nized withdrawal. Long-term use is associated with chronic neurocognitive impairment characterized by memory deficits, confusion, decreased intellectual functioning, visual disturbances, and word retrieval blocking. Memory loss and depression can persist for as long as 1 year after a chronic user has become absti-nent. Prolonged frequent ketamine use can induce *K-cramps* of intense colicky abdominal pain and abnormal hepatic function, or as severe and potentially long-lasting ulcerative cystitis that presents similar to a urinary tract infection.

Additional Management Considerations

- There is no PCP or ketamine antagonist drug.
- Vertical nystagmus is caused by PCP and no other drug of abuse; however, horizontal or rotary nystagmus also can occur. Nystagmus helps distin-guish PCP intoxication from a naturally occurring psychotic state.
- Differential diagnosis of PCP use includes head trauma, schizophrenia, acute psychosis, mania, organic brain syndrome, stroke, and other causes of altered mental status or coma.
- Ataxia and nystagmus without mydriasis in an acutely confused or agitated patient point toward PCP use and rules out stimulant drugs and LSD.

- For patients with dissociative drug use, a calm, quiet, and dimly lit environment for patient evaluation. Treatment is indicated to minimize sensory stimulation and reduce the likelihood of unpredictable, exaggerated, or violent patient reactions.
- Patients using PCP have poor judgment and require supervision.
- *Talking down* is not helpful and may exacerbate agitation.
- Oral drug ingestion mandates a prolonged clinical observation period.
- Urine drug screens usually test for PCP but not ketamine.
- Severe behavioral toxicities respond to sedation with a benzodiazepine (IM lorazepam) or haloperidol. Avoid neuroleptics, particularly with intrinsic anticholinergic properties.
- Diazepam or lorazepam IV treats status epilepticus.
- Hypertension responds to IV hydralazine or 2 to 5 mg of phentolamine.
- Hemodialysis and hemoperfusion are ineffective.
- Schizophrenic patients who are abusing PCP or ketamine are at extreme risk for severe psychiatric morbidity, including rekindling of prior symptomatology.
- Response of ulcerative cystitis to urologic care and drug use abstinence is variable.

HALLUCINOGENS

The term *hallucinogen,* meaning "producer of hallucinations," generally refers to a group of chemicals that alter consciousness without delirium, sedation, excessive stimulation, or intellectual or memory impairment.[21,22,25] LSD, psilocybin from *magic* mushrooms, MDMA, and mescaline from peyote cactus are the more commonly abused hallucinogens. All have molecular structures that closely resemble that of the neurotransmitter serotonin. Research to elucidate the mechanism by which hallucinogens cause altered perceptions has shown that these drugs act as brain and nervous system serotonin receptors, with prominent effects on the cerebral cortex and locus ceruleus. Marijuana and PCP also are hallucinogens, but they have different mechanisms of action. Although LSD is considered the prototypical hallucinogen, it is technically misnamed because it induces illusory phenomena (an illusinogen) and only rarely causes true hallucinations. An illusion is a perceptual distortion of an actual environmental stimulus, for example, someone's face seems to be melting. A person under the influence of a hallucinogen will perceive sensations that do not actually exist, such as seeing a melting face when no face is present.

LYSERGIC ACID DIETHYLAMIDE

Selected Street Names: *Acid, Blotter, Blotter Acid, Boomers, Dots, Glass, Mellow Yellow, Microdot, Pane, Paper Acid, Sugar, Sugar Cubes, Window Pane, Window Trip, Yellow Submarine, Yellow Sunshines, Zen*

Lysergic acid diethylamide (LSD) is a powerful mood-altering schedule I drug sold in tablet, capsule, and liquid forms. It usually is taken orally on sugar cubes or absorbent (blotter) paper. Its effects typically begin about 30 to 90 minutes after ingestion and last up to 12 hours. Hallucinogenic trips involve both pleasant and unpleasant effects that vary with the dose and the user's personality, mood, expectations, and surroundings. LSD and other drugs taken together do not interact to cause significant adverse reactions.

Clinical Consequences: Acute Effects and Presentations

The main effects of LSD are emotional and sensory, although some users report tachycardia, mildly elevated blood pressure and temperature, dilated pupils, dizziness, sleeplessness, anorexia, dry mouth, flushing, sweating, nausea, numbness, weakness, and a fine tremor. Intense emotions that rapidly swing from fear to euphoria may cause the user to report experiencing several emotions simultaneously. Sensory perceptions seem highly intensified and may blend, a phenomenon called *synesthesia* in which the user reports *hearing colors* or *feeling sounds*. Hallucinations change or distort shapes and movements, and may cause the LSD user to perceive that his or her body is changing shape or time is standing still. Some *trip* sensations are conducive to a sense of deeper understanding that is pleasurable or mentally stimulating. An acute dysphoric reaction, commonly called a *bummer* or *bad trip*, includes terrifying thoughts, despair, and nightmare-like feelings of anxiety and doom, such as intense fears of losing control, panic, insanity, or death. Acute paranoid states are another type of adverse response that can result from being in a hypervigilant state, manifest as overreading external cues and experiencing the bizarre thoughts that occur during hallucinations. Anxiety and paranoid reactions may last for 1 hour or a few days, and closing the eyes intensifies the reaction.

Chronic Effects and Presentations

A high tolerance to the effects of hallucinogens develops quickly as use continues, but it also quickly dissipates with drug abstinence. Tolerance that develops with LSD use generalizes to the effects of other hallucinogenic drugs such as psilocybin and mescaline, which also specifically act on serotonin receptors. Physical withdrawal symptoms have not been reported when chronic use is stopped. By some unknown mechanisms, LSD use can cause 2 long-term effects: persistent psychosis and flashbacks. LSD-induced psychosis involves a distortion or disorganization of a person's capacity to recognize reality, think rationally, or communicate with others. It can affect persons with no history or symptoms of psychological problems. It may involve dramatic mood swings ranging from mania to profound depression, vivid visual disturbances, and hallucinations. Experiencing flashbacks, or hallucinogen persisting perception disorder (HPPD) as renamed by the American Psychiatric Association (APA), involves spontaneous, repeated (and sometimes continuous) episodes of sensory distortions identical to those originally produced by LSD. Although flash-backs may include hallucinations, they typically consist of persistent visual disturbances, such as seeing false motion in the peripheral vision, or bright or colorful flashes and halos or trails attached to moving objects. HPPD events can persist unchanged for years after LSD use has terminated; however, if no such events have occurred during a year or more after the last LSD use, they likely will not recur.

Additional Management Considerations:

- Persons having acute adverse LSD reactions often do not seek care in the office practice or emergency medical setting.
- LSD toxic psychosis, which is distinct from that caused by other drugs, occurs with a clear sensorium and intact orientation along with intact recent and remote memory.
- LSD psychosis is difficult to distinguish from an acute schizophrenic psychosis. LSD hallucinations are predominantly visual, whereas schizophrenic hallucinations typically are auditory.
- Acute adverse reactions are best treated with reassurance and support through a *talk-down* in a calm and protective environment.
- When acute anxiety, panic, or paranoia is ongoing, a benzodiazepine, usually oral lorazepam, can be helpful. Severe acute reactions have responded to the combined use of lorazepam and intramuscular haloperidol.
- Neuroleptic medications can lower the seizure threshold.
- Diagnose HPPD (flashbacks) using criteria found in the *Diagnostic and Statistical Manual of Mental Disorders*, Fifth Edition. Exclude other potentially causal neurologic disorders, including brain tumors, and vascular disorders.
- There is no specific treatment for HPPD, but some patients have been helped by anxiolytic or antidepressant medications. Selective serotonin reuptake inhibitor antidepressants may initiate or exacerbate flashbacks.
- Psychotherapy is indicated whenever LSD psychosis or HPPD persists.

DESIGNER DRUGS

The term *designer drug* was coined to signify any synthetic derivative of a federally controlled substance that was illegally produced in a clandestine laboratory for illicit use and created by slightly altering the original molecular structure.[21,22] Legislation in the mid-1980s made the manufacture, sale, or possession of "amphetamine designer drugs" illegal in the United States. Other synthesized chemicals have since been added to the list of abused substances, including synthetic cannabinoids and synthetic cathinones. One key mechanism used by the DEA to decrease drug availability and use is to schedule a drug as a controlled substance, which was the process used in 2011 to ban Spice/K2, bath salts, and other related synthetic chemicals.

Amphetamine analogs remain among the most popular designer drugs on the street today. Among these designer amphetamines, the most widely used are MDMA and methamphetamine, but also methylenedioxyamphetamine (MDA) and methylenedioxyethylamphetamine (MDEA). The stimulant and psyche-delic effects of amphetamine analogs are the reason why glow-in-the-dark para-phernalia and laser light shows are popular in the rave culture. Although only MDMA and methamphetamine are discussed here, all of the drugs in this class have approximately the same acute and chronic effects, toxicities, and manage-ment considerations.

3,4-METHYLENEDIOXYMETHAMPHETAMINE

Selected Street Names: *Adam, Beans, Blue Kisses, Clarity, Disco Biscuits, E, Ecstasy, Essence, Go, Hug Drug, Love Drug, Lovers' Speed, M&M, Mercedes, Molly, New Yorkers, Peace, Roll X, Stacy, Stars, STP, White Dove, X, XTC, XE, 007s*

3,4-Methylendeioxymethamphetamine (MDMA) was developed in 1914 as a parent compound in amphetamine drug development and was tried off-label as a psychotherapeutic adjunct.[21,22,27] In 1985 it was listed as a schedule I drug, meaning there is no approved use for this drug. Although a small portion of the MDMA used in the United States is produced domestically, most is manufac-tured in Europe and smuggled into the United States through mail or courier services. MDMA (or Ecstasy) typically is ingested as oral tablets containing between 60 and 125 mg of drug. More recently, Molly, considered a purer form of Ecstasy, has become available. Molly is ingested in powder or crystal form in a capsule, but it also can be snorted or smoked. MDMA has effects similar to both the stimulant amphetamine and the hallucinogen mescaline. The effects last from 3 to 6 hours. Users commonly take a second dose as the effects of the first dose wane. However, MDMA metabolites interfere with further drug metabolism, so additional doses can produce unexpectedly high blood levels and toxic effects. MDMA tablets often contain more than MDMA; they also include adulterants and any of a number of active drugs, such as methamphet-amine, caffeine, DXM, ephedrine, ketamine, or cocaine. To modulate their *high*, users often combine MDMA with other drugs, particularly alcohol, LSD, and marijuana, or ingest 3 or more MDMA tablets at once. These patterns are called *stacking*. Ingesting MDMA and LSD together is known as *candy flipping*.

Clinical Consequences: Acute Effects and Presentations

MDMA causes a combination of effects by altering neurotransmitter activity as well as causing direct nerve cell toxicity, particularly by targeting serotonin-containing cells, but also causing norepinephrine release. Within 20 to 60 min-utes of MDMA ingestion, most users start to experience desirable drug effects, including a sense of general well-being, mental stimulation, empathy, emotional warmth, and decreased anxiety. These effects last for 2 to 3 hours before gradually subsiding. Common physical findings are dilated pupils, tachycardia, and hypertension. The hallmark effect of MDMA is the reported sensory enhancement and the distorted illusory phenomenon without overt hallucinations. In contrast, some users experience immediate anxiety, agitation, and restlessness. Many users experience insomnia with tiredness and fatigue persisting into the second day. Nausea, chills, diaphoresis, and blurred vision also occur acutely. As a selective serotonergic neurotoxin, MDMA causes muscles to ache, become tense, and spasm, commonly resulting in involuntary jaw clenching and bruxism and leading to the popular use of pacifiers in the rave setting. Using MDMA in the rave/dance club environment is associated with extended intense physical activity, which contributes to serious and potentially fatal dehydration, hyperthermia, rhabdomyolysis, and renal failure. Severe hypertension, arrhythmias, cardiac failure, fulminate hepatic failure, ataxia, syncope, panic attacks, and seizures can occur at high doses.

Chronic Effects and Presentations

MDMA effects can last a week or more after moderate use. These effects include a range of undesirable emotions, such as anxiety, aggression, sadness, irritability, and impairments to memory, information processing, sleep, appetite, or libido. Chronic use can lead to a paranoid psychosis clinically indistinguishable from schizophrenia. Drug dependence can occur, and abstinence has been associated with withdrawal symptoms.

Additional Management Considerations

- No medications work as a specific MDMA antidote.
- Most urine toxicology screening does not detect (usual) lower-dose Ecstasy use, but high-dose MDMA can be detected as an amphetamine.
- Differential diagnosis of MDMA use effects includes sudden hepatic failure.
- Evaluate MDMA users for signs and symptoms of heat injury.
- MDMA-induced hyperthermia can present like heat stroke. Depolarizing muscle relaxants (succinylcholine) for intubation can induce malignant hyperthermia.
- Avoid using β-blockers, which will exacerbate MDMA-induced hypertension.
- IV benzodiazepine treats acute agitation/panic. Haloperidol can be used adjunctively.
- IV benzodiazepine treats hypertension. If the hypertension is severe, use nitroglycerin or nitroprusside, or try a drug with combined α- and β-antagonist effects, such as labetalol.
- Many undesirable effects, particularly those affecting memory, information processing, emotions, and mood, are known to last for hours to weeks after MDMA use.

- Almost 60% of MDMA users report withdrawal symptoms, including fatigue, trouble concentrating, anorexia, and depression.
- When diagnosing paranoid psychosis and schizophrenia, rule out chronic MDMA use.

METHAMPHETAMINE

Selected Street Names: *Batu, Biker Dope, Bikers Coffee, Black Beauties, Chalk, Chicken Feed, Crank, Croak, Crypto, Crystal, Fire, Glass, Go-Fast, Hillbilly Crack, Hiropon, Ice, Meth, Methlies Quick, Pink, Poor Man's Cocaine, Rock, Shabu, Shards, Speed, Stove top, Tina, Trash, Tweak, Uppers, Ventana, White Cross, Vidrio, Yaba (pills), Yellow Bam*

Methamphetamine is a powerful amphetamine derivative and psychostimulant that is a highly addictive schedule II drug, meaning it has high potential for abuse and is available only by prescription.[22,28–31] Low-dose methamphetamine has highly limited clinical use for the treatment of certain attention deficit disorders, exogenous obesity, and narcolepsy. In the early 2000s, a spate of news stories recounted how small clandestine laboratories were using inexpensive and accessible chemicals (fertilizer, drain cleaner, starter fluid) and OTC medications, particularly those containing pseudoephedrine, to make methamphetamines until state and federal controls curtailed the supply and pharmaceutical companies changed OTC product composition. Most methamphetamine used in the United States is now fabricated in foreign or domestic superlabs. It is a white, odorless, bitter-tasting crystalline powder easily dissolved in liquids such as water or alcohol. Crystalline meth, called *ice, crystal,* or *glass,* is a higher-quality smokable form of the drug that also can be injected intravenously. Meth also can be snorted, ingested as pills, or injected rectally without a needle. Smoking meth is generally most popular because it leads to very rapid brain uptake and drug effects. IV injection and smoking both result in an immediate, intense, and very pleasurable *rush* or *flash* that lasts for minutes. Within 3 to 5 minutes of snorting meth, the user feels a euphoric high but not an intense rush. For oral ingestion, the user feels the euphoric effects after 15 to 20 minutes. Users often take additional doses in an effort to maintain the drug's effects, which wane much sooner than do the 12-hour half-life blood levels. *Binge and crash* use patterns are common and can result in a run of continuing meth use without eating or sleeping for hours or days. Women and men who engage in high-risk sexual activity, particularly homosexual men who attend circuit parties or sex clubs, have used meth to enhance sexual pleasure and performance.

Clinical Consequences: Acute Effects and Presentations

Most of the pleasurable effects are attributed to the release of very high levels of dopamine caused by meth. In addition to the rush sensation and euphoria, other short-term drug effects are increased attention, energy, alertness, and physical activity; decreased fatigue, appetite, and thirst; dilated pupils; and enhanced libido. Higher doses can cause tachypnea, tachycardia, arrhythmias, hypertension, hyperthermia, irritability, confusion, anxiety, insomnia, tremors, movement disorders, and seizures. Thus, users are at increased risk for dehydration, heat exhaustion, rhabdomyolysis, cardiovascular collapse, stroke, accidental injury, and death.

Chronic Effects and Presentations

Because methamphetamine users develop tolerance, they tend to escalate the dose or frequency of use, or they change the method of drug use in an attempt to enhance drug effects. Chronic or long-term methamphetamine abuse primarily results in addiction and dependence, plus the consequences of associated high-risk behaviors. Chronic users show signs of psychosis, including paranoia, visual and auditory hallucinations, and delusions, such as the feeling of insects (*meth mites* or *drug bugs*) crawling under the skin. Chronic scratching and picking at the skin causes a scabies-like rash that often is superinfected. Meth-associated psychosis can last for months to years after drug use has terminated and can recur in response to stress despite no further drug use. Users also exhibit mood lability, profound memory loss, compulsive behaviors, aggressive or violent behavior, depression, and general deterioration in physical health, particularly evident as significant weight loss and severe dental disease or *meth mouth*. Research on attention control has shown that the ability to ignore distractions is more profoundly affected than other aspects of attention, even after weeks of drug abstinence. Chronic use results in dramatic changes in brain structure and function that have been well documented by imaging studies. Imaging after years of abstinence has shown that damage in some brain regions is reversible and correlated with improved performance on motor and verbal memory testing, but in other brain regions, no recovery occurs. Specific functional magnetic resonance brain imaging of abstinent chronic meth users has reliably predicted relapse likelihood, based on key brain regions for decision-making, but is not yet available as a clinical tool.[32]

Additional Management Considerations

- Exposure to a meth laboratory should activate bathing and decontamination protocols as well as evaluation for other laboratory-related toxicities.
- No medications work as a specific methamphetamine antidote.
- Avoid ß-blocker use. It will exacerbate methamphetamine-induced hypertension.
- IV benzodiazepine treats acute agitation/panic. Haloperidol can be used adjunctively.
- IV benzodiazepine treats hypertension. If the hypertension is severe, use nitroglycerin or nitroprusside, or try a drug with combined α- and β-antagonist effects, such as labetalol.

- Meth-induced hyperthermia can present like heat stroke. Depolarizing muscle relaxants (succinylcholine) for intubation can induce malignant hyperthermia.
- Antibiotics may be necessary to treat infected skin eruptions.
- Specific cognitive problems need identification.
- Nutrition and dental health warrant specific attention.
- Meth-using adolescents have more emotional, psychiatric, and delinquency problems than those with other drug abuse.
- Contingency management therapy and the SAMHSA Matrix Model are the only therapeutic psychosocial approaches with known efficacy for meth dependence.
- Methamphetamine use is associated with high risk of human immunodeficiency virus (HIV) and hepatitis B and C transmission related to sexual risk taking and higher risk with injection drug use.
- Men may have residual sexual dysfunction after long-term methamphetamine use.

SYNTHETIC CATHINONES (BATH SALTS)

Selected Street Names: *Bliss, Blue Silk, Bloom, Cloud Nine, Energy-1, Hurricane Charlie, Ivory Wave, Lunar Wave, Ocean Burst, Pure Ivory, Purple Wave, Red Dove, Scarface, Snow Leopard, Stardust, Vanilla Sky, White Dove, White Lightning, Zoom*

Synthetic cathinones, most commonly known as *bath salts,* encompass a family of substances that include 3,4 methylenedioxypyrovalerone (MDPV), mephedrone, and methylone, among others that have no legitimate bathing use, but are singularly intended for substance abuse.[24,33,34] Synthetic cathinones were modeled after cathinone, the active ingredient in Khat shrub leaves, which are chewed across Africa and Asia for the stimulant effects. The ways in which these products affect the human brain are still unclear, but they function as CNS stimulants, resembling methamphetamine. MDPV is at least 10 times more potent than cocaine in its dopaminergic effects. Bath salt users report hallucinations, which are considered serotonergic effects.

Synthetic cathinone is available as white or brown crystalline products in plastic or foil packages that are labeled *not for human consumption.* They are sold for many uses, such as a bath product, research chemical, plant food, stain remover, insect repellant, and vacuum freshener, among others. Access to these products initially was legal, and they were easily obtained from the Internet, head shops, and convenience stores. After a wave of medical emergencies in 2011, these products were regulated, and, in 2012, MDPV and mephedrone became schedule I controlled substances. Related synthetic compounds remain unregulated and accessible, and they continue to emerge as the industry rapidly conforms to meet popular market demands.

Clinical Consequences: Acute Effects and Presentations

Bath salts are used orally, are inhaled, or are injected. Use causes agitation and increased energy within about 15 minutes, and the effects last from 4 to 6 hours. The user reports intense euphoria with alertness, stimulation, intensified sensory experiences, talkativeness, and sociability. Higher doses cause perceptual distortions and adverse sympathomimetic and psychiatric effects.

Sympathomimetic effects include diaphoresis, emesis, tachycardia, hypertension, hyperthermia, chest pain, headache, and seizures. Psychiatric effects include altered mental status, paranoia and panic attacks, delusions, hallucinations, and violent behavior, including self-mutilation and suicidal or homicidal activity. Data from the many emergency care cases show that individuals with underlying cardiac, neurologic, and psychiatric conditions are at the greatest risk for adverse consequences.

Chronic Effects and Presentations

The long-term effects of synthetic cathinone use are related to dependence and abuse/addiction potential. Bath salt users have reported an intense craving to use increasing amounts of the substance. The withdrawal syndrome associated with stopping use includes chills, sweats, and hallucinations, which can be severe and may require inpatient and treatment center management.

Additional Management Considerations

- Standard drug testing does not detect cathinones, but specific testing for acute intoxication can detect these chemicals, usually MDPV.
- Cathinones are often wholly or partially substituted for Ecstasy and other drugs sold in the United States and abroad.
- Cathinones are often combined with other substances, so users may be unaware that they are engaging in polysubstance use and its associated risks.

SYNTHETIC CANNABINOIDS

Selected Street Names: Black Diamond, Black Mamba, Blaze, Fake Pot, Fake Weed, K2, Mojo, Moon Rocks, Sence, Skunk, Spice, Yucatan Fire, Zohai

Synthetic cannabinoids are a category composed of a large variety of unregulated chemical compounds that are marketed as "natural herbal" and legal marijuana alternatives.[33,35] These chemicals were initially developed in the 1970s to study the cannabinoid system and receptors, so they mimic the structure of tetrahydrocannabinol (THC), the primary active ingredient in marijuana. Abuse of these products first came to attention in 2008. Spice and K2 are the most common street names.

Synthetic cannabinoid powder is dissolved in a solvent, applied to dried shredded plant material, and marketed in packets resembling potpourri. The packets are labeled *not for human consumption*. In the past, access was easy from Internet sites and head shops, but in 2011 the DEA designated the 5 most common synthetic cannabinoid chemicals as schedule I controlled substances. Synthetic cannabinoid producers stay ahead of this regulation by continually designing novel chemicals, compounds, and mixtures that offer users the desired potency and effects.

Clinical Consequences: Acute Effects and Presentations

Synthetic cannabinoids are modeled after THC, so the acute effects resemble those of marijuana. Most often, synthetic cannabinoids are used by smoking, but the preparation also can be brewed into tea and ingested. Sometimes synthetic marijuana is mixed with marijuana and smoked. Within about 4 minutes, users report feeling relaxed and sleepy, with an elevated mood and altered sense of reality that lasts from 1 to 8 hours. Synthetic marijuana acts on the same receptors as THC; however, formulations vary in strength. Synthetic marijuana has 4 to 10 times the potency of marijuana and can produce exaggerated effects such as chest pain, paranoia, delusions, and hallucinations, which are rare with marijuana use. Physiologic effects includes tachycardia, hypertension, vomiting, confusion, and agitation.

Synthetic cannabinoids frequently contain a number of other products that can be significantly more dangerous than marijuana. Although overdose of marijuana is not a consideration, overdoses have been reported with synthetic cannabinoid use and most likely are related to the noncannabinoid components in the product. Reported health outcomes related to even a single episode of synthetic cannabinoid use include seizures, myocardial ischemia, anxiety attack, suicide, and stroke with permanent residual neurologic damage.

Chronic Effects and Presentation

Similar to the acute effects, the long-term effects can be related to the cannabinoids or the contaminating substances. Synthetic cannabinoid use is considered capable of leading to addictive behaviors and dependence as well as a withdrawal syndrome, but because the drugs are relatively new, more time is needed to research their long-term effects.

Additional Management Considerations

- New synthetic cannabinoid products continue to be created and marketed.
- Both the user and the medical professional may not know what unknown substance(s) was/were used and whether the drug or contaminants are responsible for the effects.

- Synthetic cannabinoids do not result in a positive marijuana drug test. Some synthetic cannabinoids are detectable on specific urine testing.
- Smoking synthetic cannabinoids can have extreme and life-threatening effects.

INHALANTS

Selected Street Names of Volatile Solvents, Fuels, and Anesthetics: *Air Blast, Discorama, Dust, Dust Off, Hippie Crack, Medusa, Moon Gas, Oz, Poor Man's Pot*

Nitrous Oxide: *Buzz Bomb, Laughing Gas, Shoot the Breeze, Whippets*

Volatile Alkyl Nitrite: *Amys (Amyl Nitrite), Boppers, Bolt, Climax, Locker Room, Pearls, Poppers, Quicksilver, Rush, Snappers, Thrust*

Inhalants are volatile chemicals that are intentionally inhaled in order to achieve an altered mental state.[36-38] A large and pharmacologically diverse group of substances is abused as *inhalants*, a definitional term that describes the route of use. This classification method sharply contrasts with that of all other drugs of abuse, which are grouped by a common specific characteristic neurologic action or perceived psychoactive effect. Although other substances, such as nicotine, cocaine, heroin, or alcohol, can be abused through inhalation, inhalant abuse only refers to solvent or volatile substance use. Inhalants can be further subcategorized into 3 groups: volatile solvents, fuels, and anesthetics; nitrous oxide; and volatile alkyl nitrites.

Because volatile products usually are widely available, inexpensive, easily concealed, and legal (for intended purposes), these factors likely facilitate their use by younger age groups. Particular circumstances, such as occupational access to volatile substances, may promote their use in older age groups. The type, frequency, and mode of inhalant use vary according to age, product availability, culture, geography, economics, and other factors. Inhalants have been associated with isolated or impoverished living conditions, delinquency, criminal behavior and incarceration, depression and suicidal behavior, antisocial attitudes, family conflict and chaos, and a patient history of abuse, violence, or other drug abuse, including injecting drugs.

Clinical Consequences: Acute Effects and Presentations

As a group, inhalants cause a quick and generally pleasurable sensory high with rapid resolution of symptoms and little residual hangover effects. Immediate effects of inhaling volatile solvents, fuels, anesthetics, or nitrous oxide resemble early stages of anesthesia. Initial stimulation is followed by light-headedness, disinhibition, and impulsivity. Repeated breathing of inhalants extends intoxication from a few minutes to several hours. Slurred speech, dizziness, diplopia, ataxia, and disorientation occur with higher doses. After the euphoria, users commonly experience a lingering headache, drowsiness, and sleep, which effectively curtails further inhalant exposure and the risk of severe respiratory depression or coma. Very prolonged use can cause visual hallucinations. Patients may have rhinorrhea, epistaxis, sneezing, cough, excess salivation, and inflamed conjunctivae. Other patients have nausea, emesis, diarrhea, crampy abdominal pain, dyspnea, retractions, or wheezing.

Inhaled nitrites are distinct from other inhalants. They primarily cause vasodilation and smooth muscle relaxation with little CNS effect. Nitrites are inhaled to enhance sexual feelings, penile engorgement, and anal relaxation; thus, use is associated with men having sex with men. Within 10 seconds of inhalation, the user feels a floating sensation with heightened skin tactility, warmth, and throbbing, all of which wane in minutes. Nitrite use also may cause flushing, headache, light-headedness, hypotension, blurred vision, and syncope. Significant methemoglobinemia can occur, causing cyanosis and lethargy.

The diversity of types and doses of inhalants used results in diverse symptomatology and clinical presentations. Intoxication and evidence of use may be obvious, such as inhalant halitosis lasting for hours, or chemical stains or paint on clothes or skin. *Huffer rash* (perioral or perinasal eczema with pyoderma) can be evident. Inhaling aerosol computer cleaners can cause frostbite of facial skin or airway mucosa. Inhalants generally cause the user to become less inhibited, less alert, and less oriented. These effects contribute to a user's likelihood of engaging in risk behaviors that lead to accidental injury or death, such as a motor vehicle crash, drowning, fire, or falling from a height, which are the main reasons why users present to the acute clinical setting. Sudden sniffing death syndrome is a real risk each time an inhalant is used. Inhalant use sensitizes the myocardium and triggers a fatal cardiac arrhythmia. This syndrome is the primary cause of inhalant use fatality, with suffocation, aspiration, and accidental injury each accounting for about 15% of deaths. Acute mortality rates are unknown but are estimated to be at least 1%.

Chronic Effects and Presentations

Chronic inhalant abuse sequelae are as diverse as the types of volatile substances used. There is remarkable reversibility of many of the pathologic effects if inhalant use stops, but the nervous system has the least regenerative capacity. Inhalant affinity for lipid-rich tissues such as the nervous system also concentrates damage in those tissues, resulting in chronic encephalopathy, dementia, cerebellar dysfunction, tremor, and peripheral neuropathy. Decreased coordination, gait disturbance, and lower extremity spasticity can occur. Cognitive deficits have been found in memory, attention, auditory discrimination, problem-solving, visual learning, and visuomotor abilities. Specific chemicals can also cause vision loss, sensorineural hearing loss, cardiomyopathy, toxic hepatitis, distal renal tubular acidosis, metabolic acidosis, leukemia, and aplastic anemia.

Patients can present with chronic neuropsychiatric symptoms, such as confusion, poor concentration, depression, irritability, hostility, or paranoia, or they can show signs of other organ system damage. Inhalant dependence, tolerance, and withdrawal as well as toluene embryopathy and neonatal abstinence syndrome have been reported. Toxicities may occur from materials in the inhaled solvents, drugs used in combination with inhalants, and drug-drug interactions, as occurs when depressant effects are potentiated.

Chronic nitrous oxide use causes short-term memory loss and pernicious anemia-type peripheral neuropathy, both of which can improve when use ceases. Chronic volatile alkyl nitrite inhalation causes hematologic and immune system effects without causing cognitive deficits.

Additional Management Considerations

- Asking screening questions about potential inhalant use is an integral part of the primary care of young adolescent patients, male patients having sex with men, and patients with occupational inhalant exposure or availability.
- Suspect inhalant use when finding the patient's clothing, breath, mucous membranes, or skin has paint- or chemical-related odor, stains, or pathology.
- Routine urine drug screening does not detect inhalant use.
- Special urine drug testing can be part of a treatment adherence plan for benzene or toluene abuse; both have detectable metabolites after a large inhalation.
- Acute care includes decontamination of the patient's skin and clothing.
- No medications reverse acute inhalant intoxication. Pressor medications and bronchodilators are relatively contraindicated. Myocardial sensitization responds best to a calm and supportive environment.
- Acute methemoglobinemia resolves with IV methylene blue.
- Chronic inhalant use can result in organ system damage reflected as abnormal laboratory test values, such as elevated hepatic enzymes or anemia.
- Few treatment programs are designed specifically for inhalant abuse. Inhalant users may be particularly reluctant to engage in treatment and may need an extended detoxification period or "treatment readiness" preparation.
- Neuroleptics and other pharmacotherapy may be indicated to treat comorbid conditions of inhalant users.

SALVIA (SALVIA DIVINORUM)

Selected Street Names: *Diviner's Sage, Magic Mint, Maria Pastora, Sage of the Seers, Sally D, Shepherdess' Herb, Ska Pastora*

Salvia is derived from the leaves of the *Salvia divinorum* plant in the mint family.[33,39] This herb, which is used in traditional spiritual practices by Mazatec native people of Mexico, became a substance of abuse in the United States for its hallucinogenic and dissociative effects. The active ingredient, salvinorin A, is a potent agonist of the human brain kappa opioid receptors in the system regulating perception but not of the opioid receptors stimulated by heroin or the serotonin receptors activated by hallucinogens such as LSD. Neither the salvia plant nor any derivatives have any approved uses in the United States. Although federal control has not yet been applied, salvia has been scheduled as a controlled substance by nearly half of the states since 2011.

Clinical Consequences: Acute Effects and Presentations

The leaves of the salvia plant are either dried and smoked or vaporized; the fresh leaves are chewed similar to using chewing tobacco; or the leaves are eaten. When chewed, the leaf is placed in the cheek area so that the chemical is absorbed through the buccal mucosa. From chewing, the onset of effect is 5 to 10 minutes, and the effects lasting 1 to 2 hours. When smoked, the effects begin in less than 1 minute and last about 30 minutes.

Salvia provides brief hallucination experiences that mimic psychosis, so it is more often used by individuals than in social or party circumstances. Users report feeling disembodied and detached, feeling sensations of traveling through time and space, floating, flying, twisting, and spinning. They also report a highly modified perception of external reality and self with visual perception changes, including vivid lights, colors, shapes, and objects, so that it is difficult for them to interact with their surroundings. Users experience disorientation, laughter, slurred speech, dizziness, nausea, chills, slower pulse, poor coordination, swings in mood and emotions, and dysphoria. Although sometimes referred to as the *20-minute acid trip*, many users decline using salvia more than once.

Chronic Effects and Presentations

Little is established about the long-term effects of salvia, but addictive potential seems low. Rodent experiments show poor learning and memory effects. As with cannabis, many of the detrimental effects of salvia are related to behaviors and risk-taking during use, such as driving a motor vehicle while under the influence.

Additional Management Considerations

- Salvia is widely available. It is produced and sold in different strengths and formulations that vary in effect.
- Salvia is not part of standard urine drug testing, but it can be detected for a few hours if specific testing is available.
- Theoretically, naloxone could reverse the effects, but the half-life of salvia is very short, and users rarely seek acute care.

DEXTROMETHORPHAN

Selected Street Names: *Candy, Dex, DM, DXM, Red Devils, Red Hots, Robo, Rojo, Skittles, Triple C, Vitamin D*

Dextromethorphan (DXM) is a semisynthetic morphine derivative used as the active ingredient in about 150 different OTC cough and cold preparations.[40–42] Although an opioid, DXM acts as a dissociative agent, antagonizing actions at the NMDA receptor similar to ketamine and PCP. People who abuse DXM take this medication in doses much higher than those recommended for cough suppression. The rapid development of tolerance drives dose escalation by the user. Products that contain DXM have been moved behind the counter in some states to limit ease of access, including theft. A number of phrases have been coined to describe the DXM user, such as *syrup head*, or DXM use, including *Robo-tripping*, *Robo-dosing*, *Dexing*, and *sheeting* (ingesting a sheet of pills containing DXM).

Clinical Consequences: Acute Effects and Presentations

DXM is ingested orally, and gastrointestinal absorption is rapid. The neurobehavioral effects are attributed to the main active metabolite dextrorphan (DOR), which results from liver metabolism. This metabolism is highly variable because a genetically polymorphic isoenzyme determines each person's ability to metabolize DXM, so the related rate of metabolism and thus the intensity of DXM effects are quite variable. The neurobehavioral effects that generally begin within 30 to 60 minutes after ingestion and last about 6 hours have been classified into 4 intensities of effect or *plateaus*:

1. First plateau: Reached at dosages of 1.5 to 2.5 mg/kg. Includes alertness, empathy, giggling, laughing, agitation, mildly increased heart rate and temperature, euphoria, and mild intoxication.
2. Second plateau: Reached at dosages of 2.5 to 7.5 mg/kg. Includes increased intensity of first plateau effects plus changes in sensory experience leading to dissociating the mind and body, hallucinations, and perception of being in a dreamlike state.
3. Third plateau: Reached at dosages of 7.5 to 15 mg/kg. Includes difficulty recognizing people and objects, loss of coordination, ataxia and a distinctive plodding *zombie* gait, chaotic blindness, dreamlike vision, confusion, and visual and auditory hallucinations.
4. Fourth plateau: Reached at dosages higher than 15 mg/kg. Includes loss of connection with own body, altered visual perception including perceived blindness or increased hearing, hallucinations, delusions, and psychosis.

Many other symptoms occur at low levels of intoxication and escalate with dose, including tachycardia, hypertension, diaphoresis, emesis, mydriasis, nystagmus, disorientation, slurred speech, poor motor coordination, altered tactile and skin sensations, and difficulty with orgasm. DXM toxicity can cause cardiac arrhythmia, hyperthermia, cognitive deterioration, and severe serotonin syndrome in the absence of another serotonergic drug.

Chronic Effects and Presentations

Dependence and withdrawal symptoms have been reported, including fatigue, apathy, constipation, sleep disturbances, panic feelings, and flashbacks. Long-term DXM use effects include erectile dysfunction and decreased libido. Toxicity related to combination preparations, particularly acetaminophen, can be cumulative and have long-term or life-threatening consequences. Chronic use of DXM, a bromide salt, in high doses can manifest as bromism with altered mental status, neuromuscular symptoms, and bromoderma acne.

Additional Management Considerations

- Many preparations combine DXM with other active ingredients, including guaifenesin, acetaminophen, or antihistamines; thus, ingestion management must always consider the potential effects and risks from the other substances or combination of substances in addition to DXM toxicity alone.
- Polysubstance use may be more common with OTC product abuse, including DXM use, and can result in exaggerated adverse reactions and potentially life-threatening effects.
- Although severe DXM intoxication can result in hyperthermia and severe respiratory depression, coma is rarely caused by DXM overdose alone.
- Rapid propofol infusion has normalized the agitation, neuromuscular hyperactivity, and autonomic instability of severe serotonin syndrome from DXM use.[42]
- Standard drug testing does not detect DXM, but a false-positive PCP can result by liquid chromatography. GC/MS distinguishes the 2 drugs.
- Erectile dysfunction as a long-term effect may warrant specific treatment.

References

1. Johnston LD, O'Malley PM, Bachman JG, Schulenberg JE. *Monitoring the Future National Survey Results on Drug Use, 1975-2006. Volume I: Secondary School Students.* No. 07-6205. Bethesda, MD: National Institute on Drug Abuse; 2007. Available at: www.monitoringthefuture.org/pubs/monographs/vol1_2006.pdf. Accessed November 5, 2013
2. Substance Abuse and Mental Health Services Administration. *Results from the 2012 National Survey on Drug Use and Health: Summary of National Findings.* NSDUH Series H-46, HHS Publication No. (SMA) 13-4795. Rockville, MD: Substance Abuse and Mental Health Services Administration; 2013. Available at: www.samhsa.gov/data/NSDUH/2012SummNatFindDetTables/NationalFindings/NSDUHresults2012.htm. Accessed October 29, 2013
3. Johnston LD, O'Malley PM, Bachman JG, Schulenberg JE. *Monitoring the Future National Survey Results on Drug Use, 1975-2012: Volume 2, College Students And Adults Ages 19-50.* Ann

Arbor, MI: Institute for Social Research, The University of Michigan; 2013. Available at: www.monitoringthefuture.org//pubs/monographs/mtf-vol2_2012.pdf. Accessed November 12, 2013

4. *American teens more cautious about using synthetic drugs.* Ann Arbor, MI: University of Michigan News Service. Available at: monitoringthefuture.org//pressreleases/13drugpr_complete.pdf. Accessed December 20, 2013

5. Swaim RC, Beauvais F, Chavez EL, Oetting ER. The effect of school dropout rates on estimates of adolescent substance use among three racial/ethnic groups. *Am J Public Health.* 1997;87(1):5155

6. Beauvais F. Comparison of drug use rates for reservation Indian, non-reservation Indian and Anglo youth. *Am Indian Alsk Native Ment Health Res.* 1992;5(1):13–31

7. Zebrowski PI, Gregory RJ. Inhalant use patterns among Eskimo school children in western Alaska. *J Addict Dis.* 1996;15:67–77

8. Substance Abuse and Mental Health Services Administration, Office of Applied Studies. *Emergency Department Trends From the Drug Abuse Warning Network, Final Estimates 1995-2002.* DAWN Series: D-24, DHHS Publication No. (SMA) 03-3780. Rockville, MD: Substance Abuse and Mental Health Services Administration; 2003

9. Substance Abuse and Mental Health Services Administration. *Drug Abuse Warning Network, 2011: National Estimates of Drug-Related Emergency Department Visits.* DAWN Series D-39, HHS Publication No. (SMA) 13-4760. Rockville, MD: Substance Abuse and Mental Health Services Administration; 2013

10. Boyer EW, Shannon M, Hibberd PL. The internet and psychoactive substance use among innovative drug users. *Pediatrics.* 2005;115(2):302–305

11. Wax PM. Just a click away: recreational drug web sites on the internet. *Pediatrics.* 2002;109(6):e96

12. Forman RF, Marlowe DB, McLellan AT. The internet as a source of drugs of abuse. *Curr Psychiatry Rep.* 2006;8(5):377–382

13. Goldenring JM, Rosen DR. Getting into adolescent heads: an essential update. *Contemp Pediatr.* 2004;21:64–90

14. Ginsburg KR. Viewing our adolescent patients through a positive lens. *Contemp Pediatr.* 2007;24:65–76

15. American Academy of Pediatrics Committee on Substance Abuse. Substance use screening, brief intervention, and referral to treatment for pediatricians. *Pediatrics.* 2011;128:e1330–e1340

16. Kwong T, Magnani B, Rosano T, Shaw L, eds. *The Clinical Toxicology Laboratory: Contemporary Practice of Poisoning Evaluation.* 2nd ed. Washington, DC: AACC Press; 2013

17. Wu LT, Schlenger WE, Galvin, DM. Concurrent use of methamphetamine, MDMA, LSD, ketamine, GHB, and flunitrazepam among American youths. *Drug Alcohol Depend.* 2006;84(1):102–113

18. Knudsen HK. Adolescent-only substance abuse treatment: availability and adoption of components of quality. *J Subst Abuse Treat.* 2009;36(2):195–204

19. Winters KC, Botzet AM, Fahnhorst T. Advances in adolescent substance abuse treatment. *Curr Psychiatry Rep.* 2011;13(5):416–421

20. Ahuja AS, Crome I, Williams R. Engaging young people who misuse substances in treatment. *Curr Opin Psychiatry.* 2013;26(4):335–342

21. Weaver MF, Schnoll SH. Hallucinogens and club drugs. In: Galanter M, Kleber HD, eds. *Textbook of Substance Abuse Treatment.* 4th ed. Arlington, VA: American Psychiatric Publishing; 2008:191–200

22. Rome ES. It's a rave new world: rave culture and illicit drug use in the young. *Cleve Clin J Med.* 2001;68(6):541–550

23. McDonough M, Kennedy N, Glasper A, Bearn J. Clinical features and management of gamma-hydroxybutyrate (GHB) withdrawal: a review. *Drug Alcohol Depend.* 2004;75(1):3–9

24. Karila L, Reynaud M. GHB and synthetic cathinones: clinical effects and potential consequences. *Drug Testing Anal.* 2011;3(9):552–559

25. National Institute on Drug Abuse. DrugFacts: Hallucinogens—LSD, peyote, psilocybin, and PCP. Available at: www.drugabuse.gov/publications/drugfacts/hallucinogens-lsd-peyote-psilocybin-pcp. Accessed November 20, 2013

26. Morgan CJ, Curran HV, Independent Scientific Committee on Drugs. Ketamine use: a review. *Addiction.* 2012;107(1):27–38

27. National Institute on Drug Abuse. DrugFacts: MDMA (Ecstasy or Molly). Revised September 2013. Available at: www.drugabuse.gov/publications/drugfacts/mdma-ecstasy-or-molly. Accessed December 7, 2013

28. Rawson RA, Ling W. Clinical management: methamphetamine. In: Galanter M, Kleber HD, eds. *Textbook of Substance Abuse Treatment.* 4th ed. Arlington, VA: American Psychiatric Publishing; 2008:169–179

29. National Institute on Drug Abuse. Methamphetamine abuse and addiction. Research Report Series, NIH Publication No. 13-4210. Revised September 2013. Available at: www.drugabuse.gov/publications/research-reports/methamphetamine-abuse-addiction. Accessed November 5, 2013

30. Ruha AM, Yarema MC. Pharmacologic treatment of acute pediatric methamphetamine toxicity. *Pediatr Emerg Care.* 2006;22(12):782–785

31. Lineberry TW, Bostwick JM. Methamphetamine abuse: a perfect storm of complications. *Mayo Clin Proc.* 2006;81(l):77–84

32. Paulus MP, Tapert SF, Schuckit MA. Neural activation patterns of methamphetamine-dependent subjects during decision making predict relapse. *Arch Gen Psychiatry.* 2005;62(7):761–768

33. Rosenbaum CD, Carreiro SP, Babu KM. Here today, gone tomorrow...and back again? A review of herbal marijuana alternatives (K2, Spice), synthetic cathinones (bath salts), kratom, Salvia divinorum, methoxetamine, and piperazines. *J Med Toxicol.* 2012;8(1):15–32

34. Prosser JM, Nelson LS. The toxicology of bath salts: a review of synthetic cathinones. *J Med Toxicol.* 2012;8(1):33–42

35. National Institute on Drug Abuse. DrugFacts: Spice (synthetic marijuana). Revised December 2012. Available at: www.drugabuse.gov/publications/drugfacts/spice-synthetic-marijuana. Accessed October 29, 2013

36. Williams JF, Storck M; American Academy of Pediatrics Committee on Substance Abuse, & American Academy of Pediatrics Committee on Native American Child Health. Inhalant abuse. *Pediatrics.* 2007;119(5):1009–1017

37. National Institute on Drug Abuse. Inhalant abuse. Research Report Series: NIH publication number 10-3818. Revised July 2012. Available at: www.drugabuse.gov/publications/research-reports/inhalant-abuse. Accessed November 12, 2013

38. Wu LT, Schlenger WE, Ringwalt CL. Use of nitrite inhalants ("poppers") among American youth. *J Adolesc Health.* 2005;37(1):52–60

39. Drug Enforcement Administration, Office of Diversion Control. Drug & Chemical Evaluation Section. Salvia divinorum and salvinorin A. October 2013. Available at: www.deadiversion.usdoj.gov/drug_chem_info/salvia_d.pdf. Accessed October 29, 2013

40. Williams JF, Kokotailo PK. Abuse of proprietary (over-the-counter) drugs. *Adolesc Med Clin.* 2006;17(3):733–750

41. Boyer EW. Dextromethophan abuse. *Pediatr Emerg Care.* 2004;20(12):858–863

42. Ganetsky M, Babu KM, Boyer EW. Serotonin syndrome in dextromethorphan ingestion responsive to propofol therapy. *Pediatr Emerg Care.* 2007;23(11):829–831

Adolesc Med 025 (2014) 215–229

Assessment and Treatment of Substance Abuse in the Juvenile Justice Population

Elizabeth Janopaul-Naylor, BS[a]; Joanna D. Brown, MD, MPH[b*]; Elizabeth A. Lowenhaupt, MD[c]; Marina Tolou-Shams, PhD[d]

[a]Alpert Medical School of Brown University, Providence, Rhode Island;
[b]Assistant Professor (Clinical) of Family Medicine, Alpert Medical School of Brown University;
Medical Director, Rhode Island Training School; Division of Adolescent Medicine,
Hasbro Children's Hospital; Providence, Rhode Island; [c]Assistant Professor (Clinical),
Department of Psychiatry and Human Behavior, Alpert Medical School of Brown University;
Associate Training Director, Child Psychiatry Fellowship & Triple Board Residency and Director,
Medical Student Education in Child & Adolescent Psychiatry, Rhode Island Hospital/Alpert Medical
School of Brown University; Director of Psychiatric Services, Rhode Island Training School; Providence,
Rhode Island; [d]Assistant Professor (Research), Alpert Medical School of Brown University; Staff
Psychologist, Rhode Island Hospital, Bradley Hasbro Children's Research Center; Director, Rhode Island
Family Court, Mental Health Clinic and Director of Substance Abuse Treatment Services, Rhode Island
Training School, Bradley Hasbro Children's Research Center, Providence, Rhode Island

INTRODUCTION

Youth involved with the juvenile justice system face unique legal and institutional challenges and carry a disproportionate share of health risk factors.[1] Substance use-related problems are extremely common among these adolescents.[1] The primary care physician may encounter juvenile justice youth in a variety of settings: in the outpatient setting when the adolescents are on probation or living in a group home, or in a correctional setting when youth are either held in detention or incarcerated serving a sentence. Health care encounters with this population represent critical opportunities to address substance abuse: to offer support, education, screening, treatment, and appropriate referral. A recent policy statement by the American Academy of Pediatrics (AAP) points out that if youth facing substance abuse were better identified and treated in the community setting, involvement with the juvenile justice system might be prevented or reduced.[2] Whereas other

*Corresponding author:
Joanna_Brown@Brown.edu

articles in this issue focus on specific types of drugs and substance-related issues for adolescents, this article examines the pathways and demographics of this specific group of youth traversing the juvenile justice system, as well as the available evidence-based methods for assessment and treatment.

A number of health organizations offer policy statements or guidelines specifically pertaining to health care for youth involved in juvenile justice, including the screening and treatment of substance abuse. The AAP mentions widespread shortcomings in juvenile justice facilities in terms of failing to routinely screen youth for substance use and abuse or to offer adequate, on-site treatment services.[2] The National Commission on Correctional Health Care (NCCHC) recommends that youth in confinement be screened for mental health issues, including substance abuse, within 24 hours.[3] The NCCHC recommends that all adolescents with positive toxicology screens undergo further psychological evaluation. Comprehensive medical assessments are recommended within 7 days of arrival and mental health assessments within 14 days.

The American Academy of Child and Adolescent Psychiatry (AACAP) recommends that any youth with a positive initial drug screen undergo an immediate brief assessment for possible alcohol or drug withdrawal symptoms as well as a more thorough evaluation within the next 2 weeks. The AACAP practice parameter discusses how health care professionals can assist detained or incarcerated youth in understanding confidentiality as it relates to substance use and what parts of their medical record are available to their legal record. The AACAP advocates prompt transfer to more appropriate health care settings should a youth present with symptoms necessitating greater medical intervention.[4]

OVERVIEW OF THE JUVENILE JUSTICE SYSTEM

Juvenile Justice System Process

The process for youth entering the juvenile justice system is complex and includes a number of points at which substance use/abuse in youth can be recognized and addressed (Figure 1). The process outlined may vary slightly across different states, within states, and across different local/county-level jurisdictions. Involvement with the juvenile justice system starts with an offense leading to an arrest.[5] If a youth is arrested, police will bring him or her to the police station or to a juvenile detention facility. Depending on various factors, such as the severity and type of criminal offense, whether the youth is a first-time or repeat offender, the outcome of the youth's risk assessment, and whether adults are available to monitor the youth, the youth may remain in detention or be released back to the community.

If the decision is made to keep the juvenile in detention, he or she will be arraigned at court on the charge(s) as soon as possible. At court, the youth is

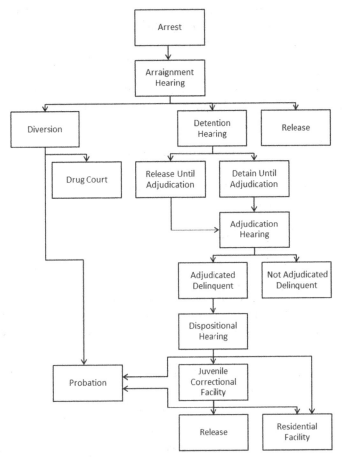

Fig 1. Juvenile justice system process. (Modeled after the Office of Juvenile Justice and Delinquency Prevention (OJJDP) case flow diagram Available at: www.ojjdp.gov/ojstatbb/structure_process/case.html. Accessed November 24, 2013.)

interviewed by a probation officer, and the judgment is made to charge, release, or divert. Diversion of an individual at this point typically means that the young offender is court mandated to complete community service, to attend counseling, or to participate in a juvenile drug court program. Drug courts were created to help people who either have a history of legal infractions that involve substances or have co-occurring legal involvement and substance use problems. Through the supervision of these courts, participants receive treatment for substance abuse as an alternative to incarceration (see Treatment section for details on drug court programs).

Three subsequent hearings play important roles in determining a youth's path through the juvenile justice system:

1. If the youth is charged with a crime, he or she will have a detention hearing. The outcome of this hearing determines whether the youth will continue to be detained before adjudication (sentencing) or if he or she can be released to the community for the interim.
2. At the adjudication hearing, the court decides whether or not the young person is found guilty or "delinquent" pertaining to his or her charges.
3. If the youth is found delinquent, the dispositional hearing determines how the youth will serve his or her sentence.

At the dispositional hearing, the youth is sentenced to a correctional facility, to a residential facility (for which there are varying levels of supervision), or to probation, which is an alternative to serving jail time during which the offender is allowed to reside in the community.

Juvenile Justice Demographics

In 2010, 1.4 million youth were arrested in the United States. Of these youth, 112,600 were adjudicated and placed into residential facilities (including detention centers; Figure 2). As of 2009, the racial makeup of the juvenile justice population was as follows: 78% white, 16% black, and 5% Asian. Current data from the Office of Juvenile Justice and Delinquency Prevention (OJJDP) does not differentiate

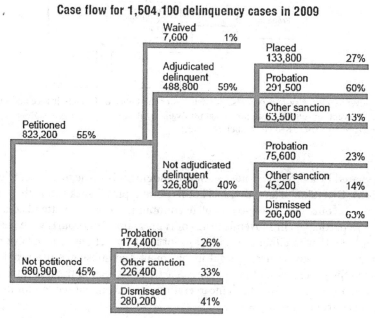

Case flow for 1,504,100 delinquency cases in 2009

Fig 2. Delinquency cases in juvenile courts, 2009. (From Department of Justice, Office of Juvenile Justice and Delinquency Prevention. Available at: www.ojjdp.gov/pubs/239081.pdf. Accessed March 19, 2014.)

Hispanic youth from white youth. Today, about 28% of arrested youth are female. The proportion of female adolescents in today's juvenile courts has doubled since 1985, whereas the number of males has increased by only 17%. In 2009, about half of all juveniles involved in the system were younger than 16 years.[6]

Juvenile Offenses

Among reasons for youths' arrests, property offenses are the most common (Figure 3). Other criminal offenses include assault, murder, prostitution, and drug-related offenses, which are the least common reason for arrest among youth.[7] Property crimes do not involve force; they include theft, vandalism, and arson. Person crimes, in contrast, do involve force; for example, robbery is defined as a person crime because it requires threatening a person with force to steal his or her property. Other person offenses include assault, murder, and rape. Public order offenses include under-age sex, prostitution, and driving while intoxicated. A status offense is a juvenile crime that would not be considered a crime for an adult, such as truancy or running away from home. Violent crimes are thought to be more frequently associated with the use of more expensive substances, such as prescription drugs and cocaine. Alcohol is more often seen in conjunction with minor and nonviolent crimes.[8]

EPIDEMIOLOGY OF SUBSTANCE ABUSE AMONG JUVENILE OFFENDERS

According to the 2010 National Survey on Drug Use and Health, rates of substance abuse among youth engaged in delinquent behavior were found to be more than 5 times greater than those of adolescents not involved with the juvenile justice system.[9] The most commonly abused substances in this population are alcohol and marijuana, but cocaine, heroin, and other illicit substances are

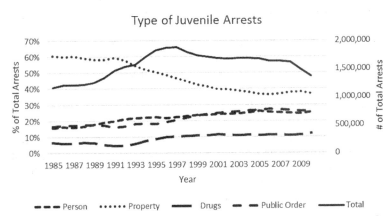

Fig 3. Data from Office of Juvenile Justice and Delinquency Prevention. *Easy Access to Juvenile Court Statistics, 1985-2010.* Available at: www.ojjdp.gov/ojstatbb/ezajcs/. Accessed March 19, 2014.

also used by juvenile offenders more frequently than by nonarrested juvenile populations. Co-occurrence of substance abuse and juvenile delinquency is associated with increased risk for recidivism, incompletion of high school, and continued and increasing substance abuse in adulthood.[10] Data from 2000 suggest that at the time of their arrest, more than half of the juvenile offenders aged 10 to 17 years tested positive for drugs or alcohol. Of those who tested negative, an additional one-fourth reported using drugs within the previous year.[11] In a study of 1829 juvenile offenders, Teplin et al[12] found that 50.7% of males and 46.8% of females met criteria for substance abuse or dependence. One-fourth met criteria for alcohol abuse and 40% for marijuana abuse. Twenty percent met criteria for abuse of multiple substances (most commonly marijuana and alcohol). In their article, Hoge et al[13] found rates of substance abuse among youth in the juvenile justice population ranged widely, from 37% to 100%.

Few data are available on the use of less commonly used substances among juvenile justice populations. One study conducted in a state's juvenile residential facilities found that more than one-third of participants reported ever having used inhalants.[14] In a study conducted in another state, at the time of arrest, 6% of boys and 4% of girls tested positive for cocaine, 2% of boys and girls tested positive for methamphetamines, and approximately 0.5% of youth tested positive for opiates.[15]

SCREENING FOR SUBSTANCE ABUSE IN THE JUVENILE JUSTICE POPULATION

Screening for substance abuse poses challenges for the juvenile justice population. Most facilities test all juvenile offenders on entry with urine drug screens. The screens vary by site, but most include testing for marijuana, heroin, barbiturates, methamphetamines, cocaine, lysergic acid diethylamide (LSD), and phencyclidine (PCP).[16] Although a primary goal of screening in the juvenile justice system may be therapeutic, most substances, whether legal (eg, alcohol) or illegal (eg, cocaine, heroin) for adults, are illegal for minors. Adolescents often choose not to reveal substance use that could be used against them in the legal setting.[17] As mentioned earlier, medical providers should understand and, when necessary, help their patients understand the limits of confidentiality with regard to urine drug screens.

Self-Report Assessment Tools

Facilities use various tools to conduct assessments of youth offenders. The most commonly used validated tools that include aspects of substance abuse but also address mental health issues more broadly include the Massachusetts Youth Screening Instrument (MAYSI), the Brief Symptom Inventory, the Million Adolescent Clinical Inventory, the Youth Self-Report, and the Diagnostic Interview Schedule for Children-Present State Voice Version. These tools are based on *DSM-IV* criteria and most likely will be updated with the implementation of the *DSM-5*.

The MAYSI, now in its second iteration, was developed in the late 1990s.[18] Designed to be administered within the first 24 hours of detention, it is the most commonly used initial screening tool across the country in juvenile detention settings. It was developed as a brief screen, with 52 yes/no questions for both males and females aged 12 to 17 years. It can be administered by a nonclinical staff member. This validated tool assesses youths' emotional status, covering a range of topics and past history, and includes questions about substance abuse. Many institutions have implemented a 2-step assessment process, in which the MAYSI-2 may be used for initial screening, followed by a more in-depth assessment tool.[19] The MAYSI-2 currently is being implemented in diversion settings, such as juvenile probation.

A commonly used, reliable, and validated screening assessment tool for substance abuse or dependence is the Substance Abuse Subtle Screening Inventory (SASSI) Adolescent Form. This 81-question measure has been widely adopted for use with juvenile justice populations because paraprofessionals can administer the tool, it is brief, and it is easy to score. It is 90% accurate for identifying youth with substance abuse or dependence disorders.[20]

SUBSTANCE ABUSE TREATMENT FOR JUVENILE OFFENDERS

Summary of Treatment Models

Current guidelines recommend 10 key elements for treatment models for youth in the juvenile justice system who abuse substances[21]:

- Integrated systems
- Assessments with tailored treatments
- Identification of comorbid disorders
- Comprehensiveness
- Experienced and trained staff
- Developmentally appropriate interventions
- Family involvement
- Efforts to engage and retain participants
- Continuity of care
- Assessment of outcomes

Despite the flexibility that these guidelines allow, the recommendations have not been fully implemented around the country. Henderson et al[22] found that facilities providing substance abuse treatment adhere on average to 5 of the 10 consensus guidelines. In 2005, Young et al[23] surveyed 141 directors of juvenile correctional facilities about their substance abuse treatment programs. Seventy-five percent reported providing drug and alcohol education. About 40% of facilities provided 1 to 4 hours of weekly substance abuse group counseling, and 20% offered 5 to 25 hours of group counseling. These groups were available only to a small portion of those with substance use disorders (SUDs). The survey also revealed that the staff-to-resident ratio was not sufficient for adequate access to individual treatment at most facilities. Fewer than half of respondents reported using a standardized assessment tool to screen for substance abuse.[23]

Pharmacotherapy

Youth may arrive at residential facilities having used substances (eg, opiates) regularly that present the potential for withdrawal. Many facilities do not have detoxification units and will transfer these youth to pediatric units until they are medically cleared.[24] In other cases, if youth are medically stable, health professionals may opt to manage withdrawal on site.

Little research has been done on the use of pharmacotherapy specifically for treating SUDs in incarcerated adolescents. In the juvenile justice setting, the use of medication to treat SUDs as well as to treat comorbid mood, anxiety, thought, or disruptive behavior disorders should be considered only as part of a comprehensive treatment plan following an appropriate biopsychosocial assessment that is sensitive to any relevant cultural, gender, family, or other youth issues.

Psychosocial Treatment Models

Several models are used for treating youth with substance abuse problems who are involved in the juvenile justice system. Most do not directly treat substance abuse but attempt to target the greater psychosocial issues affecting the youths' lives. A summary of the most common models is given in Table 1.

Individual- and Group-Based Substance Abuse Treatment
Family-based therapies are considered the most effective type of treatment for this population. However, engaging family members to participate in treatment while a juvenile is detained (and therefore not living at home) can be challenging. Therefore, individual- and group-based approaches to treatment are much more common in

Table 1
Psychosocial treatment models for youth in juvenile justice

Psychosocial treatment models	Location	Family involved?	Specific substance abuse treatment?
Motivational enhancement therapy and cognitive behavioral therapy (MET/CBT)	Residential setting or outpatient	No	Yes
Multisystemic therapy (MST)	Home	Yes	Yes
Brief strategic family therapy (BSFT)	Outpatient	Yes	No
Multidimensional treatment foster care (MTFC)	Foster care	Yes	No
Multidimensional family therapy (MDFT)	Outpatient	Yes	Yes

institutional settings. The motivational enhancement therapy and cognitive behavioral therapy (MET/CBT) model incorporates a combination of individual motivational interviewing sessions and group CBT. Initially developed by the Cannabis Youth Treatment Study as a short-term intervention, it has been used more broadly in the juvenile justice system, but it is not recommended for adolescents with severe conduct disorders. The literature identifies the need for increased supervision by providers and higher levels of intervention in this latter population.[25]

Multisystemic Therapy

Multisystemic therapy (MST), a home- and community-based treatment, was first developed in the early 1990s by Henggeler and colleagues to address the clinical and environmental needs of juvenile offenders with comorbid substance abuse and antisocial behavior traits. Through multiple randomized controlled trials that have included a variety of juvenile justice populations (eg, diversion, reentry, outpatient), this mode of treatment has been shown to be an effective model for decreasing substance use and criminal behavior in high-risk youth. Therapists maintain low caseloads and provide intensive support to youth and their families within their homes, communities, and schools.[26] Currently MST is widely disseminated for implementation with juvenile justice populations.

Brief Strategic Family Therapy

Brief strategic family therapy (BSFT) was developed in the early 1970s to address adolescent substance abuse and conduct disorders. This home/community-based intervention targets the family as a system to identify problematic patterns of relationships. The therapist then selects specific issues and works with the family to address them. BSFT has been tested in 7 randomized clinical trials and shown to be effective at reducing behavioral problems and increasing family functionality.[27]

Multidimensional Treatment Foster Care

Multidimensional treatment foster care (MTFC) was developed for delinquent youth who are at high risk for out-of-home placements. Using a foster care model, these youth are diverted from residential facilities by placement with MTFC-trained foster parents for 6 to 9 months. The goal is to reunify youth with the family of origin while remaining outside of the child welfare or juvenile justice system. The model has been shown to be effective at reducing recidivism and behavioral problems. One trial conducted to assess whether MTFC was effective for SUDs found significant reductions in substance abuse despite no formal substance abuse treatment conducted during the trial.[28]

Multidimensional Family Therapy

Like MST, multidimensional family therapy (MDFT) works in multiple domains of the participants' life: adolescent, parent, family interactional, and extrafamilial. Therapy takes place with a therapist 1 to 3 times per week for 3 to 6 months. The therapist conducts individual therapy with the adolescent and parents as well as family therapy. This intervention model focuses on substance abuse issues and has been shown to decrease substance abuse and delinquency.[29]

Comparisons of Psychosocial Treatment Models

Several meta-analyses have compared the various treatment models; all show that family-based interventions contribute the most to decreasing the rates of relapse for substance abuse. Meta-analyses and reviews conducted of adolescent substance abuse treatment interventions suggest that no single intervention has produced an effect size of substance use outcomes that suggests the superiority of any 1 particular intervention in reducing adolescent substance use. None have had sufficient effect sizes to conclude whether 1 treatment modality is superior to the others.[30,31] Additional research is needed to evaluate these treatment modalities further.

Drug Courts

Drug courts were developed as a response to the growing financial burden of the incarceration of adult offenders with SUDs. Not only was this incarceration incredibly costly, but the estimated rate of recidivism was high (about 50%). Drug courts were instituted with the goal of providing more appropriate and efficient sanctions and rehabilitation than incarceration. The first adult drug court was established in Dade County, Florida, in 1989.[32]

By the end of 2011, there were 458 juvenile drug courts (JDCs) in the United States.[33] The main attributes that differentiate JDCs from typical juvenile courts, where the approach does not focus on substance abuse-related rehabilitation, is as follows[34]:

1. Immediate intervention
2. Rehabilitation-focused adjudication
3. More direct judicial supervision
4. Access to structured treatment programs
5. Integrated team approach to the delinquent's treatment plan

Cooper and Bartlett[35] surveyed different JDCs around the country and showed that most youths were identified based on specific charges, such as drug possession, public intoxication, and theft, or by conducting drug screens of arrestees. The choice of screening tools varied across the country. Once involved in the JDC, juveniles went through phases of treatment that differed according to the level of supervision provided. Completing a phase often required the youth to fulfill tasks such as maintaining sobriety or attending school and follow-up appointments. Most programs were 12 months long, and each phase ranged from 1 to 4 months.

Extensive research has been devoted to evaluating whether drug courts have met their goals. A 1998 review by Belenko[36] was the first to conclude that adult drug courts were effective. He found that the courts provide more purposeful programming than other forms of community resources and that "drug use and criminal behavior [are] substantially reduced while offenders are participating in drug court." Drug courts, he noted, enhance accountability between the judge and the defendant because of more frequent communication. The courts led to decreases in criminal behavior both during program involvement and in the following 12 months.[36,37]

In 2007, Finigan et al[38] estimated that JDCs cost $1392 less per participant than incarceration. They calculated that with anticipated future savings from a decrease in recidivism, JDCs most likely saved $6744 per participant in taxpayer dollars.

Although many studies have found that JDCs can be effective in reducing juvenile recidivism and substance use, the implementation of drug court guidelines has been a challenge in some cases.[39,40] A number of programs have had difficulty establishing means of monitoring long-term recidivism and have had substantial numbers of participants drop out.[41,42] Youth who complete JDC programs may have fewer risk factors for relapse, dropout, or nonadherence than those who do not successfully complete JDC requirements.[43] Latessa et al[44] recently performed a meta-analysis of outcomes collected from 9 JDCs and found that recidivism rates were higher and rates of new treatment referrals were lower for those in JDCs versus formal court hearings. However, many of the courts did not appear to follow recommended guidelines for implementation and supervision.

With adequate staffing, oversight, and funding, drug courts likely are effective tools for responding to juvenile substance abusers' needs, but in practice they may face multiple barriers in providing this "specialty court" approach.

Real World Treatments

In an attempt to evaluate *real world* substance abuse treatment practices in juvenile justice settings, Chassin et al looked at 420 young males who were found guilty of a serious offense and who self-reported substance abuse. The aim was to assess *treatment as usual* (ie, the control group in many research studies). Each participant was given surveys to assess the amount of treatment they had received every 6 months for 2 years. Thirty-four percent reported receiving substance abuse treatment for the entire 2 years. More than 3 months of treatment resulted in significant reductions in reported alcohol and marijuana use. Family-involved treatment was associated with reductions in cigarette and alcohol use. The authors concluded that, despite standardized recommendations, any substance abuse treatment appeared to provide benefit to juvenile offenders.[45]

REENTRY AND AFTERCARE FOR DETAINED OR INCARCERATED YOUTH

Reentry programs (ie, those that focus on providing services during the incarceration to community reentry phase) were first established in the 1950s for adults when it was recognized that incarceration alone did not seem to deter reoffense. In the late 1980s, as rates of juvenile incarceration were increasing, there was a push to better understand how to reduce recidivism after incarceration in this population.[46]

Offenders in the early release period are at high risk for recidivism and substance use relapse and need continued support to help them refrain from criminal and substance use behaviors. For youth with a history of substance abuse, abrupt cessation of treatment may put them at risk for both relapse and recidivism. Much work in improving these transitions for youth with substance abuse problems remains to be done. In Young et al's survey of substance abuse treatment in juvenile justice systems, half (51%) of youth with SUDs in residential facilities were provided with a referral to a community-based treatment provider at discharge, whereas only 31.2% of youth in detention with substance abuse problems were given a referral.[47]

Researchers and providers are currently attempting to tackle this problem. The Criminal Justice Drug Abuse Treatment Studies (CJDATS) project has created an assessment tool to identify the substance abuse treatment needs of persons before release. It currently is being assessed for validity in predicting recidivism as well as treatment needs.[23] The CJDATS is currently conducting a study to look at effective programs for juveniles when they return to the community. The study compares 2 program models: cognitive restructuring, based on CBT, and extant aftercare services, which entails *treatment as usual* for juveniles leaving the institution. Typical aftercare primarily involves working with case management services. The study plans to evaluate participants' feedback as well as outcome measures of drug use, criminal behavior, and daily functioning.[48]

In 2009, Lipsey[49] conducted a meta-analysis of rehabilitation programs that indicated the factors that most significantly decreased juvenile recidivism included integration with school-based programs, intensive supervision, and counseling programs. The study also found no difference between outcomes within a correctional facility versus in the community. Nearly a decade later, Lipsey[50] completed another meta-analysis in which program components were analyzed separately to determine which specific factors lead to lower recidivism rates. The analysis demonstrated that counseling interventions had the highest effect on decreasing recidivism followed by the provision of multiple services for the youth as well as skill-building services. Discipline-based programs had the worst outcomes in deterring criminal behavior. The presence of a high-quality, therapeutic-based intervention targeting high-risk youth was the most important factor in reducing recidivism.[50]

CONCLUSION

Health care professionals who care for adolescents are likely to encounter youth in the juvenile justice system who have SUDs. Recognizing these problems and ensuring that these youth receive appropriate assessment and treatment can provide much-needed services for these adolescents, with potential benefits extending to multiple aspects of their lives and futures. Assessment and treatment of substance abuse in this population now benefit from a substantial body of research that has been conducted over the past 2 decades. Validated screening tools are available for juvenile offenders that identify treatment needs on entry into the system. Various intervention strategies have been developed to treat youth in the juvenile justice system, whether they are diverted, incarcerated, or reentering the community. Unfortunately, rates of recidivism and continued substance use remain high, indicating the need for ongoing development and restructuring of effective substance use interventions for this high-risk population. Treatment models that include family and tailor therapeutic approaches to specific risks and needs appear promising. Continuity of care, with access to needed services at the time of reentry into the community, is crucial in addressing substance abuse in this population. Finally, public awareness of this devastating issue remains low, and physicians can play a role in advocating for adequate services in this group of young people for whom needs are so great and effective means of treatment are available.

References

1. Golzari M, Hung SJ, Anoshiravani A. The health status of youth in juvenile detention facilities. *J Adolesc Health*. 2006;38:776–782
2. American Academy of Pediatrics Committee on Adolescence. Policy Statement: Health Care for Youth in the Juvenile Justice System. *Pediatrics*. 2011;129:128–597
3. *Standard for Health Services in Juvenile Detention and Confinement Facilities*. Chicago, IL: National Commission on Correctional Health Care; 2004
4. Penn JV, Thomas C. Practice parameter for the assessment and treatment of youth in juvenile detention and correctional facilities. *J Am Acad Child Adolesc Psychiatry*. 2005;44.10:1085–1098
5. Snyder HN, Sickmund M. *Juvenile Offenders and Victims: 2006 National Report*. Washington, DC: US Department of Justice, Office of Justice Programs, Office of Juvenile Justice and Delinquency Prevention; 2006:93–119
6. Office of Juvenile Justice and Delinquency Prevention. Easy access to juvenile court statistics. Available at: http://ojjdp.gov/ojstatbb/ezajcs/asp/display.asp. Accessed October 20, 2013
7. Knoll C, Sickmund M. *Delinquency Cases in Juvenile Courts, 2008: Fact Sheet*. Washington, DC: US Department of Justice, Office of Justice Programs, Office of Juvenile Justice and Delinquency Prevention; 2012
8. Heilbrum K, Sevin Goldstein NE, Redding R. *Juvenile Delinquency; Prevention, Assessment and Intervention*. New York: Oxford University Press; 2005
9. Mental Health Services Administration. *Results from the 2010 National Survey on Drug Use and Health: Summary of National Findings*. Rockville, MD: Substance Abuse and Mental Health Services Administration; 2011
10. *Criminal Neglect: Substance Abuse, Juvenile Justice and the Children Left Behind*. New York: National Center on Addiction and Substance Abuse at Columbia University (CASA); 2004
11. Mental Health Services Administration. *Results from the 2002 National Survey on Drug Use and Health: National Findings*. Rockville, MD: Substance Abuse and Mental Health Services Administration; 2003
12. Teplin L, Abram K, McClelland G, Dulcan M, Mericle A. Psychiatric disorders in youth in juvenile detention. *Arch Gen Psychiatry*. 2002;59:1133–1143

13. Hoge R, Guerra NG, Boxer P. *Treating the Juvenile Offender.* New York: The Guilford Press; 2008
14. Howard MO, Balster RL, Cottler LB, Wu LT, Vaughn MG. Inhalant use among incarcerated adolescents in the United States: prevalence, characteristics, and correlates of use. *Drug Alcohol Depend.* 2008;93:197–209
15. Dembo R, Belenko S, Childs K, Wareham J. Drug use and sexually transmitted diseases among female and male arrested youths. *J Behav Med.* 2009;32:129–141
16. Dembo R, Williams L, Wish E, Schmeidler J. *Urine Testing of Detained Juveniles to Identify High-Risk Youth.* Washington, DC: US Department of Justice, Office of Justice Programs, National Institute of Justice; 1990
17. Cauffman E. A statewide screening of mental health symptoms among juvenile offenders in detention. *J Am Acad Child Adolesc Psychiatry.* 2004;43:430–439
18. Grisso T, Barnum R, Fletcher K, Cauffman E, Peuschold D. Massachusetts Youth Screening Instrument for mental health needs of juvenile justice youths. *J Am Acad Child Adolesc Psychiatry.* 2001;40:541–548
19. Wasserman G, Jensen P, Ko S. Mental health assessments in juvenile justice: report on the consensus conference. *J Am Acad Child Adolesc Psychiatry.* 2003;42:752–761
20. Coll K, Iuhnke G, Thobro P, Haas R. A preliminary study using the Substance Abuse Subtle Screening Inventory—Adolescent Form as an outcome measure with adolescent offenders. *J Addict Offender Couns.* 2003;24:11–22
21. Drug Strategies. *Bridging the Gap: A Guide to Drug Treatment in the Juvenile Justice System.* Washington, DC: Drug Strategies; 2005
22. Henderson C, Young D, Jainchill N, et al. Program use of effective drug abuse treatment practices for juvenile offenders. *J Subst Abuse Treat.* 2007;32:279–290
23. Young D, Dembo R, Henderson C. A national survey of substance abuse treatment for juvenile offenders. *J Subst Abuse Treat.* 2007;32:255–266
24. Chassin L. Juvenile justice and substance use. *Future Child.* 2008;18:165–183
25. Feldstein S, Ginsburg J. Motivational interviewing with dually diagnosed adolescents in juvenile justice settings. *Brief Treat Crisis Interv.* 2006;6:218
26. Sheidow AJ, Henggeler SW. Multisystemic therapy for alcohol and other drug abuse in delinquent adolescents. In Morgan OJ, Litzke CH, eds. *Family Intervention in Substance Abuse: Current Best Practices.* Binghamton, NY: Haworth Press; 2008:125–145
27. Szapocznik J, Williams R. Brief strategic family therapy: twenty-five years of interplay among theory, research and practice in adolescent behavior problems and drug abuse. *Clin Child Fam Psychol Rev.* 2000;3:117–134
28. Smith D, Chamberlain P, Eddy J. Preliminary support for multidimensional treatment foster care in reducing substance use in delinquent boys. *J Child Adolesc Subst Abuse.* 2010;19:343–358
29. Liddle H, Rowe C, Dakof G, Henderson C, Greenbaum P. Multidimensional family therapy for young adolescent substance abuse: twelve-month outcomes of a randomized controlled trial. *J Consult Clin Psychol.* 2009;77:12–25
30. Tripodi S, Bender K. Substance abuse treatment for juvenile offenders: A review of quasi-experimental and experimental research. *J Crim Justice.* 2011;39:246–252
31. Baldwin S, Christian S, Berkeljon A, Shadish W. The effects of family therapies for adolescent delinquency and substance abuse: a meta-analysis. *J Marital Fam Ther.* 2012;38:281–304
32. *Looking at a Decade of Drug Courts.* Washington, DC: US Department of Justice, Office of Justice Programs, Drug Courts Program Office; 1998
33. National Criminal Justice Reference Service. In the spotlight: facts and figures. Available at: www.ncjrs.gov/spotlight/drug_courts/facts.html. Accessed October 25, 2013
34. Sloan J, Ortiz Smykla J. Juvenile drug courts: understanding the importance of dimensional variability. *Crim Justice Policy Rev.* 2003;14:339–360
35. Cooper C, Bartlett S. *Juvenile and Family Drug Courts: Profile of Program Characteristics and Implementation Issues.* Washington, DC: US Department of Justice, Office of Justice Programs, Drug Courts Program Office; 1998
36. Belenko S. Research on drug courts: a critical review. *Natl Drug Court Inst Rev.* 1998;1:1–42

37. Belenko S, Logan T. Delivering more effective treatment to adolescents: improving the juvenile drug court model. *J Subst Abuse Treat.* 2003;25:189–211

38. Finigan M, Carey S, Cox A. The impact of a mature drug court over 10 years of operation: recidivism and costs. Portland, OR; NPC Research; 2007. Available at: www.ncjrs.gov/pdffiles1/nij/grants/219225.pdf. Accessed March 19, 2014

39. Willard T, Wright S. *Virginia Drug Treatment Court Programs: Executive Summary.* Richmond, VA: Transformation System; 2005

40. Thompson K. *A Preliminary Outcome Evaluation of North Dakota's Juvenile Drug Court—Recidivism Analysis.* Fargo: North Dakota State University; 2001

41. Sloan J, Smykla J, Rush J. Do juvenile drug courts reduce recidivism?: outcomes of drug court and an adolescent substance abuse program. *Am J Crim Justice.* 2004;29:95–115

42. Rodriguez N, Webb V. Multiple measures of juvenile drug court effectiveness: results of a quasi-experimental design. *Crime Delinq.* 2004;50:292–314

43. Stein D, Deberard S, Homan K. Predicting success and failure in juvenile drug treatment court: a meta-analytic review. *J Subst Abuse Treat.* 2013;44:158–169

44. Latessa E, Sullivan C, Blair L, Sullivan C, Smith P. *Final Report Outcome and Process Evaluation of Juvenile Drug Courts.* Cincinnati, OH: National Criminal Justice Reference Service; 2013

45. Chassin L, Knight G, Vargas-Chanes D, Losoya SH, Naranjo D. Substance use treatment outcomes in a sample of male serious juvenile offenders. *J Subst Abuse Treat.* 2009;36:183–194

46. Altschuler D, Brash R. Adolescent and teenage offenders confronting the challenges and opportunities of reentry. *Youth Violence Juv Justice.* 2004;2:72–87

47. Farabee D, Knight K, Garner B, Calhoun S. The inmate prerelease assessment for reentry planning. *Crim Justice Behav.* 2007;34:1188–1197

48. Jainchill N. Brief report series: comparing two reentry strategies for drug abusing juvenile offenders. *Crim Justice Drug Abuse Treat Stud.* 2013. Available at: www.drugabuse.gov/sites/default/files/files/TwoReentryStrategies.pdf. Accessed February 26, 2014

49. Lipsey M. Can rehabilitative programs reduce the recidivism of juvenile offenders: an inquiry into the effectiveness of practical programs. *Va J Soc Policy Law.* 1999;6:611

50. Lipsey M. The primary factors that characterize effective interventions with juvenile offenders: a meta-analytic overview. *Vict Offender.* 2009;4:124–147

Note: Page numbers of articles are in **boldface** type. Page references followed by "*f*" and "*t*" denote figures and tables, respectively.